Health Visiting

D1245176

Health Visiting

Preparation for Practice

Fourth Edition

Edited by

Karen A. Luker

CBE, FMedSci, FQNI, PhD, BNurs, RN, SCPHN (HV), NDNCert
QNI Professor of Community Nursing
School of Nursing, Midwifery and Social Work
The University of Manchester
Manchester, UK

Gretl A. McHugh

FQNI, PhD, MSc (Public Health), BNurs (Hons), RN, SCPHN (HV)
Professor of Applied Health Research
School of Healthcare
The University of Leeds
Leeds, UK

Rosamund M. Bryar

FQNI, HonMFPH, PhD, MPhil, BNurs, RN, SCPHN (HV), NDNCert, CertEd (FE), SCM
Professor Emeritus Community and Primary Care Nursing
School of Health Sciences
City University London
London, UK

WILEY Blackwell

Library of Congress Cataloging-in-Publication Data

Names: Luker, Karen A., editor. | McHugh, Gretl A., editor. | Bryar,
  Rosamund M., editor.
Title: Health visiting : preparation for practice / edited by Karen A Luker,
  Gretl A McHugh, Rosamund M Bryar.
Other titles: Health visiting (Luker)
Description: Fourth edition. | Chichester, West Sussex ; Hoboken, NJ : John
  Wiley & Sons, Ltd., 2017. | Includes bibliographical references and index.
Identifiers: LCCN 2016012189 | ISBN 9781119078586 (cloth) | ISBN 9781119084593
  (pdf) | ISBN 9781119084556 (epub)
Subjects: | MESH: Community Health Nursing | Evidence-Based Nursing | Great Britain
Classification: LCC RT98 | NLM WY 106 | DDC 610.73/43–dc23 LC record available at
  http://lccn.loc.gov/2016012189

A catalogue record for this book is available from the British Library.

Wiley also publishes its books in a variety of electronic formats. Some content that appears in print may not be available in electronic books.

Cover image: Vicky Kasala Productions

Set in 9/12.5pt, NewsGothicStd by SPi Global, Chennai, India
Printed and bound in Malaysia by Vivar Printing Sdn Bhd

1   2017

Contents

List of Contributors

Ms Sharin Baldwin FiHV, QN, MSc, PG Dip, BSc (Hons), RN, RM, SCPHN (HV)
NIHR Clinical Doctoral Fellow and Clinical, Academic & Innovations Lead
(Health Visiting)
King's College London
and
London North West Healthcare
NHS Trust Health Visiting Clinical Academic Hub
London, UK

Professor Rosamund M. Bryar FQNI, HonMFPH, PhD, MPhil, BNurs, RN, SCPHN (HV),
NDNCert, CertEd (FE), SCM
Professor Emeritus Community and Primary Care Nursing
School of Health Sciences
City University London
London, UK

Professor Karen I. Chalmers PhD, MSc (A), BScN, RN
Honorary Professor
School of Nursing, Midwifery and Social Work
The University of Manchester
Manchester, UK

Ms Julianne Harlow MA, BSc (Hons), PGCE, SCPHN (HV), RN
Senior Lecturer
Department of Education & Childhood
University of Derby
Derby, UK

Professor Mark R.D. Johnson PhD, MA, PG Dip (HE)
Emeritus Professor of Diversity in Health & Social Care
Mary Seacole Research Centre
Health Policy Research Unit
De Montfort University
Leicester, UK

Professor Karen A. Luker CBE, FMedSci, FQNI, PhD, BNurs, RN, SCPHN (HV), NDNCert
QNI Professor of Community Nursing
School of Nursing, Midwifery & Social Work
The University of Manchester
Manchester, UK

Professor Gretl A. McHugh FQNI, PhD, MSc (Public Health), BNurs (Hons), RN, SCPHN (HV)
Professor of Applied Health Research
School of Healthcare
The University of Leeds
Leeds, UK

Professor Kate Robinson PhD, BA, RN, SCPHN (HV)
Professor Emeritus
University of Bedfordshire
Luton, UK

Mr Martin Smith MPH, FFPH, PGCert HEd, FHEA, BA (Hons), RN, DipHV, SCPHN (HV),
Consultant in Public Health
Liverpool City Council
Liverpool, UK

Dr Karen A. Whittaker FiHV, FHEA, PhD, MSc, PGCE, BNurs (Hons), RN, SCPHN (HV)
Reader in Child and Family Health
School of Nursing
College of Health and Wellbeing
University of Central Lancashire
Preston, UK

Introduction

Karen A. Luker, Gretl A. McHugh, and Rosamund M. Bryar

Our fourth edition of *Health Visiting: Preparation for Practice* is a key resource for health visitors, health visitor students, students on nursing, public health, early years, and health sciences programmes, and other health professionals working in public health, primary care, and community services. The practice of health visiting is focused on the promotion of health and the prevention of ill health. The fourth edition of *Health Visiting: Preparation for Practice* aims to inform, educate, and challenge you to deliver the most effective health visiting and so enable the promotion of health and prevention of ill health in the children, families, and communities with whom you work.

Prevention and public health have been the focus of health visiting since the early days of the sanitary visitors – the forerunners of health visitors – appointed by the Manchester and Salford Ladies Sanitary Reform Association in 1862. Since 1862, the living conditions, life expectancy, and health of the population have evolved, and alongside this there have been changes in the health challenges faced by the population. Over these more than 150 years, health visiting has responded to these changes by contributing to addressing public health issues from prevention of infectious diseases to prevention of long-term conditions; from addressing poverty and under-nutrition to working to reduce obesity in children and their parents. The aim of this edition of *Health Visiting: Preparation for Practice* is to provide you with the most up-to-date evidence to support your work on the front line of public health.

The fourth edition of this book is the latest in the line of works entitled *Health Visiting* which have aimed to support the delivery of health visiting. The first of these, *Health Visiting: A Textbook for Health Visitor Students* by Margaret McEwan, was first published in 1951. This was followed by three further editions, and, in 1977, by *Health Visiting*, edited by Grace M. Owen and written by Grace M. Owen and health visiting colleagues drawn from the health visiting programme at the Polytechnic of the South Bank (now London South Bank University). These books remind us of the changes in the preparation of health visitors during the past 60-plus years, but the statement by McEwan (1961: 17) of the purpose of health visiting is still the centre

Health Visiting: Preparation for Practice, Fourth Edition.
Edited by Karen A. Luker, Gretl A. McHugh and Rosamund M. Bryar.
© 2017 John Wiley & Sons, Ltd. Published 2017 by John Wiley & Sons, Ltd.

of today's practice: 'The health visitor is primarily a teacher and her aim is to teach the value of healthy living and to interpret the principles of health.' In addition, her observation that health visiting is: ' ... concerned with the little things of everyday life' (McEwan, 1961: 17) is also very pertinent. However, the evidence and knowledge base underpinning some of these 'little things of everyday life', such as weaning, play, and parenting, has grown enormously, as shown in the four editions of the present book. The first edition, by Karen Luker and Jean Orr, was published in 1985 and also entitled *Health Visiting*. The second edition followed in 1992 and was entitled *Health Visiting: Towards Community Health Nursing*, reflecting changes in the education of nurses and health visitors in the early 1990s. The third edition, edited by Karen Luker, Jean Orr, and Gretl McHugh, did not appear until 20 years later, in 2012, but the title, *Health Visiting: A Rediscovery*, shows the new confidence in health visiting and the role of health visitors in supporting families based on evidence concerning the importance of support for early child development and the need to reduce inequalities in health (Field, 2010; Marmot *et al.*, 2010; Allen, 2011; Dartington Social Research Unit *et al.*, 2015). The fourth edition, entitled *Health Visiting: Preparation for Practice*, builds on the third. It includes a new chapter on working with diverse communities, reflecting their multicultural make-up, and, critically, provides additional guidance on evaluation, enabling you to demonstrate the outcomes of your practice. What these books all illustrate are the ways that health visiting, over the past decades, has responded to and applied new and emerging evidence to support children, families, and communities to better promote their health.

Prevention, public health, and health visiting

Over the past 5 years, there has been investment into the education and employment of health visitors, with a subsequent increase in the number of health visitors, particularly in England and Scotland. Alongside this investment has been clarification of the health visiting service, with greater emphasis being placed on the public health role of health visitors working with children, their families, and communities. Health visitors have a long-standing role in helping communities to improve their health and well being; for example, in increasing immunisation uptake, preventing obesity, and tackling health inequalities. The Marmot Report, *Fair Society, Healthy Lives* (Marmot *et al.*, 2010), sets out a framework for tackling the wider social determinants of health, stating that health inequalities will require action on:

- giving every child the best start in life;
- enabling all children, young people, and adults to maximise their capabilities and have control over their lives;
- creating fair employment and good work for all;
- ensuring a healthy standard of living for all;
- creating and developing healthy and sustainable places and communities;
- strengthening the role and impact of ill-health prevention.

Health visitors are the lead professionals for delivery of the *Healthy Child Programme* (DH, 2009; Public Health England, 2015), and therefore have a critical role in helping to improve the life chances of current and future generations by reducing the impact of inequalities on the immediate and long-term health of the population. Recognition of the important role that prevention has to play in improving health, and also in reducing health care costs, was identified in reports undertaken by Sir Derek Wanless in England and in Wales (Wanless, 2002; Project Team and Wanless, 2003) and reiterated for England in the *NHS Five Year Forward View* (DH, 2014a). In *NHS Five Year Forward View: Time to Deliver* (DH, 2015: 7), three gaps were identified: '…the health and wellbeing gap, the care and quality gap, and the funding and efficiency gap.' Health visitors have a key role in their work with children and their families in contributing to public health outcomes that address early on the health and well being gap. The six high-impact areas show where health visitors can have the greatest influence:

- Transition to Parenthood and the Early Weeks
- Maternal Mental Health (Perinatal Depression)
- Breastfeeding (Initiation and Duration)
- Healthy Weight, Healthy Nutrition (to include Physical Activity)
- Managing Minor Illness and Reducing Accidents (Reducing Hospital Attendance/Admissions)
- Healthy Two Year Olds and School Readiness

(DH, 2014b)

Over the coming years, these areas for prevention will be the focus of health visiting services. From October 2015, local authorities took over from NHS England in the commissioning of public health services for children under 5 years (DH, 2014c). Currently, health visitors continue to be employed initially by the same employer, but service commissioning processes in coming years may see a range of new models of employment. The continued contribution of health visitors to the 0–5 years will remain key, but the greater integration of health and social care services (e.g. the Greater Manchester Health and Social Care Devolution (previously referred to as Devo Manc) project developments (Ham, 2015)) may present new opportunities, including wider integration of 0–19 services and the involvement of health visitors in population-based initiatives. In Northern Ireland, an integrated service for all children up to the age of 19 years is provided by health visitors and school nurses. There is an emphasis on working together, with a focus on delivery of child health promotion programmes and increased intensive home visiting for the 0–19 years (DHSSPS, 2010). In Wales, the recent nursing and midwifery strategy by Public Health Wales places nurses and midwives at the forefront of its public health strategy (Public Health Wales, 2014). In Scotland, in 2014, the government pledged to increase the number of health visitors by 500 over the next 4 years (The Scottish Government, 2014). Greater collaboration between services and practitioners (e.g. midwives and health visitors working with women in the antenatal period, social workers and health visitors working with families experiencing domestic violence or child safeguarding issues, school nurses and health visitors working to address obesity in 0–19 services) will be central to health visiting over the coming years. These additional resources and initiatives will assist with improving health visiting services. However, there remains a need to focus on measurable outcomes in order to evaluate these initiatives, which could lead to further changes and improvements in the methods of delivering health visiting services.

Health visiting: preparation for practice

The first and second editions of this book were pioneering in the quest for evidence to support practice and in emphasising the need for evaluation of practice. Evidence-based practice and evaluation of impact now seem to be a given, and this acknowledgement by the professional colleges, the governments of the four countries of the UK, and health visiting organisations means that our chapter on evaluating practice will be a must read and makes this an exciting time to launch the fourth edition of the book. The structure of the book is similar to that of the other editions: the content has been updated from the last edition and a new chapter has been included which focuses on the health visitor working with diverse communities. These changes have been necessary to keep pace with the developments in health policy, public health priorities, and health visiting practice. There are some new authors for this edition – some who are teaching public health and health visiting, and others who are practising as health visitors and public health specialists – ensuring that this fourth edition is relevant to meet the needs of those undergoing preparation to become health visitors and those who are practitioners working with and in the community.

Chapter 1: 'Managing Knowledge in Health Visiting' discusses the demands on the health visitor to understand the different forms and sources of knowledge in order ensure the delivery of evidence-based practice, with reference to case studies. It highlights the issues surrounding the use of guidelines and protocols in practice and looks at the concept of communities of practice (CoPs), with regard to how they can assist practitioners in working to improve their own practice. In addition, it discusses the generation and management of knowledge in practice using reflective practice and examines the perspective of the client in terms of what they know and how they know it, drawing attention to the use of social networking sites.

Chapter 2: 'Health Visiting: Context and Public Health Practice' explores the specialist and public health role of the health visitor in working with families. It examines the tensions between the public health role and the health visiting role with children and families. The public health role needs to become more clearly defined, with a focus on reducing health inequalities and giving every child in the community the best start in life (Marmot et al., 2010); this is explored in a section specifically about 'Health Inequalities'. This chapter also examines the evidence for health inequities and the contribution health visitors can bring in addressing the wider determinants of health. In addition, it highlights the importance of good leadership in public health and the challenges for health visitors in engaging in a public health role.

Chapter 3: 'The Community Dimension' explores the importance of the communities within which people live to their health and considers the range of factors impacting on people's health. It looks at the role of health visitors working with communities and the renewed focus on this area, for example as part of the health visiting service model in England. It discusses tools that health visitors can use to gain an understanding of communities through an exploration of their social history and identification and assessment of their current health needs. It looks at the development of the skills required to work with communities, making use of health promotion theory and building on the skills that health visitors have in working with individuals and collaborating with other services, with reference to national and international learning resources and tools. Working with communities to achieve better health is a long-term process, but health visitors, with their access to all families with children under 5 years of age, are in a unique position to support the building of healthier communities.

Chapter 4: 'Approaches to Supporting Families' explores different approaches to supporting families and evaluates several child health programmes that are currently in existence. It discusses the evidence for successful interventions to support families, including the findings from evaluations of these programmes, and considers the influence of policies on health visitors' work in supporting families. Finally, it examines the competing challenges faced by health visitors in trying to work with families, including the public health agenda, the level of evidence, and the availability of resources.

Chapter 5: 'Safeguarding Children: Debates and Dilemmas for Health Visitors' focuses on safeguarding and the enhanced child protection role of the health visitor. It defines the key concepts, such as 'child abuse' and 'significant harm', and highlights the incidence and prevalence of child abuse. It discusses the policy and legislation relevant to safeguarding practice, as well as the assessment of vulnerable children using the Common Assessment Framework (CAF) and the Graded Care Profile (GCP) for neglect. It looks at the issues and dilemmas around safeguarding children that students will encounter in their practice and discusses how the utilisation of supervision to support critical reflection and thinking can provide a supportive mechanism. It also highlights examples of published inquires into child deaths and serious case reviews. Overall, this chapter will assist with the development of leadership in practitioners working in the safeguarding arena.

Chapter 6: 'Working with Diverse Communities' is a welcome addition to the fourth edition. It outlines the changes in the ethnic makeup of the UK population and discusses their implications for health care in general, with a specific consideration of religious issues. It introduces the concepts of 'cultural competence' and 'institutional discrimination', and considers what we mean by 'diverse'. It discusses cultural practices relevant to health visitor practice, including matters around pregnancy, diet, customs relating to birth and naming, and mental health, and provides some examples. Finally, it considers safeguarding in a multicultural setting, with a special focus on genital cutting or female genital mutilation (FGM). Throughout the chapter, communication is addressed, and the case is made that increasing cultural competency will help in developing communication skills to support work with diverse communities.

In the previous editions, **Chapter 7: 'Evaluating Practice'** was always ahead of its time, insofar as everyday health visitors seldom formally evaluated the impact of their work. This chapter has been updated and explores the importance of evaluation in health visiting practice, which is a necessity in today's economy, to ensure that what health visitors are doing is effective and of value. It discusses key sources of evidence available to health visitors in the evaluation of their practice. It examines the different types of evaluation and suggests ways to approach them. It is important to ensure that health visitors and other practitioners have the skills and knowledge to identify and critique the available evidence and information in their role in supporting families and communities. Health visitors need knowledge about where to get the best information and the skills to be able to access up-to-date resources for the delivery of evidence-based practice; this chapter helps to provide this.

As in previous editions, the reader is encouraged to engage in learning activities at various points throughout the text; these can be found at the end of each chapter. It is anticipated that these activities will help students, health visitors, and others to reflect upon and develop their practice.

Health visitors will face many challenges over the coming years, but the vision for high-quality care and improved service provision makes it an exciting time for the profession. We hope that this new edition will assist with 'preparation for practice' and improve the contribution health visitors can make to the health and well being of children, their families, and communities, which will ultimately lead to better health outcomes for the whole population.

References

Allen, G. (2011) Early Intervention: The Next Steps. Department for Work and Pensions and Cabinet Office, London.

Dartington Social Research Unit, University of Warwick & Coventry University (2015) The Best Start at Home. Early Intervention Foundation, London. Available from: http://www.eif.org.uk/publication/the-best-start-at-home/ (last accessed 30 March 2016).

DH (2009) Healthy Child Programme: Pregnancy and the First Five Years of Life. Department of Health, London. Available from: https://www.gov.uk/government/uploads/system/uploads/attachment_data/file/167998/Health_Child_Programme.pdf (last accessed 30 March 2016).

DH (2014a) NHS Five Year Forward View. Department of Health, London. Available from: https://www.england.nhs.uk/ourwork/futurenhs/ (last accessed 30 March 2016).

DH (2014b) Overview of the Six Early Years High Impact Areas. Department of Health, London. Available from: https://www.gov.uk/government/uploads/system/uploads/attachment_data/file/413127/2903110_Early_Years_Impact_GENERAL_V0_2W.pdf (last accessed 30 March 2016).

DH (2014c) Transfer of 0–5 Children's Public Health Commissioning to Local Authorities. Department of Health, London. Available from: https://www.england.nhs.uk/ourwork/qual-clin-lead/hlth-vistg-prog/ (last accessed 30 March 2016).

DH (2015) NHS Five Year Forward View: Time to Deliver. Department of Health, London. Available from: https://www.england.nhs.uk/wp-content/uploads/2015/06/5yfv-time-to-deliver-25-06.pdf (last accessed 30 March 2016).

DHSSPS (2010) Healthy Futures 2010–2015: The Contribution of Health Visitors and School Nurses in Northern Ireland. Department of Health, Social Services and Public Safety, Belfast.

Field, F. (2010) The Foundation Years: Preventing Poor Children Becoming Poor Adults. The Report of the Independent Review of Poverty and Life Chances. Cabinet Office, London. Available from: http://webarchive.nationalarchives.gov.uk/20110120090128/http:/povertyreview.independent.gov.uk/media/20254/poverty-report.pdf (last accessed 30 March 2016).

Ham, C. (2015) What Devo Manc could mean for health, social care and wellbeing in Greater Manchester. The King's Fund, London. Available from: http://www.kingsfund.org.uk/blog/2015/03/devo-manc-health-social-care-wellbeing-greater-manchester (last accessed 30 March 2016).

Luker, K.A. & Orr, J. (eds) (1985) Health Visiting. Blackwell, Oxford.

Luker, K.A. & Orr, J. (eds) (1992) Health Visiting: Towards Community Health Nursing, 2nd edn. Blackwell, Oxford.

Luker, K.A, Orr, J. & McHugh, G. (eds) (2012) Health Visiting: A Rediscovery, 3rd edn. Wiley-Blackwell, Chichester.

Marmot, M., Atkinson, T., Bell, J., Black, C., Broadfoot, P., Cumberlege, J., Diamond, I., Gilmore, I., Ham, C., Meacher, M. & Mulgan, G. (2010) Fair Society, Healthy Lives: The Marmot Review. Marmot Review Team, University College, London. Available from: http://www.instituteofhealthequity.org/projects/fair-society-healthy-lives-the-marmot-review (last accessed 30 March 2016).

McEwan, M. (1951) Health Visiting: A Textbook for Health Visitor Students. Faber & Faber, London.

McEwan, M. (1961) Health Visiting: A Textbook for Health Visitor Students, 4th edn. Faber & Faber, London.

Owen, G.M. (ed.) (1977) Health Visiting. Bailliere Tindall, London.

Project Team & Wanless, D. (2003) The Review of Health and Social Care in Wales. The Report of the Project Team advised by Derek Wanless. Welsh Assembly Government, Cardiff. Available from: http://www.wales.nhs.uk/documents/wanless-review-e.pdf (last accessed 30 March 2016).

Public Health England (2015) Rapid Review to Update the Evidence for the Healthy Child Programme 0–5. Public Health England, London. Available from: https://www.gov.uk/government/uploads/system/uploads/attachment_data/file/429740/150520RapidReviewHealthyChildProg_UPDATE_poisons_final.pdf (last accessed 30 March 2016).

Public Health Wales (2014) Raising the Profile: The Public Health Wales Nursing and Midwifery Strategy Working towards a Healthier, Happier and Fairer Wales. Public Health Wales, Wales.

The Scottish Government (2014) 500 New Health Visitors. The Scottish Government, Edinburgh. Available from: http://news.scotland.gov.uk/News/500-new-health-visitors-ddc.aspx (last accessed 30 March 2016).

Wanless, D. (2002) Securing Our Future: Taking a Long-Term View. HM Treasury, London. Available from: http://webarchive.nationalarchives.gov.uk/+/http:/www.hm-treasury.gov.uk/consult_wanless_final.htm (last accessed 30 March 2016).

1
Managing Knowledge in Health Visiting

Kate Robinson
University of Bedfordshire, Luton, UK

Introduction

The mantra of evidence-based practice (EBP) is now heard everywhere in healthcare. This chapter will explore what it might mean, both theoretically and in the context of everyday health visiting practice. Is it a way of enhancing the effectiveness of practice or yet another part of the new managerialism of guidelines, targets, and effectiveness? Why might EBP be an important ideal? When a practitioner intervenes in a client's life, the outcome should be that the client is significantly advantaged. In health visiting, that advantage can take many forms: the client can have more and better knowledge, they might feel more capable of managing their affairs, they might better understand and be able to cope with difficult thoughts, feelings, and actions – the list is extensive. Later chapters will detail the ways in which health visiting can lead to better outcomes for clients and communities. However, the proposition that there should be an advantage derived from the practitioner's intervention is particularly important in the context of a state-financed (i.e. taxpayer–funded) healthcare system. If an individual wishes to spend their money on treatments or therapies of dubious or unexplored value offered by unregulated practitioners, then that is entirely a matter for them, provided that they have not been misled or mis-sold! However, when the state decides to invest its resources in the provision of a particular service and associated interventions then arguably there has to be some level of evidence or collective informed agreement which gives confidence that the choice is justified. In addition, of course, every health visitor must be able to account for what she does and doesn't do to the Nursing and Midwifery Council (NMC), if required.

Chapter 7 explores how health visiting might be assessed, measured, and evaluated. The emphasis in this chapter is on how we choose, individually or collectively, to develop particular services and perform particular actions which we know with some degree of certainty should lead to better outcomes for the client. But how do

Health Visiting: Preparation for Practice, Fourth Edition.
Edited by Karen A. Luker, Gretl A. McHugh and Rosamund M. Bryar.
© 2017 John Wiley & Sons, Ltd. Published 2017 by John Wiley & Sons, Ltd.

we know things with any certainty? What sort of knowledge do we need to make good choices? Although there are very many different ways of categorising or describing forms of knowledge, for our purpose here it will be sufficient to make some simple distinctions. We might categorise knowledge by type. For example, Carper's (1978) categorisation of knowledge as empirical (largely derived from science), aesthetic (or artistic), ethical, or personal is well known and is used in nursing. Or we might categorise it by source, and ask where it comes from (books, journals, other people, personal experience, etc.). Or we might use the simple but important distinction between knowing *that* and knowing *how* (McKenna et al., 1999). For example, I can know that swimming pools are places people go to engage in swimming and other water sports without ever having been to a swimming pool, but I can only say I know *how* to swim if I can do so. In the former case, I can probably explain how I came by the knowledge, but in the latter, I may not be able to explain how I know how to swim or what I am doing when swimming; the knowledge statement *I know how to swim* is dispositional: its truth is determined by my ability to swim. Such 'knowing how' knowledge is sometimes called 'tacit knowledge', in contrast to 'explicit knowledge' or 'knowing that'. Our concern here is less about how theoretically we might define knowledge than about the question of what sort of knowledge health visitors *could* and *should* be using – and who says so – and what sort of knowledge they *are* using. There is substantial controversy here, as various factions argue that *their* type or source of knowledge is the most important. And the outcome of what might be argued to be a fight to define the 'proper' knowledge basis for practice is important as it has the potential to impinge directly on the health and safety of the client and on the degree to which health visiting can be said to 'add value' to clients.

In later sections of this chapter, we will look more closely at EBP, which is currently the dominant knowledge protocol in the National Health Service (NHS), and try to establish what forms of knowledge it valorises – and what forms it discounts – and why. The chapter will also look at reflective practice (an alternative protocol for generating and managing knowledge about practice that is supported by many institutions and individuals within nursing) and at the idea of knowledge being generated and managed within communities of practice (CoPs) (an idea that is popular in education and some other public sector areas); each of these can be viewed as a social movement, with enthusiastic advocates trying to 'capture' the support of key health organisations and institutions, as well as the hearts and minds of individual practitioners. We will also look at what is known about the types and sources of knowledge that healthcare practitioners actually use in practice – which prove to be somewhat different from any of the 'ideals' promoted by these social movements.

But before examining any of these 'ideal' types of knowledge management, it will be useful to remind ourselves about the practice of health visiting. For evidence-based health visiting or reflective health visiting or any other imported concept to be a reality, it must be integrated into the taken-for-granted, existing ways in which health visitors go about their business. But defining or describing health visiting is not simple. If we start by looking at what the government thinks it is, then we must recognise that, in the UK, health visiting is practised in four nations (involving two assemblies and two parliaments), each of which has a different idea of what health visitors should do, and to what ends. We then have the view of the profession as a whole, which is expressed through various collective means. But when we try and look at the actual practice of health visiting, we find that there is a lack of shared knowledge about what goes on in the very many interactions which lie outside of the public domain of hospitals and clinics. Despite these difficulties, the next two sections will look briefly at the contexts in which health visitors manage knowledge.

Defining health visiting practice

The Department of Health commissioned a review of health visiting, *Facing the Future* (DH, 2007), aimed at highlighting key areas of health visiting practice and skills. This is not a wholly research-based document – and makes no claims to be – although there are some references to research. Rather, 'this review is informed by evidence, government policy and the views of many stakeholders' (DH, 2007: §1). Decisions about what health visiting should be about are therefore largely presented as decisions for the community of stakeholders in the context of stated government priorities. Key elements of the decision-making process can be seen as pragmatic and commonsensical – in the best sense. For example, the review argues that the health visiting service should be one which someone will commission (i.e. pay for), one that is supported by families and communities (i.e. acceptable to the users of the service), and one that is attractive enough to secure a succession of new entrants (i.e. it has a workforce of sufficient size and ability).

In terms of the future skills of health visitors, the review is clear that they will be expected to be able to translate evidence into practice – although it is less specific about what sort of evidence will count and how the process will be managed. However, at the national level, it recommends that the relevant research findings to support a 21st-century child and family health service be assembled. There is also some indication that future practice will be guided by clear protocols: 'Inconsistent service provision with individual interpretation' will be replaced by 'Planned, systematic and/or licensed programmes' (DH, 2007: recommendation 8). As we shall see, the reduction in variations in practice is one of the key aims of the EBP movement. In terms of evidence underpinning practice, the document also draws specific attention to the expanding knowledge base in mental health promotion, the neurological development of young children, and the effectiveness of early intervention, parenting programmes, and health visiting. Clearly, this is a very broad base of evidence, derived from a range of academic and practice disciplines.

So, while the review is not specifically about the evidence or knowledge base of health visiting and how it might be used, many of the relevant themes in debates about EBP begin to emerge. For example:

- What is the role of the practitioner in assembling and assessing evidence?
- How can evidence be translated into practice?
- What counts as evidence?
- How can other bodies support the practitioner by generating and assembling evidence?

- How can any practitioner be conversant with developing knowledge bases in a wide variety of other disciplines?
- What will be the role of protocols, guidelines, and 'recipes' for practice?

These questions all remain relevant, and health visiting commissioners, managers, and practitioners attempt to answer and reconcile them at all levels of practice. However, at the highest level of government, where the health visiting service is created and defined, significant changes in the knowledge base have been used to refocus the purpose and practice of health visiting. The new knowledge largely stems from the neurosciences and developmental psychology, and not from within health visiting itself, and is concerned with how and when brain development occurs. It underpins the premise that early intervention in every child's life – starting from conception – to optimise brain development is a key plank in strategies aimed at improving educational attainment, reducing crime and antisocial behaviour, reducing obesity, and improving health. Perhaps the most robust expression of what might be called the 'early intervention movement' is the first of two government reports by the Labour MP Graham Allen: *Early Intervention: The Next Steps* (Allen, 2011a). The context of Allen's report is the UK fiscal deficit and the Conservative/Liberal Democrat coalition government's agenda of addressing this deficit by making substantial reductions in public spending. Indeed, Allen's second report (Allen, 2011b) is entitled *Early Intervention: Smart Investment, Massive Savings*. In order to emphasise the need for early intervention, his first report starts with two images of a child's brain: one from a 'normal' child and one from a child who has suffered significant deprivation in early childhood. The differences in neurological development are obvious and striking, even to a lay reader, but the important conclusion from the evidence is that such damage is caused by poor parenting, is largely permanent, and is the cause of significant problems in the child's behaviour, which both impede the well being of the child and damage society. These are claims which stem from research that is not easily accessible to health practitioners or their clients. It is also research that is ongoing, with claims being contested and disputed: work by Noble *et al.* (2015) identifies family income and parental education as being the prime correlates to neurological development, for example.

While the claims about neurological development in Allen's first report remain deeply contested, they have been accepted at the highest levels of government, so the questions of what to do and who will do it become acute. In terms of what to do, policy makers look to evidence-based, precisely defined packages of action that have been robustly evaluated to provide the most secure way forward. Allen (2011a: ch. 6) identifies 19 programmes (e.g. the Family Nurse Partnership (FNP)) which he believes should form the basis of early intervention because of their targets and proven efficacy. Such intervention packages have been developed in many countries, often by private agencies, and need either to be incorporated into 'traditional' ways of working – or to replace them (see Chapter 5). So we now have complex bodies of evidence about both a perceived problem *and* a systematic solution used to prescribe practice. Such packages do not just say what must be done but also define *how* it must be done, and we will look at some of the issues raised by them in a later section. In practice, the responses to the early intervention imperative have varied between the UK's nations, each having to answer such questions as: To what degree should intervention be targeted, and at whom? Who should carry out the intervention, and do they have the capacity and capability? and How should we ensure that the work is carried out consistently and effectively?

The Department of Health in England responded with the creation of a revitalised and expanded health visiting profession. The Health Visitor Implementation Plan 2011–15 (DH, 2011) proposed that health visitors provide a four-level service, with services allocated according to the needs of the child and family. There was also to be increased recruitment and training, including an emphasis on leadership development. While this was welcomed by the profession, there were dissenting voices. *The Lancet*, for example, posted a commentary by a public health doctor who supported the emphasis on early years intervention but argued that 'This policy takes a narrow approach, concentrating investment in expanding professional capacity in a service which can only provide part of the solution' (Buttivant, 2011). And the Department of Health itself commissioned a major literature review (Cowley *et al.*, 2013, 2015) to try and identify evidence to support the policy. In the other nations of the UK, different approaches were taken. In Scotland, for example, health visiting as such remained comparatively marginalised until in 2013 the Chief Nursing Officer required that 'the current Public Health Nursing (PHN) role … should be refocused and the titles of Health Visitor and School Nurse be reintroduced' (Moore, 2013: summary). The health visitor was to work with children aged 0–5 using 'targeted' interventions. Part of the rationale for the change was evidence that the public understood and preferred these 'traditional' titles. In Wales and Northern Ireland, too, there was increased focus on early years, although local policies reflected local traditions and ambitions. So, while no-one was disputing the knowledge base of an early intervention strategy, there have been considerable differences in the way this translates into policy for practice. High-level policy makers have their own ideological commitments and knowledge of local history, which mediate between knowledge and policy (for practice). Research rarely dictates policy, but it does inform it.

In England, the three key policies of early intervention, evidence-based pathways, and health visitor leadership remained throughout the defined years of the Health Visitor Implementation Plan 2011–15. The National Health Visiting Service Specification 2014/15 (NHS England, 2014) continued to make explicit reference to the evidence base of the Allen (2011a) report: 'Research studies in neuroscience and developmental psychology have shown that interactions and experiences with caregivers in the first months of a child's life determine whether the child's developing brain structure will provide a strong or a weak foundation for their future health, wellbeing, psychological and social development' (NHS England, 2014: 1.1.3 p. 5). The four levels of intervention remained in place and explicit reference was made to care pathways. Additional specifications for practice come in the form of required assessment protocols. This national specification is reflected in local practice handbooks. As an example, a practice handbook for health visiting team members published in 2012 by the Shropshire County Primary Care Trust (PCT) (Langford, 2012) ran to 43 pages of prescription concerning when visits were to be made and what should be done in each. The document is rich in references – 'Evidence/Rational' (*sic*) – but these are largely not to original research but to recipes for action; for example, it specifies 10 assessment tools. So, by 2015, the idea that health visiting was an innovation technology rather than an individualistic practice was well established, at least in England and some other parts of the UK. Health visiting practice was conceived of as something which could be prescribed to solve defined national problems. Such policy prescriptions are not confined to health problems but can also be found elsewhere in social care, education, and the justice system – usually in areas where governments are particularly concerned to achieve particular outcomes. For example, a similar approach was taken in the case of another perceived threat to society – (Islamist) terrorism – where schools were encouraged to use packaged interventions designed to prevent the radicalisation of children.

From the point of view of the profession as a whole, the resurgence of health visiting was seen as an opportunity to raise its profile and consolidate its gains. A new body, the Institute of Health Visiting (iHV), was founded in 2012 with the avowed core purpose of raising 'professional standards in health visiting practice … By promoting and supporting a strong evidence base for health visiting and offering CPD [continuing professional development] and professional training' (iHV, 2012). In other words, it sought to improve practice not by telling health visitors what to do but by improving their knowledge and skills. A central part of the work of the iHV is therefore the development of various 'tools' to help practitioners enhance their practice and guide them through an increasingly complex world of guidelines, pathways, programmes, and protocols and an expanding research base involving many disciplines. These tools are not 'prescriptions' of good practice but rather provisions of access to learning opportunities, case studies, publications, and Web-facilitated channels for practitioner–practitioner and practitioner–expert interaction. You could characterise this as a 'bottom-up' process of using evidence to improve practice, in contrast to the 'top-down' process of prescription based on policy, but as we shall see, both models remain part of the EBP ideology. Within EBP, there is also a substantial body of work exploring how knowledge management fits into the everyday realities of practice. So, what do we know of actual practice in health visiting – its opportunities and constraints?

What do health visitors do – and where do they do it?

Against the background of the government seeking to prescribe health visiting practice as a remedy for society's ills, it is important to review what is known about the actual practice of health visiting; that is, what health visitors do on a day-to-day basis. Unfortunately, relatively little is known – other than tacitly by those who do it – about the realities of everyday health visiting. That it is rarely seen as a valid subject either for scientific research or for practice narratives is also true of a similar practice: social work. In the case of social work, however, we find an interesting research programme conducted by Harry Ferguson (2008, 2010), which aims to bring to light the essential nature of its practice. Ferguson argues that current research is focused on systems and interprofessional communication, which 'leaves largely unaddressed practitioners' experiences of the work they have to do that goes on beyond the office, on the street and in doing the home visit' (Ferguson, 2010:1100). Ferguson is trying to refocus on actual practice; he further argues:

> Reclaiming this lost experience of movement, adventure, atmosphere and emotion is an important step in developing better understandings of what social workers can do, the risks and limits to their achievements, and provides for deeper learning about the skilled performances and successes that routinely go on.
>
> (Ferguson, 2010:1102)

Of course, this is just as true for health visiting, where a significant part of the practice is leaving the office, driving to the client, thinking about how the visit will work, knocking on the door, and so on. Ferguson's account of the excitement and fear of walking through disadvantaged neighbourhoods and of negotiating home visits with disobliging clients is focused on social workers working in child protection, but it must resonate with all practising health visitors. The way in which he conceptualises the home visit is of particular interest: 'All homes and the relationships within them have atmospheres and how professionals manage stepping into and negotiating them is at the core of performing social work and child protection and managing risk effectively' (Ferguson, 2010:1109).

So how would the ever-useful Martian sociologist describe health visiting practice? They would be bound to notice that it is largely about doing things with words. Note the emphasis on *doing*; talk isn't just something which surrounds the doing, it *is* the doing – praising, blaming, asking, advising, persuading: every utterance is an action produced for a purpose, although the speaker is rarely consciously aware of this. The skills involved in talking are so deep that, just like with walking, they are not normally subject to constant ongoing analysis. Most of us do not consciously think about how to walk – we just do it. But talk is the health visitor's key performative skill, and because doing things with talk is a primary skill, health visitors need a more profound understanding of how it works – just as a ballet dancer would need a more profound understanding of how her body works than would the person taking the dog for a walk. Of course, as well as talking, health visitors also make notes and write reports, but this is still doing things with language in order to interact with others.

In the 1980s, there was considerable interest within sociology in researching how interactions, largely based on talk, could constitute various forms of institutional practice. This idea was rather neatly defined in an edited volume of studies called *Talk at Work*. The editors argue:

> that talk-in-interaction is the principal means through which lay persons pursue various practical goals and the central medium through which the daily working activities of many professionals and organisational representatives are conducted.
>
> (Drew & Heritage, 1992: 3)

Health visiting is one such profession, and a number of studies have been conducted within that sociological tradition (see, for example, Dingwall & Robinson, 1990; Heritage & Sefi, 1992). The focus is on making available what happens in the 'private' world of the home visit. Cowley *et al.* (2013), in their extensive review of health visiting literature, reinforce the centrality of the home visit in health visiting, arguing that it is one of the three key components of practice (the other two being the health visitor–client relationship and health visitor needs assessment).

Health visitors also work in clinics, general practitioner (GP) surgeries, children's centres, church halls, social services departments, and so on. So a further defining characteristic of health visiting is that it does not have a fixed locality or place of work. There is an interesting literature on the issue of place in healthcare (see, for example, Angus *et al.*, 2005; Poland *et al.*, 2005), and of course it relates to the issue of mobility which is central to Ferguson's (2008, 2010) work. Poland *et al.* (2005) argue that, while practitioners are sensitive to issues of place, this has largely been ignored in debates about best practice and EBP. They further assert that:

> Interventions wither or thrive based on complex interactions between key personalities, circumstances and coincidences … A detailed analysis of the setting … can help practitioners skilfully anticipate and navigate potentially murky waters filled with hidden obstacles.
>
> (Poland *et al.*, 2005: 171)

By 'place', Poland *et al.* (2005) mean a great deal more than mere geography. The concept includes a range of issues, notably the way power relationships are constructed and the way in which technologies operate in and on various places. Alaszewski (2006) draws our attention to the risk involved in practising outside 'the institution'. While there are ways in which physical institutions mitigate the risks from their clientele:

> The institutional structure of classification, surveillance and control is significantly changed in the community. Much of the activity takes place within spaces that are not designed or controlled by professionals, for example the service user's own home.
>
> (Alaszewski, 2006: 4)

The discussion in this section draws on concepts and evidence from a number of sources, which can be used as vehicles for thinking about health visiting. But, as Peckover (2013) points out, we do not have a coherent body of research on the reality of health visiting practice. Cowley *et al.* (2015: 473), in their review of the literature, acknowledge that their work has revealed the concepts and theories underlying health visiting but not 'the forms of practice that exist in reality.' We know what health visitors *aim* to do but not what they *actually* do. Peckover argues that this lack of a 'meta-narrative' for health visiting is both a weakness and a strength: a weakness because it struggles to explain itself to policy makers and to establish a strong base in higher education, but a strength in that it seems to be able to adapt to changing demands. Given the complexity of health visiting, we need to look at the top-down prescriptions for practice and ask, first, how we can reconcile the practice prescriptions of the policy makers and managers with what we know about what Ferguson calls 'the fluid, squelchy nature of practices …' (Ferguson, 2008: 576), and, second, how we can source evidence to support the parts of practice which do not, or do not yet, fall within the realm of defined practice. Can the concepts and practices of EBP and knowledge management help?

Evidence-based practice

In order to understand the importance of the EBP movement, you need to take yourself back in time about 30 years. Back then, doctors and nurses did what they had been taught to do; experienced practitioners became teachers and passed on what they had learned in their years of practice. There was almost no reference to research findings, but lots of reference to both 'facts' and 'proper ways of doing things'. That is not to say that there was no innovation: new drugs became available and there were surgeons trialling procedures we now take for granted, such as joint replacements. But the idea that the way to do things in healthcare was passed on from previous practitioners was prevalent. So the idea of EBP was really revolutionary – and there was considerable opposition to it.

What has come to be known as EBP had its foundations in the evidence-based medicine (EBM) movement, which started in the UK in the early 1990s. The NHS was interested in funding and promoting research, and there was a research infrastructure. However, there was increasing dissatisfaction among some key individuals in the medical profession – notably Dr (now Sir) Muir Gray, who was an NHS Regional Director of Research and Development – over the fact that, within medicine, treatments which had been proven to be effective were not being used, while treatments which had been shown to have no or little beneficial effect continued to be used. This was despite considerable efforts to change practice; for example, the Getting Research into Practice and Purchasing (GRIPP) project, developed in the Oxford NHS region, looked at four treatments:

- the use of corticosteroids in preterm delivery;
- the management of services for stroke patients;
- the use of dilation and curettage (D&C) for dysfunctional uterine bleeding;
- insertion of grommets for children with glue ear.

Good research evidence was available to underpin decisions in all these areas of practice, and health authorities within the Oxford region sought to ensure that practice adhered to the research-based recommendations. However, variations in practice proved difficult to eradicate, and it was felt that more needed to be done. Did the practitioners not understand the research? Did they need motivation to change from their traditional ways of practice? Perhaps a more widespread and coordinated effort to base practice on research needed to be developed.

The fundamental proposition of the subsequent EBM movement was that practice should take account of the latest and best research-generated evidence to underpin both individual clinical decision making and collective policy making. At the heart of EBM is the idea that it provides a vehicle by which the practitioner can continually examine and improve their individual practice by testing it against scientifically validated external evidence and importing proven treatments. Activity 1.1 will help you to explore the evidence around interventions delivered by health visitors.

Sackett *et al.* (1997) define EBM as consisting of five sequential steps:

1. Identifying the need for information and formulating a question.
2. Tracking down the best possible source of evidence to answer that question.
3. Evaluating the evidence for validity and clinical applicability.
4. Applying the evidence in practice.
5. Evaluating the outcomes.

So, for example, a doctor faced with a patient with a severe infection might ask, 'Which antibiotic will best cure this infection?' and look to the literature on drug trials for an answer. Thereafter, they would evaluate the validity of the trial and its relevance to their patient, administer the drug (or not), and see what happened. Or, to use one of the examples from the GRIPP project, a doctor treating a child with 'glue ear' might ask, 'Will surgery to insert grommets make a difference in the long term compared with conservative treatment?' A search of the literature would indicate that surgery to insert grommets is not necessarily cost-effective in the long run in terms of outcome. But this example illustrates a complexity that the rational model of EBM does not necessarily deal with. At the point that the doctor opts for conservative treatment, what message is conveyed to the parent with a child who has suddenly gone deaf and who is losing both speech and friends? The research evidence on cost-effectiveness may not fully acknowledge the social issues surrounding the clinical problem. EBM is essentially a linear model for change which assumes that clinicians should make rational choices based on the scientific evidence available to them. It does not necessarily take into account the choices that clients would make, which might be equally rational for them. Activity 1.2 will be helpful in gaining some experience in the practice of EBM.

EBM defines the best source of evidence as the randomised control trial (RCT), or better still a group of RCTs, which can be systematically reviewed and analysed. Early on in EBM, the idea was that clinicians would get involved in all stages of the process, including the search for and evaluation of the evidence, and there were – and are – various manuals and training programmes to help them do that. This can be defined as the simple linear model of practitioner-based EBP, which is still espoused by some. But, in practice, a cadre of specialist and largely university-based 'experts' has grown up to manage the search for and evaluation of the scientific evidence and to produce specifications for practice, which are then disseminated through various fora. These specifications are known by a number of names, including 'clinical guidelines' and 'care pathways', and their use will be explored later in the chapter. The degree to which any specification will constitute a suggestion or an instruction to practitioners largely depends on the importance of the topic and the costs of that area of practice. The contrast between two propositions found in EBM – that individual practitioners should evaluate the evidence and change their practice accordingly and that evaluating evidence is an expert skill requiring considerable resources – remains important. Research evaluation is a key component of many healthcare curricula, but the degree to which it might or should be a key component of practice remains contested.

So, the EBM movement has been, and continues to be, subject to considerable debate and criticism. However, there is a danger that it is criticised for ideas which it does not wholly espouse.

First, its initial proponents did not suppose that the use of research evidence would entirely override clinical judgment, but rather that it would work in conjunction with it:

> External clinical evidence can inform, but can never replace, individual clinical expertise and it is this expertise that decides whether the external evidence applies to the individual patient at all and, if so, how it should be integrated into a clinical decision.
>
> (Sackett *et al.*, 1997: 4)

Second, while it is true that a hierarchy of evidence was proposed, which placed that derived from RCTs at the top as the 'gold standard', it did not assert that other forms of evidence were not of some value, and neither did it entirely ignore evidence derived from qualitative research (Glaszious *et al.*, 2004).

Early EBM was an enthusiasts' movement, but a whole industry has since grown up around it, and it is now central to government health policy and is spreading into other occupations. So, who is supporting the development of EBM and its promotion in new disciplines such as nursing, social work, and education – and why?

First, there is a lobby from researchers. After all, if no-one uses their work then why should government continue to fund it? Healthcare research is now a substantial industry, forming a significant part of many university budgets. New journals have sprung up to explore the issues, and, of course, publication is the lifeblood of academics. Gerrish (2003), citing Estabrooks (1998), argues that EBM has generated a shift in power and prestige in healthcare from experienced expert clinicians to researchers.

Second, there is the government, which is increasingly committed to the development of evidence-based policy making in many spheres, certainly including health. A range of organisations have been established to support EBM and fund research designed to feed directly into practice, including the Cochrane Collaboration (which exists to produce systematic reviews), the National Institute for Health and Care Excellence (NICE), and a number of university-based units, such as the University of York Centre for Reviews and Dissemination. Within government-funded research programmes, there has been an increased emphasis on 'impact', in addition to validity, reliability, and so on. Activity 1.3 will help you to explore elements of effective health visiting practice.

Third, there are the nurses, social workers, and teachers themselves. Although there was (and is) some concern within medicine that EBM would erode the importance of clinical judgment, in these professions the idea of developing a strong formal and recognised evidence base was seductive. A few decades ago, the theory that a profession needed to have certain characteristics became popular in occupations such as nursing, social work, and teaching. While the theory itself was deeply flawed, as it largely ignored issues of power and prestige based on class and gender, it did inspire a section of nursing to fight for an independent regulatory body – now the NMC – and for graduate entry to the occupation, which has now been realised with the 2010 change in NMC regulations. This professionalising agenda has extended to a belief that a 'proper' profession will have – and use – an extensive evidence base gleaned from research; that is, it should aspire to be an 'evidence-based' profession. Consequently, some nursing constituencies have vigorously championed the development of nursing research and the inclusion of nursing in multidisciplinary research – and indeed there has been a very rapid expansion of nursing research, although much of it remains small-scale (Cowley et al., 2013, 2015).

Fourth, there is the consumer, who increasingly wants the 'best' treatment available and is intolerant of variations in practice – or 'postcode lotteries'. This may in part be fuelled by media reports of research 'breakthroughs'. However, the consumer's attitudes are at best ambivalent – the extensive and growing use of 'alternative' therapies, many of which have a research evidence base which is slight at best, shows that the consumer also wants to decide for themselves what works. Activity 1.4 will help you to explore this further.

So, we can conclude that powerful forces have fuelled the development of the EBM movement and have vested interests in its success. More fundamentally, like any social movement, it had to be in the right place at the right time. A number of factors seem to have been crucial. Importantly, the oil crisis of the mid 1970s forced Western industrial societies into financial panic. Muir Gray acknowledges the importance of this economic crisis in the development of EBM (cited in Traynor, 2002). Never again would the price of something not matter, and state-funded healthcare represents a massive part of government expenditure. When doctors undertook operations for glue ear with no proven benefit, that was no longer just their decision. And partly as a result of the economic crisis, society was also changing. Traynor (2002) defines key products of this new emphasis on fiscal control to be the rise of managerialism, the increased use of audit, and an increased emphasis on research and development (R&D). In addition, society was increasingly conscious of risk but wary of the power and authority of both science and professions to provide solutions. How did EBM fit into this landscape? In theory, having sufficient research evidence to specify 'best practice' allowed managers greater control over individual practitioners, and audit systems ensured that this control was maintained. Although EBM is based on a science embedded in experimental work, it was not a scientific 'grand narrative'; rather, it provided 'recipes' for best practice, which would, in theory, reduce variations in practice and control risk. A further key element in the success of EBM – and in making it a worldwide phenomenon – is the exponential growth in information technology. Without the ability to search digital databases worldwide, EBM would be a much reduced enterprise.

The concepts behind EBM have spread to other healthcare occupations, and subsequently beyond healthcare into management, education, and social work; it is commonplace now to describe the movement as EBP. In 2008, NICE was given a remit for work in public health, including disease prevention and health promotion. Changes have thus had to be made to the way in which EBP operates even within the heartland of medicine. Kelly et al. (2010) offer an 'insider's' perspective on some of these challenges as they work within NICE on the public health agenda – which of course goes beyond healthcare into education, social welfare, and so on, and depends on disciplines such as psychology, sociology, and anthropology. In moving into new areas, institutions such as NICE have had to travel beyond biomedicine, with its relatively simple causal models, and engage with very different academic and practice disciplines with their own distinct ways of generating and validating knowledge. A fundamental problem is that the EBM methodology for generating evidence, which gives superiority to RCTs, is not going to work. Few such trials are conducted outside of biomedicine, and much of the knowledge in social science disciplines is generated by the use of theories and models, which are not amenable to the sort of meta-analysis to which trials can be subjected:

> Theories and models require a different way of encapsulating their form and content, their provenance, their ideological dispositions and so on. They are not facts in the sense that someone's occupation or systolic blood pressure are facts. Theories are ways of organising ideas, usually designed to make observable facts clearer or more coherent, or to offer some kind of explanation for the particular way the facts are, or appear to be.
>
> (Kelly *et al.*, 2010: 1059)

If these differences in the way in which knowledge is generated and validated cannot be acknowledged then much of the knowledge of these disciplines will be disregarded as being of lower status or as including bias.

A further problem is that in many public health issues there is a long causal pathway between an intervention and the change it is designed to create, and this creates conceptual complexity not encountered when testing drug A against drug B. Kelly *et al.* (2010) outline some of the ways in which they are engaging with these issues, which include both creating new methodologies (e.g. developing logic models to manage methodological pluralism) and trying to use experts in the field to generate consensus.

Issues underlying the use of primary research were highlighted in 2015 when an extensive study by leading academics within psychology published data showing that 'many psychological papers fail the replication test' (Open Science Collaboration, 2015). The ability to repeat an experiment and get the same results is a cornerstone of the scientific method, so clearly this called into question the original results. This study is part of an ongoing debate about how we conduct not just psychology but *all* science and whether issues such as a pressure to publish positive results skew the literature. A key contribution to the debate (Ioannidis, 2005) is entitled 'Why most published research findings are false' and a commentary by Richard Horton (2015) in *The Lancet* argues that the situation is deteriorating. Horton suggests that many aspects of research culture are contributing to 'bad science': 'The apparent endemicity of bad research behaviour is alarming. In their quest for telling a compelling story, scientists too often sculpt data to fit their preferred theory of the world' (Horton, 2015: 1380).

So, despite its success in embedding itself into national structures and in spreading into new fields, EBP remains a highly contested concept and an evolving practice. Even within EBM, there were many concerns, which were articulated early on in a useful summary document titled *Acting on the Evidence* (Appleby *et al.*, 1995), produced by the University of York. This document summarises EBM as 'the movement away from basing healthcare on opinion or past practice and towards grounding healthcare in science and evidence' (Appleby *et al.*, 1995: 4). It raises a number of issues. First, it argues that insufficient account is taken by EBM of the uncertainty of clinical practice. Second, it says that it is impossible to generate information on everything – a key issue for health visiting, which exists in a highly complex epistemological and social context. Third, it notes that information about clinical effectiveness generated by RCTs is about populations, whereas clinicians deal with individuals:

> How rigid do we expect the doctor to be in reconciling the scientifically derived probabilities of clinical effectiveness with the situation of the individual patient?
>
> (Appleby *et al.*, 1995: 30)

The current landscape of EBP

As we look across the new occupations engaging in EBP, we can see three interesting responses to the original concept, each of which will be explored more fully in the following sections. First, there are those who make theoretical objections to EBM, and particularly to its export into other areas. This is probably best exemplified in a published 'dialogue' between Iain Chalmers, a key figure in the EBM movement, and Martyn Hammersley, a leading figure in the sociology of education and research methods, which will be described shortly. Second, there are those who are quite enthusiastic about EBP but dismayed that it just doesn't seem to change practice. This has produced what might be called the 'barriers' literature, which attempts to identify and eradicate the reasons why EBP doesn't work and has developed into an industry devoted to what has become known as 'implementation science'. Third, there are those who embrace the concept of EBP but who want to redefine the notion of what counts as evidence – largely because it doesn't seem to resonate with the realities of their practice. Nursing in particular has criticised the technological model of knowledge used in EBM, and has argued that the linear model of research evidence utilisation may not be wholly appropriate to nursing practice.

From within the discipline of education, Martyn Hammersley has produced one of the most accessible critiques, engaging directly with the arguments of major supporters of EBP – notably Iain Chalmers, who wrote an article in support of EBM entitled 'Trying to do more good than harm in policy and practice: the role of rigorous, transparent, up-to-date evaluations' (Chalmers, 2003). Hammersley's response is direct: 'Is the evidence-based practice movement doing more good than harm? Reflections on Iain Chalmers' case for research-based policy making and practice' (Hammersley, 2005). He seeks first to establish common ground, suggesting that there should be broad agreement about the following propositions:

- Practitioners occasionally do harm in their professional work.
- Research can help provide practitioners and policy makers with useful information.
- Not everything presented as research is either reliable or, indeed, research.

Further, Hammersley agrees with Chalmers that research needs to be mediated before it can be used by individual practitioners:

> the results of research should be presented to lay audiences through reviews of the available literature, rather than the findings of individual studies being offered as reliable information.
>
> (Hammersley, 2005: 87)

However, he goes on to argue, first, that the methodologies favoured in EBP – the RCT and the systematic review – are themselves subject to methodological critique and should not be assumed to produce bias-free evidence: 'research findings must always be interpreted and are never free from potential error' (Hammersley, 2005: 88). This is not an argument about quantitative and qualitative methods, but rather an argument that *all* forms of research are socially constructed and that all research is generated and read within a particular context of experience and judgment.

Second, he argues that Chalmers, and by extension other EBP proponents, believes that research can *arbitrate* in areas where there are debates about what counts as good practice. By implication, he suggests that Chalmers has gone beyond the originally proposed 'partnership' between external research evidence and clinical judgment to valorise the external evidence. He rejects the idea that RCTs should have a privileged status above other kinds of knowledge and be used to resolve disputes.

Third, he argues that judgment is fundamental to good practice because 'practice is necessarily a matter of judgment, in which information from various sources (not just research) must be combined' (Hammersley, 2005: 88). He asserts that that the role of professional judgment may differ between different forms and arenas of practice and argues that downplaying the importance of professional judgment in favour of research evidence could, in some contexts, reduce the quality of practice rather than enhance it.

The dialogue continues with Chalmers' (2005) response, 'If evidence-informed policy works in practice, does it matter if it doesn't work in theory?', which claims that Hammersley misrepresents his views. Interestingly, Chalmers cites a specific example, familiar to health visitors, of research findings changing the previous 'commonsense' recommendations about the way a baby should sleep – on its front or back – as one of the key pieces of evidence supporting the importance and impact of EBP:

> These and countless other examples should leave little doubt that it is irresponsible to interfere in the lives of other people on the basis of theories unsupported by reliable empirical evidence.
>
> (Chalmers, 2005: 229)

Hammersley is not the only critical commentator of the EBM movement. For example, Kerridge *et al.* (1998), writing from a basis in health ethics, argue that EBM has serious ethical flaws. First, while EBM is concerned with outcomes, there are many aspects of outcomes which cannot be properly measured; they cite as examples pain, justice, and quality of life. Second, it is difficult in EBM to decide between the competing claims of different stakeholders. While EBM potentially downgrades the power and authority of individual doctors, who should replace them in the power position? Is it managers? Is it patients? And if the latter, how can that be managed? Third, EBM interventions may transgress common morality because they are concerned only with evidence of efficacy. Kerridge *et al.* raise issues about the ethical status of trials: on the one hand, there are now strict criteria which might be seen as 'good', but on the other, these criteria shift over time. They also argue that RCTs in themselves are subject to ethical questions about 'the selection of subjects, consent, randomisation, the manner in which trials are stopped, and the continuing care of subjects once the trials are complete' (Kerridge *et al.*, 1998: 1152).

The literature on EBM and practice is full of such claims and counter claims. But while such debates may be exciting and energising for those involved in them, they can be somewhat bewildering or even daunting to lay (i.e. non-research) practitioners. But they are important in terms of practice. Kerridge *et al.* cite Dr Michael Wooldridge, then Australian health minister, who said that '[we will] pay only for those operations, drugs and treatments that according to available evidence are proved to work' (Kerridge *et al.*, 1998: 1153). By implication, governments will only support those activities which can be shown to have an effect – and an effect which the government wants.

From a purely practical point of view, what is the evidence that research findings, even when expertly mediated through the Cochrane Collaboration, NICE, or other guideline systems, are – or, indeed, can be – directly applied to practice in the linear model implied by evidence-based practitioners? There is considerable evidence that it is not being applied directly as anticipated, which suggests that we need to think of the relationship between research and practice in more complex terms. In order to examine and explain these problems, a literature developed exploring what were known as the 'barriers' to utilising research. If we could just identify and remove those barriers, the argument went, all would be well. Grimshaw and Thomson argued that, 'Despite the considerable resources devoted to biomedical science, a consistent finding from the literature is that the transfer of research findings into practice is a slow and haphazard process' (Grimshaw & Thomson, 1998: 20). Grol & Wensing found the same thing:

> One of the most consistent findings in health services research is the gap between best practice (as determined by scientific evidence), on the one hand, and actual clinical care, on the other.
>
> (Grol & Wensing, 2004: §57)

These authors studied barriers to change and proposed that they occur at different levels: the nature of the innovation itself, the individual, the social context, the patient, the wider context – really, just about anything. In the UK, Gerrish (2003) explored some of the barriers to introducing research into nursing based on a study within a large acute hospital; she groups them into factors relating to the organisation, the way research is communicated, the quality of the research, and the nurse. Again, it seems difficult to identify anything which might not constitute a barrier. Clearly, some of these factors may include barriers to introducing any kind of change; healthcare organisations are very large and complex, and the healthcare sector is highly regulated and risk-averse. Others are specific to research-based knowledge, and Gerrish argues that the way in which research is conducted and the type of knowledge it generates may be important. The traditional model of EBP, as we have seen, assumes the superiority of acontextual, disembodied technological knowledge and a linear model of utilisation. Gerrish argues that other research models, such as the enlightenment model or action research, might have substantial value. However, the practitioners of implementation science have pursued the idea that barriers to implementation *must* be overcome and have generated a whole research domain dedicated to exploring not what ought to be done but rather how to ensure that it is done in practice. This work has become another 'industry' supporting healthcare, generating its own journals, conferences, and research units. The aim of these practitioners is to create an effective implementation infrastructure. This represents a substantial step beyond the work of the EBM pioneers, who used the language of *promoting* and *disseminating* research, assuming that all right-minded practitioners could and would alter their practice in response. Implementation science acknowledges the complex world in which practice takes place and seeks to investigate how programmes can be designed and presented such that they can be *implemented* in practice. Activity 1.5 explores barriers to implementing research evidence in health visiting.

There is a substantial constituency in nursing which has embraced the concept of EBP, and a supportive base of journals, professional bodies, and university units has been established. This might seem surprising in an occupation which has fought to defend the importance of qualitative research and does not have a substantial tradition of conducting RCTs or systematic reviews (important exceptions in the context of health visiting include Elkan *et al.* (2000), who systematically reviewed the evidence on the effectiveness of domiciliary health visiting, and Cowley *et al.* (2015)). Judith Parker, former director of the Victoria Centre for Evidence Based Nursing in Melbourne, provides an interesting perspective on why nursing should embrace EBP in an editorial in *Nursing Inquiry* (Parker, 2002), in which she feels she has to defend her personal support for EBP, not least because she has a reputation for engaging in research in a different epistemological tradition, which focuses on experience and narrative. She argues that its time has come as the result of a range of economic, political, and market imperatives. She draws attention to the way in which it helps society manage risk, reduce costs, and provide accountability. In addition, she argues that:

> It provides investigative and justificatory tools to manoeuvre the morass of uncertainty in situations where decisions must be made without knowing the consequences and where many of the comforting routines of the past have fallen away.
>
> (Parker, 2002: 140)

But other researchers have taken a somewhat different path in reconciling engagement with EBP with their value base. Rycroft-Malone *et al.* (2004), in an interesting study titled 'What counts as evidence in evidence-based practice?', suggest that nurses can reconceptualise EBP by greatly broadening the kinds of evidence which are embraced by the movement in order to make it both more acceptable and more useful. They explore the potential for using four types of evidence: that derived from research; clinical experience; the knowledge of patients, clients, and carers; and the local context and environment. The last is somewhat of a 'catch-all' term and includes information from audit and performance, as well as patient narratives, organisational knowledge, local policies, and so on. The authors pose two challenges. First, whatever the source, for knowledge to count as evidence it needs to be examined and tested in some way. So, for example, 'in order for an individual practitioner's experience and knowledge to be considered credible as a source of evidence, it needs to be explicated, analysed and critiqued' (Rycroft-Malone et al., 2004: 84). Second, they argue that we need to develop our collective understanding of how these various evidences are integrated to generate effective practice. It is important to note that this reconceptualising of acceptable evidence goes far beyond the work to expand the evidence base outlined by Kelly et al. (2010). While they are looking to see how other 'sciences' can be incorporated, Rycroft-Malone et al. (2004) are developing the concept of useful evidence as coming from outside traditional science.

In the next section, these themes are further explored through case studies of practice, showing real instances of how knowledge is generated and used by practitioners at all levels. However, before we move on, it may be helpful to note an important paper which defines the sources of knowledge currently used by nurses and illustrates some of the themes raised in the last two sections. Estabrooks et al. (2005) explored the sources of nurses' knowledge through two major ethnographic studies in hospitals in Canada, finding that nurses categorise them into four broad groupings: social interactions, experiential knowledge, documentary sources, and a priori knowledge. Importantly, the category of social interactions dominates their findings. They report that when nurses have immediate and practical concerns, they will turn first to their peers, who can give both information and reassurance, as illustrated by one of their respondents: 'If one of my colleagues says you know what, D, I have seen that happen time and time again … don't worry about it, I will be reassured by that' (Estabrooks et al., 2005: 464). The nurses have a hierarchy of knowledge, but it is not consistent with EBP:

> The high regard for experience also caused nurses occasionally to reject advice from clinical nurse specialists, educators, and physicians when they believed that the advice was inconsistent with their own experiential knowledge. Also nurses sometimes rejected evidence-based patient care protocols in favour of those practices they consider effective based on experience.
>
> (Estabrooks et al., 2005: 468)

Hopefully, this sets the scene for a discussion of how knowledge is managed in particular instances.

Managing knowledge and evidence in practice

Much of the debate in both EBM and EBP utilises an 'ideal' model of the linear movement of research findings into practice. But how is knowledge actually managed in practice? In this section, we examine four 'case studies' which look at how evidence is used for decision making in practical situations (although not all of them are defined as such by their authors). The first is at the national policy level, the second describes the development of local guidelines by GPs, the third looks at the use of protocols by nurses in a diabetic clinic and a cardiac medical unit, and the fourth looks at the practice level within primary care, mainly focusing on GPs and practice nurses.

Case study 1.1:   Introducing new technology

May (2006) examined the potential introduction of telehealthcare systems and explored how policy makers and researchers engaged with each other over this practical issue. The data in May's case study are derived from a series of public and private meetings held between 1998 and 2004 and from two sessions of the UK House of Commons Health Committee in 2001 and 2005. The meetings involved a very wide range of participants: senior health service managers from every NHS level, social care managers from the public and voluntary sectors, policy makers from a number of UK government departments and from the Welsh Assembly and the Scottish Office, university researchers, and representatives of service providers and manufacturers. May was involved in the meetings as a participant – as an expert advisor from a sociological perspective.

At the beginning of the process, the proponents of telehealthcare, the NHS managers, and the policy makers were all agreed that they needed the robust evidence that RCTs and systematic reviews could provide. However, as time went on there was increasing dissatisfaction with the use of trials. A senior clinician said:

> Trials are vital, they give us the evidence, but the evidence is always arguable and it doesn't influence policy makers as much as we would like. *They suffer from evidence fatigue* …
>
> (May, 2006: 519; emphasis in original)

The trials were disparaged for one of their defining characteristics: they are acontextual, in order that they are generalisable, so by definition they cannot provide evidence about the practicalities of innovation in a specific service context. As respondents noted, trials may advantage researchers but they do not reflect what happens in 'normal' practice.

So, while researchers wanted to conduct clinical trials – they got funding to do them and published their results, which could lead to further funding – the managers who actually wanted to get on and solve their problems were disenchanted. Clinical trials did not provide the 'workability' evidence that they needed. By the time of the meeting in 2004, clinical trials had ceased to be of interest and managers and policy makers were looking to work with service providers to set up local demonstration projects. Interestingly, the providers themselves had moved away from providing telehealthcare, which involves clinical practice at a distance, to telecare, which involves safety systems that support people in their own homes; there was thus a commensurate reduction in the need for research evidence on clinical safety and levels of risk.

May (2006) identified a number of issues in the organisation and reception of knowledge produced within a Health Technology Assessment model of formal quantitative knowledge generation. He argued that:

> In practical terms the division between research elites and local managers is expressed by the latter seeking more flexible modes of knowledge production … In the world of service provision, such highly medicalised models of research practice have been by-passed or displaced by different kinds of institutional actors as they seek to rapidly implement new models of service provision.
>
> (May, 2006: 528–9)

He also argued that formal research methods provide a 'flavour' of science to support decisions which are essentially political. In terms of the science, he concluded that evidence is always socially constructed within specific contexts.

Case study 1.2: Creating guidelines in primary care

McDonald & Harrison (2004) looked at the process of developing local clinical guidelines on the treatment by GPs of patients with actual or potential heart disease. At the time of their study, the GPs were linked into a Primary Care Group (PCG) (PCGs were later replaced by PCTs, which have since been replaced in turn by commissioning groups of GP practices). This was a participant observation study, as one of the authors was an expert adviser to the group, in the field of economics and finance. The study was largely based on field notes made at a series of meetings between 1997 and 1999.

The impetus for the development of the local guidelines was in part the imminent publication of the National Service Framework on Coronary Heart Disease and in part concern about the costs of existing practice. Statins, used to treat or prevent heart disease, are relatively cheap drugs, but the number of potential recipients is large, so their overall cost can be significant. The PCG had an existing cardiac focus group, which included the Health Authority's pharmaceutical advisor, the local consultant cardiologist, and a number

(Continued)

Case study 1.2: (*Continued*)

of GPs. This group was charged with making recommendations to all the GPs about managing patients with cardiovascular disease.

The first part of the work focused on developing a statin prescribing guideline. The group used a number of sources of evidence, including the results from several significant RCTs (which clearly showed statins could be effective in reducing mortality), an article from the *BMJ* (which discussed the cost-effectiveness of prescribing strategies in relation to statins), guidelines published by the Standing Medical Advisory Committee (SMAC), and information from pharmaceutical companies.

What issues concerned the group? First, the GPs complained that they didn't understand the SMAC guidelines or the RCT results: 'There was general agreement on the difficulties of making informed choices, particularly when faced with "evidence" from pharmaceutical company representatives' (McDonald & Harrison, 2004: 228). They were confused by the risk tables attached to the SMAC guidelines and felt there were key issues missing, such as family history. The pharmaceutical advisor – who was presumably keen to limit prescribing – suggested that it might be best to concentrate on patients with coronary heart disease, because they were high-risk. The group then debated what constituted a high risk, with a number of GPs giving examples from their own patient populations; importantly, 'The discussions of risk perception revealed that GPs each had their own ideas about what constituted risk' (McDonald & Harrison, 2004: 228), which largely centred around their views on the importance of lifestyle and smoking. A major discussion focused on the age cut-off for prescribing statins. While the pharmaceutical advisor urged a focus on younger patients, a number of the GPs cited particular cases of elderly patients whom they believed 'deserved' statin therapy, and the pharmaceutical advisor's advice was not taken. Further debates included one about what test should be used to establish cholesterol levels. At one point, the economic advisor produced a substantial paper modelling the costs and benefits of options for change, but she was politely told that the GPs were 'simple souls' who couldn't understand it. The group did eventually agree a guidcline, but it was clear that it was guidance rather than prescription. The result of all the work is interesting: before the guideline was produced, there was huge variation in prescribing; afterwards, there was huge variation in prescribing!

McDonald & Harrison (2004) were interested at the start of the study in whether guidelines were the tools of management or of a professional elite. Their conclusion was that it is really more complicated than that: localities, people, and histories all play a part. The GPs relied on reference to individual cases: 'I had a patient in the other day' (McDonald & Harrison, 2004: 228); managers who were concerned about the outcomes of the project tended to move on to other jobs before the work was complete; and while the GPs agreed with the consultant when he was there, they ignored his views after he had left. However, McDonald & Harrison (2004) argued that while these guidelines did not seem to alter practice, an increased government focus on guidelines subsequent to this study may have made adherence more likely. In terms of the way in which local guidelines might be developed, a conclusion from this study must be that the introduction of technical research solutions into practice is not a simple linear process and practitioners rely heavily on their own knowledge and experience.

Case study 1.3: Protocol-based decision making in nursing

Rycroft-Malone *et al.* (2009) looked at nurses' decision making in two contexts: a diabetic and endocrine unit and a cardiac medical unit. Using a variety of data collection methods, including participant and nonparticipant observation, interviews, field notes, and existing documentation, they sought to determine how nurses reached decisions, and in particular whether and how they used protocols. As noted by the authors, standardised care approaches can have a variety of names, including 'protocols', 'care bundles', 'care pathways', and 'clinical guidelines'. However, they all have the similar aim of standardising practice through the provision of a 'best care' recipe. This is intended to ensure that 'best care' is given but also to simplify decision making for practitioners. At each of the research sites, a number of protocols were available, although interestingly, a number of them were put away in the office.

The authors found that there were four major sources of information used in decision making: interaction with colleagues, standardised care approaches, instinct, and interaction with patients. They found that 'Decision making was a social activity, especially during a shift with nurses of mixed experience and knowledge' (Rycroft-Malone *et al.*, 2009: 1494) and that nurses would often look to senior or more experienced nurses for advice. While protocols were used, this was not in an obvious and systematic way. The nurses in the cardiac medical unit thought they were too busy to refer to protocols, and in any case, they believed that they were impersonal and did not necessarily define best practice. In the diabetic clinic, the nurses were aware that the patients had a lot of knowledge about their own conditions and that any protocol would have to be 'flexed' to accommodate this. In general, the knowledge derived from the protocol became 'intertwined with experience' and indistinguishable from it in everyday decision making. Where protocols were thought to be useful was in teaching, in 'new' situations, and in supporting the nurses' decision making post hoc, in case of a query.

Importantly, the study noted that nurses make a lot of decisions, on subjects ranging from medication and treatment to time management, and that protocols could not possibly be available for every one. It found that:

(Continued)

Case study 1.3: (*Continued*)

Some nurses described the mental processes during decision-making as following steps or a mental flowchart or checklist, not necessarily linked to a particular guideline or protocol.

(Rycroft-Malone *et al.*, 2009: 1494)

As we shall see, this concept, as well as the notion of authority figures, resonates with some of the conclusions of the final case study.

Case study 1.4: Knowledge management in primary care

Gabbay & le May (2004, 2010) conducted a substantial ethnographic study looking at knowledge management in primary care based in two practices. They were interested in how research evidence might pass into practice, and particularly in how – and if – this was managed at the level of the individual practitioner and/or the level of the collective. They were also interested in how the two were connected. They did not find evidence to suggest that research findings were feeding directly into decision making:

We found that the individual practitioners did not go through the steps that are traditionally associated with the linear-rational model of evidence based health care – not once in the whole time we were observing them. Neither while we observed them did they read the many clinical guidelines available to them

(Gabbay & le May, 2004: 3)

In contrast, they found a more complex picture of practitioners using a variety of sources of information, notably professional journals (not research journals) and networks of other practitioners, to build up their knowledge. Within their professional networks, some people were thought of as 'authorities' who could be relied on to give good advice – the local PCT pharmaceutical advisor was considered such a reliable source. In one practice, a local protocol for heart failure was generated. The doctor who was asked to develop it used the local hospital guidelines (where the cardiologist was another respected 'authority'), integrating them with two other published guidelines and with her own experience. The result was presented to the practice team, which largely left the scientific basis unquestioned – after all, it was based on trusted sources. Their concerns were much more about whether the protocol was workable and would advantage the practice both in terms of financial and quality measures.

Gabbay & le May (2004) coined the term 'mindlines', in contrast to 'guidelines', to convey the way in which practitioners use such sources, as well as their training and experience, to generate personal internalised tacit knowledge that guides their practice. These 'mindlines' are not static but will be progressively negotiated and changed through various interactions (e.g. practice meetings, discussions with colleagues, interactions with patients). They argued that, if research is to affect practice, it will be via these processes and not through an idealised model of rational adoption. Further, they drew attention to the importance of locality: clinicians practice in a particular context of colleagues, managers, and histories. Consequently, they proposed that:

> the real skill of the practitioner might be expected to be that of learning reliably from the knowledge of trusted sources either individually or through working in a community of practice.
>
> (Gabbay & le May, 2004: 6)

These brief summaries cannot do justice to the richness of data and analysis contained in each case study, which would reward further reading. They paint a rich picture of how things get done – in effect, telling 'stories' about how the participants make sense of their world. The studies all relate to key issues of importance to health visiting: How is national and local policy determined? How are guidelines constructed and used? How does a group of people on the 'front line' manage its knowledge base? This literature does not support the concept of a linear model of research being unproblematically imported into practice. But, while a debate raged about the theoretical, political, and practical aspects of EBP, the actors in these cases simply went about their business in ways that seemed sensible to them and would achieve the outcomes they wanted. That is not to say that they did not understand that knowledge is both contested and situated. Key messages from the case studies include the notion that research is never value-free; that its relevance and applicability are as important as issues of research design; and that in practice, both managers and practitioners have to decide what to do in conditions of uncertainty and in the context of patient expectations. Because knowledge is contested, so must be one of its important manifestations in healthcare: the protocol or guideline. Hutchinson & Shakespeare argue that:

> Wherever a protocol is generated – and it may be at the highest governmental level of standard setting and regulation – it is operationalised by individuals working in contexts that shape their own practice and identity. Therefore, while protocols may appear to be straightforward unambiguous statements of practice matters, there is an infinite range of possible application.
>
> (Hutchinson & Shakespeare, 2010: 75)

The nurse respondents in Traynor et al.'s (2010) study also referred to protocols when describing their decision making. This study, which is based on nurses' accounts of their practice, describes a dichotomy between technical and indeterminate knowledge. Clearly, the former relates to formal sources of knowledge, including protocols, whereas the latter is related to terms such as 'instinct' and 'intuition'. The nurses' descriptions of technical knowledge – guidelines, manuals, protocols, and evidence – acknowledge them as valid but of little use in practice. Traynor *et al.* suggest that:

> participants constructed a balanced, but professionally defendable position. On one hand, they acknowledged and appreciated formalised instruments for being helpful and in some cases necessary in clinical decision-making ... On the other hand, the instruments were also something obviously (in practical and ethical terms) impossible to adhere to fully in practice, and therefore they need constant modification according to the clinical situation.
>
> (Traynor *et al.*, 2010: 1589)

Activity 1.6 enables you to explore the use of guidelines in practice. Whether protocols, guidelines, care pathways, and so on are locally or nationally constructed, they will be mediated by the practitioner and, Hutchinson & Shakespeare (2010) argue, by the context in which the practitioner is operating.

A further study (Kyratsis *et al.*, 2014) of the use of evidence in practice focused on managers' decision making. This study was carried out in nine NHS hospitals in England and focused on decision making around infection prevention and control. The authors found that a variety of sources of evidence were used, including research, local trial data, and peer reports. However:

> different forms of evidence were not simply accessed and applied 'at face value' by the decision-makers. It was necessary to continuously interpret and (re)construct the evidence in some way, according to one's own professional identity, organisational role, team members and audience, and organisational objectives. Far from being merely technical or 'scientific', we found this process to be highly iterative and 'messy'. Many questioned what counted as evidence.
>
> (Kyratsis *et al.*, 2014: xxiii)

A key part of their finding was the importance of professional identity. Managers from different professional backgrounds used and valued sources of information differently. The authors proposed that three 'evidence templates' were used: biomedical-scientific, practice-based, and rational policy. Doctors valorised the biomedical-scientific way of making sense of evidence, nonclinical managers mainly used the other two, and nurses used all three. The authors concluded:

> An evidence-based management approach that inflexibly applies the principles of evidence-based medicine, our findings suggest, neglects how evidence is actioned in practice and how codified, systematised knowledge generated from research inter-relates with other forms of evidence that are also valued by decision-makers.
>
> (Kyratsis *et al.*, 2014: xxiv)

So where does this leave us in terms of EBP? Clearly, the issues are much more complex than the pioneers of EBM thought, and the idea of just 'disseminating' research findings and seeing practice change was unrealistic – as was the idea that frontline practitioners had either the time or the skills to review complex bodies of knowledge before deciding what to do. However, the pressure to ensure that expensive research findings changed practice remained. As evidence mounted of the 'failure' of EBP to achieve the required outcomes, especially in areas of complex human activity, a new way of approaching the problem became prominent: the idea of 'disseminating' research findings gave way to the concept of 'implementing' them and a new area of systematic research activity came into being, known as 'implementation science'. This is devoted to exploring why research findings are not translated into the sort of practice that achieves desired outcomes and how the gap can be successfully bridged.

One example of the changing emphasis can be seen in the Scottish Intercollegiate Guidelines Network (SIGN). SIGN has been producing evidence-based national clinical guidelines for best practice since 1993. Since 2009, it has focused on using research on implementation to improve the use of these guidelines, with the aim of becoming a world leader in guideline implementation. El-Ghorr et al. (2011) describe how SIGN generated ideas on effective implementation support activities by engaging with users, implementers, and stakeholders. A key part of the strategy is the involvement of patients as champions for change, initially through patient groups and voluntary organisations.

Two concepts are particularly important in implementation science: fidelity and adaptation. Fidelity is really about control. The argument is that if we develop an evidence-based intervention and test it in practice and show that it works, then in order to replicate that effect elsewhere we need to control as much of the intervention as possible so that it is delivered 'with fidelity' to the original. We saw earlier that Allen (2011a) was enthusiastic about the idea of precisely defined interventions – such as the 19 pathways of early intervention which he wanted to see implemented – and argued that the greatest barrier to achieving the required outcomes was lack of fidelity. Of course, this idea is not new: it closely resembles the sort of retail franchise arrangements which we see in every high street. And, just as in retail, these specified interventions will be owned by a corporation or a university or a practice organisation which franchises both the right to replicate the practice intervention and a range of accompanying training and evaluation programmes. The development of franchised programmes is now big business.

Wiggins et al. (2012) of the Childhood Wellbeing Research Centre have, on behalf of the Department for Education, produced a very useful review of how such evidence-based programmes are to be implemented They assert that 'Evidence suggests that a carefully planned and well-resourced implementation is key to better outcomes and programme success' (Wiggins et al., 2012: 4). The process to be followed for a successful programme implementation is defined, following Fixsen et al. (2009), as:

- exploration and adoption;
- installation;

- initial implementation;
- full operation.

Throughout these stages, careful attention must be paid to the development of new systems, policies, and practices, the training and coaching of staff in new ways of practice, and the establishment of monitoring and evaluation systems. It is the totality of all these systems and policies together which is sometimes called the 'infrastructure' of implementation. Throughout this process there is likely to be considerable contact with the organisation holding the franchise, because 'Programmes have been found to be more effective if the local model remains faithful to the original programme design' (Wiggins et al. (2012: 13). But, of course, this is extremely difficult, as 'the core components have to be built into the daily performance of thousands of practitioners in the diversity of provider organisations functioning within different types of systems' (Wiggins et al. (2012: 13). We saw earlier (and you will know from your own experience) how complex that performance is. So, a contrary view is that programmes will be most successful if they are adapted to the local context, and, of course, it is the practitioner – individually and collectively – who has the knowledge about local clients, local practices, and local histories and value systems necessary to inform any adaptation strategy. And as Fixsen et al. (2009: 532) recognise, 'In human services, the practitioner is the intervention'. So, each health visitor's knowledge of her own practice and how it might interact or conflict with new ways of working is important. However, this is not to suggest that a 'pick and mix' approach to a programme will be effective; nor will the use of elements of one programme in the context of a different client group. Health visitors involved in such programmes need to be clear about how it was developed – and why – and to be alert to 'mission creep'. Cowley et al. (2012) point out that such programmes are targeted at specific needs, whereas health visiting offers a universal service, and ask whether the two ways of working are compatible.

Whatever the difficulties, practitioners have to function in the complex world of EBP, including implementation science. While they may not be required to understand the totality of the research underpinning their practice directly, it is important that they understand the nature of the vehicles now used to package research for them: guidelines, research reviews, programmes, protocols, and so on. Two useful concepts are reliability and relevance. Some sources are highly reliable – a guideline from NICE, for example, will be based on the highest quality of research evidence expertly evaluated. However, a guideline locally constructed by colleagues in response to local needs may be more relevant. A further important concept is risk. The consequences of not following a guideline or of using a guideline inappropriately will vary. Health visitors have to operate in conditions of uncertainty. In this context, they need to ask whether it is better to complete a given assessment tool or stop and listen to their client's narrative. Richards (2015) offers a useful reminder via a case study of how interactions can be negative as well as positive. Professional interaction, however well meaning and evidence-based, is always related to issues of power. But practitioners do not need to resolve these conflicts alone. We have already noted the development of the iHV, which provides many resources to assist practitioners. In the following two sections, we will look at two different ways of helping practitioners manage their knowledge in practice and their knowledge about practice.

Communities of practice

The current interest in the concept of CoPs comes largely from the work of Lave & Wenger (1991). An accessible introduction to CoPs is provided by Wenger-Trayner & Wenger-Trayner (2015), who state that 'Communities of practice are groups of people who share a concern or a passion for something they do and learn how to do it better as they interact regularly' (Wenger-Trayner & Wenger-Trayner, 2015: 1). The primary focus, and the reason CoPs are of interest and of potential use in healthcare, is on how we learn and how learning can take place in ways that are not dependent on 'teaching'. CoPs therefore have the potential to create a mechanism through which practitioners can learn to improve their own practice. A CoP can occur in any sphere of social activity, but it will always have the following attributes:

- a shared domain of knowledge;
- a group willing to share ideas and to interact;
- a shared practice.

So, a classroom could be a CoP, as could the staff working in a GP practice, as could a group of health visitors and nurses working around a clinic. Such communities do not need to correspond to institutional boundaries – for example, although all the health visitors in a particular district or city might be brought together in a meeting organised by management, this does not automatically constitute a CoP, although it might be managed so that it does. Key to a CoP is the mutual engagement of the participants and their willingness to work together in developing their practice through a variety of activities, the end result of which will be a shared repertoire of ideas, commitments, and memories (Lave & Wenger, 1991). Activity 1.7 will help you explore activities relevant to your own practice.

While it is obvious that such communities are arenas of shared learning and development, it should not be assumed that they will have the same interests and goals as either other communities or their employers. For example, Wenger (1998) refers to schools in which CoPs organise their knowledge in opposition to that proposed by institutional curricula. Each community will have its own ideas about what constitutes knowledge and competence. Neither should it be assumed that all the participants think and act the same way; rather, they are engaged in a shared enterprise. Each participant might have a very different view of what constitutes valid knowledge, but they are prepared to discuss and negotiate until they achieve workable solutions. Communities are also not just about managing knowledge: they are vehicles for social engagement, meaningful work, and the development of identity. The resources which a community will use are not all, or even largely, locally generated. Language is the most obvious example of a resource which is imported from outside, although communities may nuance language to reflect their particular history and circumstances. Research knowledge and national and local protocols for practice will also be imported, but because a community is a negotiated enterprise, their meaning and use will differ between communities.

There are many CoPs, which together generate a *landscape* of practice. These communities intersect and interact in various ways. Wenger (1998) argues that the participant at the periphery of a community can sometimes bring new ideas into it because she or he is still able to see beyond the knowledge it takes for granted. Newly qualified practitioners can take this role, bringing resources from their 'old' CoP – the classroom or placement – into their 'new' community of work.

Hutchinson & Shakespeare (2010) draw our attention to Wenger's ideas about the ways in which sources of professional knowledge and expertise have been associated with particular institutions:

- Universities are connected with theory and research.
- Workplaces are connected with experience and local practice.
- Regulatory agencies produce prescriptions of best practice.
- Professional bodies are concerned with local management and professional identity.

Each of these institutions will have many CoPs. Researchers in universities largely enjoy similar contractual obligations and rights related to their employment, but they are likely to belong to different CoPs related to their research interests and methodological affiliations. Academics interested in reflective practice, for example, may be more likely to be in a CoP with practitioners using reflective practice than with fellow academics who embrace RCTs. Negotiation takes place within communities about what sort of knowledge is to be valorised. Practitioners may despise 'university' knowledge as irrelevant to practice; university practitioners may see health service practice as largely a source for recruitment to research. However, Andrew *et al.* (2008) offer a very practical example of a working CoP in nursing which crosses these institutional boundaries. They describe how a group of 30 practising nurses and university academics throughout Scotland operated as a CoP within the framework of the Gerontological Nursing Demonstration Project. They interacted regularly, both online and in the real world, and explored their practice in an environment of mutual respect and support. A number of best-practice statements were produced, which have since been disseminated widely. Andrew *et al.* argue that:

> In nursing, CoPs have the potential to allow practitioners and academics to collaborate to challenge and change practice … this way of working has the potential [to] create a vibrant work and learning environment. The fluidity of the framework encourages practitioners and academics, to integrate incrementally, the dimensions of research, education, clinical practice and user experience, to respond to the increasing demand for wider institutional and professional awareness.
>
> (Andrew *et al.*, 2008: 251)

Despite this optimism, a review of the evidence on CoPs in healthcare published in 2011 could conclude only that they 'may' have a role in improving practice in healthcare (Ranmuthugala *et al.*, 2011). One of the issues is that CoPs vary greatly in terms of their membership, organisational structure, and focus, so it is hard to generalise.

Within health visiting, the development of a uni-professional CoP was hindered by the geographical realities – even with recent increases in numbers, it is a relatively small professional group scattered throughout the country and constantly on the move. Face-to-face interaction beyond the immediate district is therefore difficult and costly in terms of time. A research project based at the University of Hertfordshire trialled the idea of a *virtual* community interacting online. This allows for asynchronous inter-action, which is helpful for busy professionals. The project set up the Health Visitors' Community of Practice Evidence Hub, which 'allowed health visitors to articulate professional knowledge to support and implement evidence-based practice' (Ikioda *et al.*, 2013). Members could raise questions and share evidence and good practice. The project team managed the development of the CoP, offering training sessions and materials to the participants and structuring the website around pre-arranged topics. In terms of creating a successful CoP, Ikioda *et al.* (2013) note that:

- The role of the moderator is key.
- The degree of involvement by the participants varies considerably.
- New members are important in reinvigorating the CoP.

The CoP for health visitors has been adopted by the iHV and can be accessed via its website (iHV, 2015). Evidence from the project shows that, of its 16 topics, parenting attracted the most postings, followed by infant feeding/child nutrition and professional issues in health visiting, while building community capacity attracted the least. Ikioda *et al.* (2013) conclude that topic relevance is important to the success of a virtual CoP, especially because topics in health visiting may quickly become outdated as the context for practice changes.

Reflective practice

Another way of both generating and managing knowledge in practice is through what is known as 'reflective practice'. Just like EBP, reflective practice started as an enthusiasts' movement but has now become institutionalised within nursing – and is used in other occupations, particularly within healthcare. The basic concept is relatively simple:

> Reflection is more than just thinking, it is an intentional practice based learning activity that focuses on improving future actions in clinical practice by looking back at what has already happened or is happening.
>
> (Driscoll & Teh, 2001: 102)

It is intended to help the practitioner unearth and explore her knowledge about her practice, with a view to moving beyond routinised actions into new ways of thinking and doing. Because it is not easy to 'just reflect' on one's practice, various methodologies have been produced to assist the practitioner. These essentially offer a series of 'prompts' or questions to help her structure her thinking. In addition, prac-titioners are encouraged to keep a reflective diary or journal in which they describe and explore their practice. Reflective practice has been adopted by institutions within nursing as a way of ensuring and evidencing that practitioners continue learning and are therefore eligible for re-registration, and it is being taken up within medicine and other healthcare occupations for the same reason. It has also been adopted by many universities and associated regulatory agencies and built into many education curricula at both pre- and post-registration levels. In Scotland, for example, it is a major part of the Flying Start Programme for newly qualified practitioners. The National Preceptorship Framework for Health Visiting (McInnes et al., 2014), which was developed by the iHV on behalf of Health Education England and the Department of Health as a transition support programme for new health visitors, identifies reflection as an important tool for learning. New health visitors (or preceptees) are required to keep a personal reflection log and to provide a written reflective account and evaluation after 12 months of practice. The document is not prescriptive about the process of reflection, although it does reference Kolb's (1984) learning cycle model and Johns' (2013) model of reflective practice.

However, while its proponents and supporters remain enthusiastic about the power of reflective practice, it has not been without its critics. Jennifer Greenwood (1998), of the University of Western Sydney, wrote an editorial entitled 'On nursing's "reflective madness"'. She argues that reflection requires adequate time and proper training and that, in the absence of these, it will result in poor learning. More profoundly, she argues that although the theories supporting reflection were intended as an antidote to the valorisation of technical rationality, they themselves support the idea that 'intelligent action requires conscious thought' Greenwood (1998: 3) and fail to understand that much of the tacit knowledge the practitioner uses to deal with complex practice is inherently unavailable to them. Mackintosh (1998) argues that the theoretical basis of reflective practice remains unclear despite acknowledged links to educational theorists, particularly Schön (1983). A further issue is that reflection has come to focus on the individual practitioner's thoughts, values, and beliefs. So, for example, Somerville & Keeling say that:

> Reflection is the examination of personal thoughts and actions. For practitioners this means focusing on how they interact with their colleagues and with the environment to obtain a clearer picture of their own behaviour. It is therefore a process by which practitioners can better understand themselves in order to be able to build on existing strengths and take appropriate future action.
>
> (Somerville & Keeling, 2004: 42)

Consequently, such models tend to downplay a number of important aspects of practice. First, by focusing on the non-technical–rational aspects of knowledge, such as the personal and ethical, they may not help practitioners understand how they might integrate technical–rational knowledge into practice. Second, the patients and clients may in these accounts become passive recipients of practice rather than active participants in a joint enterprise. Third, by focusing on the personal, they may ignore the social aspects of knowledge management. And fourth, and perhaps most importantly, they do not focus on the outcomes for the patient or client. Nevertheless, Ferguson argues, in the context of social work, that it is important to create 'opportunities for stillness, to slow things down, moments for reflection on the entire experience' (Ferguson, 2008: 576). He also uses a phrase which may not accord with bureaucratic thinking but might resonate with seasoned practitioners: the need for 'decoding the smell of practice' (Ferguson, 2008: 576).

Looking back at Case Study 1.4 and the discussion on CoPs, it could be argued that we need to focus more on how groups and communities manage knowledge; even within individual reflection, we could ask the practitioner to reflect explicitly on her CoP and her place within it. Is it a community which encourages managed innovation? Is it a community which values knowledge coming from external sources – and, if so, which ones? Is it a community which values the knowledge base of the client and looks at their individual circumstances? How are protocols discussed and integrated into practice by the community? In each of these examples – and many others – the practitioner can explore her relationship with the group, deciding whether she is satisfied that it is a CoP that supports her learning and what she might do to improve her practice. Poland *et al.* (2005), in their discussion of place, suggest that reflection could usefully see practice through the 'lens' of place, which again would offer a fuller understanding of the social environment of practice.

A further important criticism of reflective practice is that the resources available to the individual practitioner through recollection cannot reflect the reality of practice. Recall is rarely accurate. Here we need to return to the comments at the beginning of the chapter about the complexity of health visiting practice and the focus on the central importance of language. Taylor & White (2000), writing about social work and community nursing practice, agree with reflective practice insofar as it provides a potential response to the technical–rational approach embedded in EBP, which they agree cannot deal with the complexities and ambiguities of practice. However, they propose that engaging in *reflexive* practice offers a remedy to the problems of memory and recall. They argue that:

> We are not interested simply in what we have done and how we have gone about things when we reflect on our practice, we must also concern ourselves with the (tacit) assumptions we are making about people, their problems and their needs when we apply knowledge about child development, mental health, learning disability and so forth.
>
> (Taylor & White, 2000: 35)

By this, they mean that practitioners must produce hard evidence (they propose audiotape recordings) about their practice in order to analyse it rigorously. This will allow them to determine what they have actually done, rather than what they can recall. Their 'tacit' knowledge may not be available for recall but it will appear and will be available for analysis in the record of what they said. Taylor & White propose that practitioners can themselves undertake the kind of analytic work about institutional practices which can be seen in Drew & Heritage (1992):

> by analysing transcripts of their own talk as part of a regular self-audit, professionals can be made more aware of the embedded alternative readings, so that they may judge for themselves whether those readings are or were worth pursuing.
>
> (Taylor & White, 2000: 135)

Taylor & White provide useful ideas about how this transcript analysis can be done; for example, they suggest a number of analytic questions concerning how authority is conveyed, how control is managed, how facts are defined and by whom, and so on. And while clients may be relatively absent in reflective practice, within reflexive practice they become both visible and expert practitioners in their own right:

> Patients are not docile and passive recipients of advice and treatment. They use the resources at their disposal to show their moral adequacy, to resist being undermined, to attempt to define 'the facts' and to make themselves worthy of sympathy.
>
> (Taylor & White, 2000: 115)

Clearly, reflective practice is a useful but contested concept. However, it has been adopted as an important element of preceptorship – the process by which the new entrant to health visiting is guided to become a competent practitioner. The Preceptorship Charter, which was developed by the iHV on behalf of the Department of Health, requires the preceptee to follow a reflective process when working with the preceptor 'to become increasingly self-aware, able to see the salient points in any situation and use their past experience to make judgments and decisions in practice' (iHV, 2013: 2). The National Preceptorship Framework makes substantial reference to reflective diaries or logs as well as to using reflection within ongoing supervision. As part of the NMC revalidation process, introduced in 2016, for health visitors, nurses and midwives, reflective practice is a central part of this process.

Clients: what do they know and how do they know it?

So far, the focus has largely been on how the practitioner accesses and assembles knowledge and what might be useful sources of valid and reliable evidence. In the past, access to such knowledge would have been mostly limited to practitioners, and this created an important differential between practitioner and client and arguably was part of the power base of the practitioner, who was seen as the 'expert'. However, this differential has largely been eroded by the explosion of online media. In terms of text-based knowledge, clients have *access* to the same sources of knowledge as most practitioners. Whatever is on the Web is available, potentially, to everyone. Wilson tells us that 'A poll in August 2001 concluded that almost 100 million Americans regularly go on line for information about health care' (Wilson, 2002: 598). She also tells us that over 100 000 sites offer health advice – and this was in 2001. Health visitors can see this as a threat or a challenge – but either way, they cannot ignore its near-ubiquitous presence.

The general public can now access a range of formal sources of knowledge: the Cochrane Library, NICE guidelines, other guidelines, original research reports, and all the media responses to the same. Many research and professional journals are also now open access: they are freely available online. Government websites provide national and local data on public health statistics (see Chapter 7). Access is also free to a number of less formal sources of knowledge, such as wikis, media reports, advertising sites, and so on. There is absolutely no possibility that access to these data sources can be controlled. Any search engine will provide lists of both these knowledge sources – formal and informal – together. Wikipedia is one of the best known knowledge access sites and – despite the ritual wringing of hands by academics as to its unreliability – is as reliable a source of information as any.

There is, as you might predict, a lively debate about the quality of the advice on these sites and whether they should be quality controlled in some way. A study of health information in relation to managing fever in children at home (Impicciatore *et al.*, 1997) found 41 relevant Web pages (there will be more today), but only four which adhered closely to published guidelines for the home management of childhood fever. Wilson (2002) suggests that there are a number of possible mechanisms for 'controlling' information:

- a self-applied code of conduct or quality label;
- user guidance systems;
- filtering tools which accept or reject sites;
- quality and accreditation labels applied by third parties.

Codes of conduct do exist, but it is one thing to write a code and another to enforce it. Third-party accreditation systems are extremely expensive.

An alternative approach is to say that the general public copes with books and will learn to cope with the Internet. So, one argument is that:

> The greatest challenge is not to develop yet more rating tools, but to encourage consumers to seek out information critically, and to encourage them to see time invested in critical searching as beneficial.
>
> (Wilson, 2002: 600)

What is the role of the health visitor in this debate? What advice should she give clients about the information on the Web? How might she explain the relative validity of various websites?

Social networking and the media

Social networking and the media now represent a major source of information for a number of client groups – especially mothers. Online communication has allowed clients to move away from the role of a passive recipient of information and into that of an active participant in a dialogue. There are a huge number of social networking resources, which may be used synchronously or asynchronously. An internet forum (or message board, Usenet group, etc.) is essentially asynchronous: it is not a live conversation. Two of the most obvious examples are Mumsnet and Netmums. Whereas once the new mother might have depended on the local mother and toddler group – and she may well still – today she also has access through such websites to a vast community of people experiencing the same rites of passage and tackling the same problems as herself. Not only can she access that knowledge, she can specifically seek answers to her questions – and is very likely to get responses – and can contribute her own experiences. It can be argued that these sites are essentially large CoPs: they are clearly focused on the practice of motherhood, and many participants are keen to engage and contribute, although many others may be content to watch from the periphery. Certainly, both Mumsnet and Netmums provide enormous resources of advice and experience, which may not be verified in any formal fashion but are undoubtedly very influential.

If access to online sources of information is a major part of how knowledge is transmitted and acquired in the 21st century, it might be argued that the role of the health visitor is twofold: first, to ensure that all her clients have access to these sources; and second, to help each client understand their use and validity. With regard to the first, the government has made it clear that access to digital information is a right of every citizen. With regard to the second, the practitioner needs a sophisticated understanding of how all kinds of evidence are promoted and disseminated online.

Kata (2010) has called the Internet 'A Postmodern Pandora's Box'. She looked at Internet sites in the USA and Canada that were opposed to vaccination and found that they offered only one version of 'truth': that vaccination is unsafe, ineffective, unnatural, and a threat to civil liberties (in some parts of the USA, vaccination is required for entry into the public school system). Furthermore, some sites asserted that the diseases which vaccination was designed to prevent were either not serious – an example was smallpox – or were caused by other agents – polio, for example, was thought to be caused by eating too much sugary food: notably ice cream, hence its prevalence in the summer. In terms of the style of the websites, personal testimonies – mostly narratives from parents who felt their children had been damaged by vaccines – were the most common means of generating a response.

Given that such sites will continue to proliferate in a democratic society increasingly dependent on online communications, an obvious response might be to offer a strong refutation based on the scientific evidence and to increase the focus on educating parents. Kata argues strongly that this cannot be effective:

> The post-modern perspective questions the legitimacy of science and authority. Traditional controversy dynamics, with 'audiences' needing to be 'educated' by 'experts' no longer apply. Confidence in the power of expertise has sharply declined; appeals to experts are often considered manipulative.
>
> (Kata, 2010: 1715)

She asserts that we need to understand the discourses and ideologies which underpin people's beliefs in order to enter into a meaningful dialogue with them.

The controversy over the measles, mumps, and rubella (MMR) vaccine offers a useful example of how some of these issues are managed by parents in a real-world situation. In the late 1990s, a research paper was published which suggested a link between the MMR vaccine and the development of autism and inflammatory bowel disease (Wakefield et al., 1998). While not many parents read The Lancet, the media picked up on the potential importance of the issue and it became headline news. The take-up of the combined vaccine fell from over 90% to a low of 58% in some parts of the country and there were outbreaks of measles and mumps (Hilton et al., 2007). Evidence from a study of parental views using focus groups (Hilton *et al.*, 2007) demonstrates that parents had serious concerns about who to trust in this situation. A number of sources of information were cited, but their credibility varied. The government had little, possibly because of its position on previous public health scares, including the bovine spongiform encephalopathy (BSE) outbreak. The degree to which the media was trusted varied widely, but the shear amount of media coverage and the fact that it tried to show both sides of the story – and thereby raised the profile of Wakefield *et al.*'s (1998) work – fuelled concerns about the vaccine's safety. Views about the trustworthiness of healthcare professionals were again mixed, but doubts were raised as they were perceived to be part of 'the system' and therefore bound to support the government 'line' – and possibly also secured a financial advantage by meeting targets. A common theme in the parents' responses was that they:

> did not know to what extent their own GP or health visitor was acting in their child's best interest, as opposed to acting in their role as an advocate of public heath policy.
>
> (Hilton *et al.*, 2007: 8)

Biss (2015), in her illuminating monograph, *On Immunity*, reminds us that debates about vaccination are about power and trust as well as science, and that vaccination has been promoted as a way of preventing the spread of contagion from the poor to the wealthy. While health professionals were often seen as having entrenched positions, Wakefield himself was admired by some as having dared to bring the issue out into the open. He was seen as a principled 'whistleblower'. Interestingly, the most trustworthy source was defined as other parents, who were perceived as 'just telling it like it is'. Even within the media coverage:

> Parents spoke of feeling particularly drawn to anecdotal stories involving real people, and spoke about finding other parents' stories more convincing than statistics and reassurances from scientists and politicians
>
> (Hilton *et al.*, 2007: 9)

As we have seen, parents can now access a rich source of other parents' stories and concerns online.

Hilton *et al.* (2007) also raise the issue of the expectations parents may have of health services, which can be different from those of the health visitor. The BBC News health website quotes a mother as saying she wants a guarantee that there is no danger; specifically, she wants 'Some documentation, or reliable medical information from GP surgeries or the government to prove that there is no link whatsoever' (BBC News, 2008). While clients may want certainty, very little research can provide it, particularly at the level of the individual. This issue has been well explored by the proponents of EBM: see, for example, Gray (1997), who acknowledges that RCTs can only ever deal in generalities over a given population. The fact that in a study population of, say, 2000 there is 1 case of negative effects cannot be extrapolated to define the risk to any single individual as 1 in 2000. The specific risk to the individual is largely unknowable, so in all one-to-one discussions with a client the practitioner must rely on her own experience and skills, as well as on evidence 'imported' from outside. She should also take into account the experience, beliefs, and skills of her client.

The debate

At various points in this chapter, we have looked at how we can obtain and use evidence *for* practice, evidence *about* practice, evidence about *your* practice, and the *client*'s evidence base. Two of these have received much more attention than the others because they are supported by substantial groups of enthusiastic followers and, more importantly, have become embedded in institutions and policies at every level. EBP focuses on evidence *for* practice and, despite serious critiques from both those willing it to succeed and those opposed to it in principle and practice, it is fully embedded into the NHS quality assurance systems at all levels, even though it absorbs considerable resources. While, in general, the emphasis is now on the prescription of protocols for practice – the use of which may determine the funding formula of providers – some nurses are still enjoying the spirit of the early days of EBP when individual practitioners were exhorted to find and evaluate the evidence and change their practice. An anecdotal review of curricula for health visiting suggests that despite the critiques – and the lack of actual success in changing practice – the focus remains on evidence *for* practice, and the idea that individual practitioners can and should review and evaluate the validity and relevance of research studies and decide to change their practice on the basis of the same remains a prevalent model. Hopefully, it is clear from the preceding argument that, for a number of reasons, this is not a sustainable or indeed a safe model for practice. First, it is impossible for any practitioner, or even group of practitioners, to keep up with the range and volume of relevant research. Second, evaluating research is a very skilled and specialised undertaking, and the methodological variety of relevant studies makes evaluation of the full range impossible. Third, very many of the studies in nursing and health visiting are conducted on a small scale and, while often stimulating and interesting, cannot provide the evidence needed to underpin practice change.

However, practitioners are the focus of a massive array of protocols. Protocols are a way of communicating between all the different layers of practice, management, and regulation (Hutchinson & Shakespeare, 2010). Those protocols which come, or purport to come, from rigorous scientific research assert that they have a particular scientific warrant that gives them a privileged status. But, as has been shown, they may in fact be of dubious scientific provenance and embedded in particular political or managerial positions. Practitioners should always explore – and, if necessary, challenge – these prescriptions for practice.

The other focus, certainly within nursing but increasingly in other groups, has been on generating evidence about *your* practice through use of reflective practice. As with EBP, a whole industry of journals, books, and 'experts' has flourished around reflective practice, and the movement – evangelical, again – has become embedded in curricula and re-accreditation processes.

Within nursing curricula, the two great knowledge ideologies of EBP and reflective practice tend to be separated, perhaps because those who support the one rarely support – and probably would find it difficult to teach – the other. This is unfortunate, because we should be bringing them together as different facets of evidence in practice and generating a dialogue between them.

The two most neglected aspects of evidence in practice are evidence *about* actual practice and the *client*'s evidence base. With regard to the latter, there is a very substantial body of work in sociology about how prospective or actual patients and clients think about health, illness, and care (see, for example, Radley & Billig, 1996). There is some interest from researchers – for example, Rycroft-Malone *et al.* (2004) argue that knowledge from patients, clients, and carers is one of the four important sources of evidence for practice. However, within much of current practice it has lost the conceptual depth and clarity of the sociological literature and has been conceptualised as 'the patient experience', which is largely captured through routinised satisfaction surveys and reviews of complaints, and used by managers as evidence of good practice (or not).

With regard to evidence *about* practice, at the very beginning of this chapter it was argued that we have very little primary evidence about practice: about what it looks like and where and how we might have expected this body of evidence to grow and it has not. There may be a number of reasons for this. It is often difficult to get ethical permission to record – using audio or video – actual practice. While this is understandable, it is interesting in a country where CCTV cameras follow your every move! Where recording does take place, the rich data which it produces provide a real challenge to researchers, both in the time they take to analyse and in fitting them in to published accounts. But the vision of Taylor & White (2000) of a workforce continually recording and analysing its practice is a compelling one. Traynor *et al.* (2010) suggest that a parallel strategy may be useful – that of asking practitioners to produce narratives about their practice and then subjecting these to the sort of rigorous discourse analysis which Taylor & White use for primary data. Certainly, the health visiting knowledge base lacks rigorous narratives about practice for analysis and debate.

Summary

A central theme of this chapter has been that all knowledge is contestable. While the example of the anti-vaccination websites might constitute an extreme case of the rejection of scientific evidence, it is clear from the case studies that in everyday practice all kinds of experience and knowledge are brought forward alongside science as justification for practice. As May notes:

> Struggles about the facts – what they are, who they are made and recognised by, and how they are played out in different kinds of political arena – are ubiquitous in the conditions of late modernity.

(May, 2006: 513)

Practising in a post-modern world, therefore, demands of the practitioner a sceptical and sophisticated understanding of the different forms and sources of knowledge generation, from the national to the local level. However, a further key theme has been that the practitioner need not, and indeed should not, grapple with these issues alone. Practice takes place in a complex social environment of networks, 'authorities', experienced practitioners, client experiences, and so forth, all of which can be effectively utilised as rich sources of knowledge. The effective practitioner, it can be argued, is not one who adheres to simple models for practice derived from any source, but rather one who works with colleagues in examining, contesting, negotiating, and exploiting all the knowledge sources available to her – and contributes generously to the knowledge needs of others.

References

Alaszewski, A. (2006) Managing risk in community practice: nursing, risk and decision-making. In: Risk and Nursing Practice (ed. P. Godin). Palgrave, London. pp. 24–41.

Allen, G. (2011a) Early Intervention: The Next Steps. Cabinet Office, London.

Allen, G. (2011b) Early Intervention: Smart Investment, Massive Savings. Cabinet Office, London.

Andrew, N., Tolson, D. & Ferguson, D. (2008) Building on Wenger: communities of practice in nursing. *Nurse Education Today*, **28**, 246–52.

Angus, J., Kontos, P., Dyck, I., McKeever, P. & Poland, B. (2005) The personal significance of home: habitus and the experience of receiving long-term home care. *Sociology of Health and Illness*, **27**(5), 161–87.

Appleby, J., Walshe, K. & Ham, C. (1995) Acting on the Evidence. National Association of Health Authorities & Trusts, Birmingham.

BBC News (2008) MMR: mothers divided. Available from: http://news.bbc.co.uk/1/hi/health/1804665.stm (last accessed 30 March 2016).

Biss, E. (2015) On Immunity: An Inoculation. Fitzcarraldo Editions, London.

Buttivant, H.M. (2011) The health visitor improvement plan 2011–2015. *The Lancet UK Policy Matters*, 6 May 2011. Available from: http://ukpolicymatters.thelancet.com/policy-summary-the-health-visitor-improvement-plan-2011-2015/ (last accessed 30 March 2016).

Carper, B.A. (1978) Fundamental patterns of knowing in nursing. *Advances in Nursing Science*, **1**(1), 13–23.

Chalmers, I. (2003) Trying to do more good than harm in policy and practice: the role of rigorous, transparent, up-to-date evaluations. *Annals of the American Academy of Political and Social Science*, **589**, 22–40.

Chalmers, I. (2005) If evidence-informed policy works in practice, does it matter if it doesn't work in theory? *Evidence and Policy*, **1**(2), 227–42.

Cowley, S., Kemp, L., Day, C. & Appleton, J. (2012) Research and the organisation of complex provision: conceptualising health visiting services and early years programmes. *Journal of Research in Nursing*, **17**(2), 108–24.

Cowley, S., Whittaker, K., Grigulis, A., Malone, M., Donetto, S., Wood, H., Morrow, E. & Maben, J. (2013) Why health visiting? A review of the literature about key health visitor interventions, processes and outcomes for children and families. (Department of Health Policy Research Programme, ref 016 0058). National Nursing Research Unit, Florence Nightingale School of Nursing and Midwifery, King's College London.

Cowley, S., Whittaker, K., Malone, M., Donetto, S., Grigulis, A. & Maben, J. (2015) Why health visiting? Examining the potential public health benefits from health visiting practice within a universal service: a narrative review of the literature. *International Journal of Nursing Studies*, **52**(1), 465–80.

DH (2007) Facing the Future. *A Review of the Role of Health Visitors.* Department of Health, London.

DH (2011) Health Visitor Implementation Plan 2011–15. Department of Health, London.

Dingwall, R. & Robinson, K. (1990) Policing the family? Health visiting and the public surveillance of private behaviour. In: The Home Care Experience: Ethnography and Policy (eds J. Gubrium & A. Sankar). Sage, Newbury Park. pp. 253–74.

Drew, P. & Heritage, J. (eds) (1992) Talk at Work. Cambridge University Press, Cambridge.

Driscoll, J. & Teh, B. (2001) The potential of reflective practice to develop individual orthopaedic nurse practitioners and their practice. *Journal of Orthopaedic Nursing,* **5**, 95–103.

El-Ghorr, A., James, R. & Twaddle, S. (2011) SIGN is customising implementation support to every guideline. Available from: http://www.guidelinesinpractice.co.uk/may_11_ghorr_sign_may11#.VaJThZPF8s0 (last accessed 30 March 2016).

Elkan, R., Kendrick, D., Hewitt, M., Robinson, J.J., Tolley, K., Blair, M., Dewey, M., Williams, D. & Brummell, K. (2000) The effectiveness of domiciliary health visiting: a systematic review of international studies and a selective review of the British literature. *Health Technology Assessment,* **4**(13), i–v, 1–339.

Estabrooks, C. (1998) Will evidence based nursing practice make practice perfect? *Canadian Journal of Nursing Research,* **30**, 15–36.

Estabrooks, C.A., Rutakumwa, W., O'Leary, K.A., Profetto-McGrath, J., Milner, M., Levers, M.J. & Scott-Findlay, S. (2005) Sources of practice knowledge among nurses. *Qualitative Health Research,* **15**(4), 460–76.

Ferguson, H. (2008) Liquid social work: welfare interventions as mobile practices. *British Journal of Social Work,* **38**, 561–79.

Ferguson, H. (2010) Walks, home visits and atmospheres: risk and the everyday practices and mobilities of social work and child protection. *British Journal of Social Work,* **40**, 1100–17.

Fixsen, D., Blase, K., Naoom, S. & Wallace, F. (2009) Core implementation components. *Research on Social Work Practice,* **19**(5).

Gabbay, J. & le May, A. (2004) Evidence-based guidelines or collectively constructed 'mindlines?' Ethnographic study of knowledge management in primary care. *British Medical Journal,* **329**, 1013.

Gabbay, J. & le May, A. (2010) Practice-based Evidence for Healthcare: Clinical Mindlines. Routledge, Abingdon.

Gerrish, K. (2003) Evidence-based practice: unravelling the rhetoric and making it real. *Practice Development in Health Care,* **2**(2), 99–113.

Glaszious, P., Vandenbroucke, J. & Chalmers, I. (2004) Assessing the quality of research. *British Medical Journal,* **328**, 39–41.

Gray, J.A.M. (1997) Evidence-based Healthcare. Churchill Livingstone, Edinburgh.

Greenwood, J. (1998) On nursing's 'reflective madness'. *Contemporary Nurse,* **7**(1), 3–4.

Grimshaw, J.M. & Thomson, M.A. (1998) What have new efforts to change professional practice achieved? *Journal of the Royal Society of Medicine,* **S35**(91), 20–5.

Grol, R. & Wensing, M. (2004) What drives change? Barriers to and incentives for achieving evidence-based practice. *The Medical Journal of Australia,* **180**, S57–60.

Hammersley, M. (2005) Is the evidence-based practice movement doing more good than harm? Reflections on Iain Chalmers' case for research-based policy making and practice. *Evidence and Policy,* **1**(1), 85–100.

Heritage, J. & Sefi, S. (1992) Dilemmas of advice: aspects of the delivery and reception of advice in interactions between health visitors and first-time mothers. In: Talk at Work (eds P. Drew & J. Heritage). Cambridge University Press, Cambridge. pp. 359–417.

Hilton, S., Petticrew, M. & Hunt, K. (2007) Parents' champions vs. vested interests: who do parents believe about MMR? A qualitative study. *BMC Public Health,* **7**(42).

Horton, R. (2015) Offline: what is medicine's 5 sigma? *The Lancet*, **385**, 1380.

Hutchinson, S. & Shakespeare, P. (2010) Standard setting, external regulation and professional autonomy: exploring the implications for university education. In: Education for Future Practice (eds J. Higgs, D. Fish, I. Goulter, S. Loftus, J. Reid & F. Trede). Sense, Amsterdam. pp. 75–84.

iHV (2012) Frequently Asked Questions November 2012. Institute of Health Visiting.

iHV (2013) Preceptorship charter. Institute of Health Visiting. Available from: https://www2.rcn.org.uk/__data/assets/pdf_file/0006/530655/Preceptors_Charter_Final7.pdf (last accessed 30 March 2016).

iHV (2015) HV Community of Practice Evidence Hub. Available from: https://cophv.evidence-hub.net/ui/pages/login.php?ref=https%3A%2F%2Fcophv.evidence-hub.net%2F (last accessed 30 March 2016).

Ikioda, F., Kendall, S., De Liddo, A. & Buckingham Shum, S. (2013) Factors that influence healthcare professionals' online interaction in a virtual community of practice. *Social Networking*, **2**, 174 – 184.

Impicciatore, P., Pandolfini, C., Casella, N. & Bonati, M. (1997) Reliability of health information for the public on the world wide web: systematic survey of advice on managing fever in children at home. *British Medical Journal*, **314**, 1875.

Ioannidis, J.P.A. (2005) Why most published research findings are false. *PLoS Medicine*, **2**(8), 696–701.

Johns, C. (2013) Becoming a Reflective Practitioner. 4th edn. Wiley, Chichester.

Kata, A. (2010) A postmodern Pandora's box: anti-vaccination misinformation on the internet. *Vaccine*, **28**, 1709–16.

Kelly, M., Morgan, A., Ellis, S., Younger, T., Huntley, J. & Swann, C. (2010) Evidence based public health: a review of the experience of the National Institute of Health and Clinical Excellence (NICE) of developing public health guidance in England. *Social Science & Medicine*, **71**, 1056–62.

Kerridge, I., Lowe, M. & Henry, D. (1998) Ethics and evidence based medicine. *British Medical Journal*, **316**, 1151–3.

Kolb, D. (1984) Experiential Learning as the Science of Learning and Development. Prentice Hall, Englewood Cliffs.

Kyratsis, Y., Ahmad, R., Hatzaras, K., Iwami, M. & Holmes, A. (2014) Making sense of evidence in management decisions: the role of research-based knowledge on innovation adoption and implementation in health care. *Health Services and Delivery Research*, **2**(6).

Langford, C. (2012) Helping Parents to Enjoy their Under 5s. Shropshire Community Health NHS Trust. Available from: http://www.shropscommunityhealth.nhs.uk/content/doclib/10802.pdf (last accessed 30 March 2016).

Lave, J. & Wenger, E. (1991) Situated Learning, Legitimate Peripheral Participation. Cambridge University Press, Cambridge.

Mackintosh, C. (1998) Reflection: a flawed strategy for the nursing profession. *Nurse Education Today*, **18**(7), 553–7.

May, C. (2006) Mobilising modern facts: health technology assessment and the politics of evidence. *Sociology of Health and Illness*, **28**(5), 513–32.

McDonald, R. & Harrison S. (2004) The micropolitics of clinical guidelines: an empirical study. *Policy and Politics*, **32**(2), 223–39.

McInnes, E., Page, A. & Marsh, M. (2014) A national preceptorship framework for health visiting. Institute of Health Visiting. Available from: http://ihv.org.uk/wp-content/uploads/2015/09/iHV_preceptorshippack_V16-WEB.pdf (last accessed 30 March 2016).

McKenna, H., Cutliffe, J. & McKenna, P. (1999) Evidence-based practice: demolishing some myths. *Nursing Standard*, **14**(16), 39–42.

Moore, R. (2013) Public health nursing services – future focus. *Directorate for Chief Nursing Officer, Patients, Public and Health Professionals, Edinburgh, Chief Executive Letter 13 (2013)*. 28 June 2013.

NHS England (2014) National Health Visiting Service Specification 2014/15. NHS England, March 2014.

Noble, K., Houston, S., Brito, N., Bartsch, H., Kan, E., Kuperman, J., Akshoomoff, N., Amaral, D. Bloss, C., Libiger, O., Schork, N., Murray, S., Casey, B., Chang, L., Ernst, T., Frazier, J., Gruen, J., Kennedy, D., Van Zijl, P., Mostofsky, S., Kaufmann, W., Kenet, T., Dale, A., Jernigan, T. & Sowell, E. (2015) *Nature Neuroscience*, **18**, 773–8.

Open Science Collaboration (2015) Estimating the reproducibility of psychological science. *Science*, **349**(6251).

Parker, J.M. (2002) Evidence-based nursing: a defence. *Nursing Inquiry*, **9**(3), 139–40.

Peckover, S. (2013) From 'public health' to 'safeguarding children': British health visiting in policy, practice and research. *Children and Society*, **27**, 116–26.

Poland, B., Lehoux, P., Holmes, D. & Andrews, G. (2005) How place matters: unpacking technology and power in health and social care. *Health and Social Care in the Community*, **13**(2), 170–80.

Radley, A. & Billig, M. (1996) Accounts of health and illness: dilemmas and representations. *Sociology and Health and Illness*, **18**(2), 220–40.

Ranmuthugala, G., Cunningham, F., Plumb, J., Long, J., Georgiou, A., Westbrook, J & Braithwaite, J. (2011) A realist evaluation of the role of communities of practice in changing healthcare practice. *Implementation Science*, **6**(49).

Richards, K. (2015) Understanding the potential negative impact of interventions on children: a SCPHN student's perspective. *Journal of Health Visiting*, **3**(4), 210–14.

Rycroft-Malone, J., Seers, K., Titchen, A., Harvey, G., Kitson, A. & McCormack, B. (2004) What counts as evidence in evidence-based practice? *Journal of Advanced Nursing*, **47**(1), 81–90.

Rycroft-Malone, J., Fontenla, M., Seers, K. & Bick, D. (2009) Protocol-based care: the standardisation of decision-making? *Journal of Clinical Nursing*, **18**, 1490–500.

Sackett, D.L., Richardson, W.S., Rosenberg, W. & Haynes, R.B. (1997) Evidence Based Medicine. How to Practice and Teach EBM. Churchill Livingstone, Edinburgh.

Schön, D. (1983) The Reflective Practitioner: How Professionals Think in Action. Temple Smith, London.

Somerville, D. & Keeling, J. (2004) A practical approach to promote reflective practice within nursing. Available from: http://www.nursingtimes.net/204502.article (last accessed 30 March 2016).

Taylor, C. & White, S. (2000) Practising Reflexivity in Health and Welfare. Open University Press, Buckingham.

Traynor, M. (2002) The oil crisis, risk and evidence-based practice. *Nursing Inquiry*, **9**(3), 162–9.

Traynor, M., Boland, M. & Buus, N. (2010) Autonomy, evidence and intuition: nurses and decision-making. *Journal of Advanced Nursing*, **66**(7), 1584–91.

Wakefield, A.J., Murch, S.H., Anthony, A., Linnell, J., Casson, D.M., Malik, M., Berelowitz, M., Dhillon, A.P., Thomson, M.A., Harvey, P., Valentine, A., Davies, S.E. & Walker-Smith, J.A. (1998) Ileal-lymphoid-nodular hyerplasia, non-specific colitis, and pervasive developmental disorder in children. *Lancet*, **351**, 637–41.

Wenger, E. (1998) Communities of Practice, Learning, Meaning and Identity. Cambridge University Press, Cambridge.

Wenger-Trayner, E. & Wenger-Trayner, B. (2015) Communities of practice: a brief introduction. Available from: http://wenger-trayner.com/wp-content/uploads/2015/04/07-Brief-introduction-to-communities-of-practice.pdf (last accessed 30 March 2016).

Wiggins, M., Austerberry, H., & Ward, H. (2012) Implementing evidence-based programmes in children's services: key issues for success. Research Report DFE-RR245, Department for Education, London.

Wilson, P. (2002) How to find the good and avoid the bad or ugly: a short guide to tools for rating quality of health information on the internet. *British Medical Journal*, **324**, 598–602.

Activities

Activity 1.1

Finding the supportive evidence

Identify two common health visitor interventions and provide the evidence that a commissioner would use in deciding whether to pay for them. Do you find the evidence convincing? If the commissioner had to choose between them, which one should take priority?

Activity 1.2

Practising EBM

Identify the best treatment for sore nipples by completing Table 1.1 using EBM.

Table 1.1 Practising EBM

Step	Example
Identify the need for information and formulate a question	What is the best treatment for sore nipples?
Track down the best possible source of evidence to answer the question	
Evaluate the evidence for validity and clinical applicability	
Compare the evidence you have with the practice you have seen	
Does the evidence support the practice? If not, how would you argue for a change?	
How would you evaluate the outcome?	

Activity 1.3

Assessing the effectiveness of your practice

Identify a question concerning the effectiveness of health visiting practice. Search organisational websites (e.g. NICE, www.nice.org.uk; SIGN, www.sign .ac.uk; the Cochrane Collaboration, www.cochrane.org) to collect your evidence. How easy are they to use? Do they help you answer your question?

Activity 1.4

Identify and evaluate the evidence base

Think of an alternative therapy (e.g. reflexology) and explore the evidence base. If a client asked about the effectiveness of this treatment, what would you tell them?

Activity 1.5

Implementing research evidence

Using the categorisation suggested by Gerrish (2003) (i.e. factors relating to the organisation, the way research is communicated, the quality of the research, and the practitioner), explore the barriers in your own practice context.

Activity 1.6

Use of guidelines

Identify a guideline currently in use in your practice. Discuss the sources of evidence that underpin it. You might like to use the the Appraisal of Guidelines for Research & Evaluation (AGREE) Instrument (available from www.agreetrust .org) to appraise the quality of the guideline, asking such questions as: Has the overall objective of the guideline been described? Have the clients' views and preferences been taken into account? Have the criteria for selecting the evidence been clearly described?

Activity 1.7

Communities of practice

CoPs develop their practice through a variety of activities. Wenger-Trayner & Wenger-Trayner (2015: 3) provide a table listing a few typical activities, accompanied by examples. Access this table and identify those activities that would be relevant to your own practice. For each activity you identify, give an example from your own practice. Are there any activities that are relevant to your own practice that are not included in the table?

2

Health Visiting: Context and Public Health Practice

Martin Smith

Liverpool City Council, Liverpool, *UK*

Introduction

Health visiting has long been recognised as providing a model for public health nursing in the UK. However, for a number of decades it has found itself having to respond to a fast-moving world of policy change and contrasting political views of public health, which has left the profession constantly having to adapt to the prevailing political ideology in order to ensure its survival. To its credit – if not relief – the profession has responded well to these challenges. Indeed, since the late 1990s there has been an implicit assumption in UK policy that health visitors have a key public health role to play in the support of children and families (Home Office, 1998; DH, 1999, 2010, 2011; HM Government, 2006). It could be argued that such policies arose less in the interests of health visiting and more as a means of securing the economic potential of the future adult population, as Glass (1999) suggested was the case with Sure Start. Nevertheless, these and a plethora of other policies at both the global and national level have resulted in health visiting becoming increasingly associated with an early years intervention model for practice and framed within a public health context through working with individuals, families, and communities (DH, 1999, 2003, 2011; NHSE 2014).

What is less clear is exactly what the public health context means for health visiting. The origins of health visiting are said to be firmly rooted in a public health approach (Adams, 2012), and indeed, its beginnings as an occupation are said to have aligned closely with the public health movement (Cowley & Frost, 2006; Cowley *et al.*, 2013). However, public health itself is recognised as a contested concept (Verweij & Dawson, 2009; Dawson, 2011), with different and often conflicting interpretations of its meaning. This chapter aims to articulate the concept of public health for the practice of health visiting. To do so will expose public health as a social construct, with a range of perspectives on what it means and on some of the consequent tensions and ambiguities that exist between policy and practice. It is therefore an

Health Visiting: Preparation for Practice, Fourth Edition.
Edited by Karen A. Luker, Gretl A. McHugh and Rosamund M. Bryar.
© 2017 John Wiley & Sons, Ltd. Published 2017 by John Wiley & Sons, Ltd.

analytical text rather than a description of 'how to do' public health nursing. This is important for two reasons. First, as Craig (2000) highlighted and Dahl & Clancy (2015) have shown, the range of perspectives on the nature of public health nursing has a direct impact on how it is practised. Second, it is essential for practitioners to consider these tensions, because their own understanding of public health, and of their role as specialist community public health nurses (SCPHNs), will frame the decisions they make concerning their own health, the approach they take to the interpretation of policy, and the promotion of health with others.

This exploration of the connection between health visiting and public health is particularly relevant for contemporary practice and a policy context which focuses the role on families and young children. This analysis will therefore take account of a broad child health policy framework that covers both international and national policy and legislation. Globally, UNICEF has reported continuing concerns over the plight of children subjected to the forces of poverty and inequities in health (UNICEF, 2009). This comes 20 years after the United Nations Convention on the Rights of the Child (UNCRC) (UNICEF, 1989), which highlights children's right to life and health, and yet globally 1 billion children are still deprived of food or shelter, clean water or health-care, with thousands under the age of 5 dying every day from preventable causes (UNICEF, 2009). More recently, UNICEF has highlighted the continuing – and in some respects, widening – inequities for children from the poorest households compared to those from the most affluent (UNICEF, 2015). The UNCRC is the world's most ratified convention, with the UK government among its signatories. The UK government was also a signatory, along with other UN member states, to the Millennium Declaration in 2000 (UN, 2000), which set out eight goals to be achieved by 2015, two of which were concerned with reducing child mortality (reduce by two-thirds between 1990 and 2015) and improving maternal health (reduce maternal mortality by three-quarters between 1990 and 2015). A more recent worldwide consultation undertaken by the UN has reconfirmed how central 'health' is to any future development agenda (UNDG, 2013). As the 2015 limit on the Millennium Development Goals (MDGs) beckoned, and with poverty and inequality still very evident for many nations, there were moves by the UN to build on these goals through the promotion of a more inclusive, sustainable development approach (UNDP, 2015a). It is clear that despite the goal-setting aspirations of governments, and perhaps as a consequence of the limited power and authority of the UN, there is still much work to be done.

A concern for the health and well being of children is also important nationally at a time when the UK government grapples with recovery from a global recession and implements a political strategy to stimulate economic growth through a reduction in public services and the institution of welfare reforms. Indeed, recession or not, the constant pressure for cost-efficiency within health and social care services means that the ongoing political rhetoric around reducing child poverty and improving the health and life chances of children presents significant challenges – as well as opportunities – for health visiting. This was clearly evident in the Marmot Review of health inequalities, which laid out the disproportionate impact of poverty on the lives of children and called for a policy objective of 'Giving every child the best start in life' (Marmot et al., 2010 p. 15) as the highest priority, with health visitors having a key role. From a policy perspective, health visitors are clearly at the forefront of supporting this goal, both by leading the Healthy Child Programme (DH, 2009) and through strong links to Children's Centres (Lansley, 2010). There is a requirement for there to be 'A named health visitor on every Children's Centre Management Board' (NHSE, 2014: 21). Additionally, in October 2015 the movement from the National Health Service (NHS) to local authorities of the commissioning responsibility for services for children aged between 0 and 5 years, which includes health visiting and Family Nurse Partnership (FNP), is clearly focused on a role designed to give children and their families a healthy start (DH, 2015).

In addition to analysing public health as a construct, this chapter will also provide an analysis of the health visiting role in relation to children and families and will consider how this sits within a public health approach to practice. This is important as it has been argued that a focus on children rather than the whole population does not fit a public health approach (Symonds, 1991). However, children are a distinct population and, as will be demonstrated from a lifecourse perspective, poor social circumstances in early life can have lasting influences on population health (Davey Smith et al., 1997; Blair et al., 2010). Lifecourse theory suggests that exposure to the cumulative impact of health and environmental factors during childhood is connected to the development of disorders, disability, and death in adults. Health visitors are in a prominent position to maximise the health and well being of this future adult population, which will one day have children of its own.

The Marmot Review (Marmot et al., 2010) recognised this and saw health visitors as critical to the success of any programme that aimed to improve the life chances of children, highlighting concerns over the falling numbers of health visitors. The review was not a lone voice in this regard, with calls for significant investment (HSC, 2009; UKPHA, 2009; Unite, 2009). However, despite these calls and an expedient political rhetoric on the importance of health visiting (DH, 2007, 2009; DH/DCSF, 2009), future prospects remained bleak.

The advent of a new UK coalition government in 2010 brought significant changes for health visiting and the subsequent policy direction has seen the commissioning of health visiting and family nurse partnership becoming the responsibility of local government since 2015 (DH, 2015). At a time of economic and social austerity, the profession found itself at the dawning of a new era, with significant investment from 2011 resulting in a major increase in the workforce of more than 4000 additional health visitors (Bennett, 2015a). However, this investment comes at a price, with health visitors facing challenges in enacting government policy which, it will be argued, diverges from the four principles that underpin health visiting (CETHV, 1977; Cowley & Frost, 2006). Meeting these challenges will mean making full use of each of the principles in order to gain any possibility of success. These four principles are explored in detail later in the chapter.

Throughout the discussion, the terms 'health visiting' and 'public health nursing' will be used interchangeably. This is not to assume that the terms mean exactly the same thing. Indeed, Craig (2000) has already given an enlightening deconstruction of the concept of 'public health nursing' and what it means for UK health visiting. However, for the purposes of this chapter, the analysis will remain focused on the context of health visiting for a public health role and not on the relationship between health visiting and nursing *per se*.

Public health

Before examining the relationship between health visitors and the public health function, it is important to consider and understand what is meant by 'public health' and the language and frameworks commonly used to describe it. 'Public health' is widely recognised to be a contested concept (Orme *et al.*, 2007; Verweij & Dawson, 2009; Baggott, 2011). As a result, several terms are used to describe or help explain the need for it. In the first instance, and to support the analysis, it may be useful to consider the two underlying terms separately: 'public' and 'health'.

Defining 'public'

Verweij & Dawson (2009) suggest the term 'public' may be interpreted in two ways. First, as an aggregate (sum) of the experiences of individuals within a given population. Examples of populations in this context are given in Box 2.1. You may also find Activity 2.1 useful. And second, as collective and organised action either by the state or by groups of people. Therefore, 'both the interventions and objectives of public health are "public" and go beyond the level of individuals' (Verweij & Dawson, 2009: 21). The concept of 'public' is important for health visitors as much of their work is with individuals, and an understanding of the health of those individuals can be aggregated to a population level to support a broader understanding of health need and the social context within which they live their lives.

> **Box 2.1   Examples of defined populations for health visitors**
>
> - Geographically determined: general practitioner (GP) registered practice list, geographical area, etc.
> - Settings: prisons, nurseries, children's centres, etc.
> - Characteristics: homeless, travelling families, asylum seekers, etc.

Furthermore, the notion of collective or organised action can mean two things for health visitors:

- The *organisation* of a response for care, based on the health visitor understanding the aggregate need within the 'population' of clients (e.g. the development of a postnatal support group in response to an increasing demand for postnatal mental health support).
- Facilitating and supporting *collective* action either with or on behalf of groups or communities to tackle local issues that affect health (e.g. supporting a resident's association in articulating the health impact of poor housing in a community or seeking political support to prevent the closure of a nursery).

Understanding the concept of 'public' through work that is substantially with individuals presents challenges for health visitors. The process of contact and care with one individual or family followed by another fragments the perception of population in day-to-day practice. SmithBattle *et al.* (2004) found such difficulty among inexperienced public health nurses (PHNs) in Canada[1] as they came to terms with the transition from nursing to public health nursing. This finding arose from a qualitative study of knowledge and skill acquisition among PHNs, which demonstrated how, through experiential learning, the PHNs developed a perceptual grasp of the 'bigger picture'. There was a shift from a reliance on a nurse-focused agenda, with predetermined frameworks and protocols to follow, to a 'situated understanding of practice' (SmithBattle *et al.*, 2004: 96). In other words, through their experiences with individuals and families, the PHNs were increasingly able to recognise the larger patterns and subtle cues embedded within the social context of their clients' lives. They demonstrated a shift from viewing client contact as a narrow, clinical situation to one in which there were patterns that required a community response. As one of the PHNs stated, 'Individuals in a community are as healthy as their community is, and vice versa … You can't address one without addressing the other' (SmithBattle *et al.*, 2004: 99). The study was therefore clear in its view that 'individual and family level experience was a crucial foundation for aggregate-level practice' (SmithBattle *et al.*, 2004: 99). The challenge of taking a population approach for those entering health visiting is still very real, as illustrated in guidance from the Royal College of Nursing (RCN, 2012) which encourages all nurses to work 'upstream' and provides illustrative cases studies to help them recognise and participate in 'public' health work.

So, for health visitors, the concept of 'public' as something that reflects collective and organised action (Verweij & Dawson, 2009) may develop with experience, as they gain a perceptual understanding of and readiness to respond to the broader issues surrounding complex situations within families.

Defining 'health'

Defining 'health' is equally complex. It depends on the underlying perspectives and values of those that seek to explain what it is. Earle (2007) highlights how health can be categorised into three broad areas:

- Health as the absence of disease. This reflects a negative (i.e. absence of disease) narrow biomedical interpretation of health.
- Health as well being, in its widest, most positive sense. For example, the World Health Organization (WHO) defines health as a 'state of complete physical, social and mental wellbeing, and not merely the absence of disease and infirmity' (WHO, 1946).
- Health as a resource. This suggests that health is embedded in the processes and actions of everyday life. For example, the WHO (1986) defines health as 'a resource for everyday life, not the object of living. It is a positive concept emphasising social and personal resources as well as physical capabilities'.

[1] PHNs in Canada have a similar role to health visitors in the UK.

Cowley & Frost (2006) note the challenges of attempting to define the value of health. They refer to work by health visitors in 1992 that considered the value of health and its practicability through health promotion from a health visiting perspective. This working group identified seven underpinning beliefs informing health visiting practice:

1. *Rights and responsibilities*: As everyone has a fundamental right to an optimum state of health, health visitors take on a responsibility to address health inequality and inequity.
2. *Health in context*: Health cannot be separated from the socioeconomic and cultural context in which it is experienced. It is the health visitor's understanding of individuals, their families, and their communities that takes account of the wider influences on health.
3. *Choice and blame*: Health must be regarded in broad holistic terms, encompassing individuals and families within their personal situations. Health visitors need to utilise their skills to promote an environment in which individuals, families, and communities are able to make healthy choices. They will need to consider who in society has responsibility for health beyond the individual, in order to minimise the risk of 'blaming the victim' (Ryan, 1976).
4. *Positive health*: Health promotion involves finding ways to create resources for health. This requires health visitors to think innovatively with families and communities about how to maximise their social and personal resources in order to effect health improvement.
5. *Health improvement*: Health visitors work to enable people to make full use of their physical, emotional, and social capacities to improve health. The focus is on working with the active participation of clients to address those factors that influence their health in the broader context.
6. *Empowerment*: Health visitors enable people to recognise that through active participation, they have the power to achieve health for themselves and to shape their own lives and those of their families. They therefore need to recognise the importance of facilitating people to engage in decision making about their health, particularly those groups who are frequently marginalised and excluded and are known to make less use of services (e.g. those on low incomes, from ethnic minority groups, or with mental illness).
7. *Community partnership and participation*: Healthcare services should be readily acceptable and accessible, and involve full community participation. This requires health visitors to work together with individuals, families, and communities and alongside other professionals in order to maximise their opportunities and capabilities to improve health.

(adapted from Cowley & Frost, 2006: 13–14)

From the analysis undertaken by the working group to which Cowley & Frost refer, it is evident that the concept of health requires health visitors to be adaptable and responsive to the needs of the most disadvantaged and socially excluded in society. In a review of research literature concerning health visiting, Cowley et al. (2013) found evidence supporting a health creating or salutogenic approach to health visiting practice. The health visitor role becomes one that seeks out ways to promote health, taking account of the environment in which people live and enabling people to actively participate in and shape their own lives. Activity 2.2 may be useful in helping you to explore your own underpinning values concerning health promotion.

Defining 'public health'

Recognising the diverse natures of 'public' and of 'health' and the competing perspectives that can occur in their explanations, it is not surprising that to interpret 'public health' presents significant challenges. Verweij & Dawson (2009) highlight how interpretations of public health fall into two main categories – narrow and broad – much as the definitions of health do. The narrow perspective sees public health in terms of how long people can remain free from disease. In contrast, the broad perspective sees public health not only in terms of protecting the health of the population but also in a broader role of health promotion and disease prevention (Verweij & Dawson, 2009). This broader view is said to be 'anticipatory, geared to the prevention of illness rather than simply the provision of care and treatment services' (Baggott, 2011: 1). However, taking a broad approach presents a key difficulty for the concept of public health. Perspectives that are packaged to be inclusive and capture the broad issues across society result in a concept that is so ambiguous they risk collapsing into a confusing set of ideas that are devoid of any useful purpose. The temptation to define public health in narrow terms – to address a specific problem or disease – is strong, but this risks focusing on treatment and provision of care without taking account of the broad range of factors that can influence health. You may wish to undertake Activity 2.3 at this point.

Different perspectives on public health will reflect what society sees as the prevailing priorities for improving the health of the public (Baggott, 2011). Baggott highlights that 'Different interests favour their own particular interpretations of public health and their interplay establishes its meaning … it is essentially a political process' (Baggott, 2011: 2). As mentioned in the introduction, the political process of public health has clearly had an impact on health visitors and their health promoting work with children and families in recent decades. Baggott goes on to suggest a number of broad ideological perspectives on public health that reflect the key debates surrounding freedom and responsibility between the individual and the state. You may wish to undertake Activity 2.4 at this point.

It is clear from these perspectives that the prevailing political environment has an impact upon how services for families with children are delivered. Indeed, current UK policies are designed to cope with the global recession through a reduction in welfare and public sector spending. This will have an impact on children and families, with cutbacks in services and benefits. Health visitors will therefore increasingly be working with families with reduced or limited incomes who have no access to family support. It is important at this point to consider public health more specifically in relation to health visiting.

A frequently cited definition of public health is that of the UK Commission for Inquiry into the Public Health Function, undertaken in the late 1980s: public health is 'The science and art of preventing disease, prolonging life and promoting health through the organised efforts of society' (DH, 1988; Faculty of Public Health, 2010). This is often referred to as the 'Acheson definition', as Sir Donald Acheson, the Chief Medical Officer at the time, chaired the committee. It clearly presents a broad interpretation of public health and encompasses some of the difficulties in interpretation highlighted in this section. It also reflects a collectivist ideology (Baggott, 2011). Beaglehole & Bonita (1997) have suggested that it emphasises the main components of public health:

- population perspective;
- collective responsibility for health and prevention;
- the role of the state, linked to a concern over underlying socioeconomic determinants of both health and disease;
- a multidisciplinary basis, incorporating quantitative and qualitative approaches;
- an emphasis on partnership with the populations served.

These components see health improvement through action with populations that take account of the wider social determinants of health, much as Cowley & Frost's (2006) seven beliefs underpinning health promotion in health visiting seek to demonstrate. One of the key phrases within the Acheson definition is the 'science and art of preventing disease'. This not only reflects a scientific perspective that uses epidemiological evidence and research to determine the causes of ill health, but also suggests that public health is concerned with innovation and action through health delivery. For health visitors, this is a key aspect of practice, involving understanding not only the needs of the population through the process of health needs assessment (HNA) (see Chapter 3), but also how to 'create' a response to those needs in practice at a local level (e.g. following cuts within the welfare system, working jointly with local welfare rights agencies to make welfare rights and benefits information accessible in a local clinic).

Human rights and public health

Beaglehole & Bonita's (1997) analysis of the Acheson definition highlights collective responsibility, concern over socioeconomic determinants of health, and the importance of partnerships for public health. It also suggests human rights have an underlying significance for health. Sirkin et al. (2005: 538) are very clear that healthcare professionals 'have a responsibility to protect and promote human rights'. The reasons for this are twofold. First, those human rights that are violated (e.g. being subjected to torture or deprived of an education) can have health consequences. And second, the process of promoting and protecting human rights can be the most effective means to securing health (Sirkin et al., 2005). Health visitors therefore have a responsibility to protect and promote human rights as a means of optimising the health of communities and reducing the impact of health inequalities. Indeed, as employees of a public service, health visitors are required to comply with the UK Human Rights Act 1998 and with international legislation ratified by the UK government. This includes:

- the Universal Declaration of Human Rights (UDHR) (UN, 1948);
- the International Covenant on Economic, Social and Cultural Rights (ICESCR) (UN, 1966);

- the European Convention on Human Rights (ECHR) (Council of Europe, 1950);
- the UNCRC (UNICEF, 1989).

These declarations of human rights contain series of 'articles' that reflect rights of freedom and rights of protection – what Fromer (1981) refers to as option rights and welfare rights, respectively. As Sirkin *et al.* (2005) allude to, if the ideal health outcomes in the WHO definition of health are to be acknowledged, then health will underpin all human rights. Conversely, there could be an occasion when, in the interests of public health, other human rights might be restricted (e.g. when someone is detained against their will because they have a highly infectious disease or are at risk of causing harm to themselves or others).

Despite the UK government having ratified these conventions, the Human Rights Act 1998 is the only agreement relating to human rights that has been enshrined in UK law, and this is therefore the framework that makes the government directly accountable for human rights. Recently, a repeal of the Human Rights Act has been suggested (Conservative Party, 2014). Whether repealed or not, international covenants of human rights are referred to in legal processes and are accepted as part of legal argument in determining case law. Interestingly, the UK Human Rights Act and its parent human rights framework, the ECHR, do not contain a specific article on the right to health, meaning there is no explicit accountability for that right in the current national legislation. If health visitors wish to use any human rights legislation to argue the right to health, therefore, they need to articulate that right in terms of deprivation of other rights under a range of available articles, much as Sirkin *et al.* (2005) highlight in the process of promoting and protecting human rights.

Box 2.2   Article 24 of the United Nations Convention on the Rights of the Child (UNICEF, 1989)

1. States Parties recognise the right of the child to the enjoyment of the highest attainable standard of health and to facilities for the treatment of illness and rehabilitation of health. States Parties shall strive to ensure that no child is deprived of his or her right of access to such health care services.
2. States Parties shall pursue full implementation of this right and, in particular, shall take appropriate measures:
   (a) To diminish infant and child mortality;
   (b) To ensure the provision of necessary medical assistance and health care to all children with emphasis on the development of primary health care;
   (c) To combat disease and malnutrition, including within the framework of primary health care, through, *inter alia*, the application of readily available technology and through the provision of adequate nutritious foods and clean drinking-water, taking into consideration the dangers and risks of environmental pollution;
   (d) To ensure appropriate pre-natal and post-natal health care for mothers;

(Continued)

Box 2.2 *(Continued)*

> (e) To ensure that all segments of society, in particular parents and children, are informed, have access to education and are supported in the use of basic knowledge of child health and nutrition, the advantages of breastfeeding, hygiene and environmental sanitation and the prevention of accidents;
>
> (f) To develop preventive health care, guidance for parents and family planning education and services.
>
> 3. States Parties shall take all effective and appropriate measures with a view to abolishing traditional practices prejudicial to the health of children.
>
> 4. States Parties undertake to promote and encourage international cooperation with a view to achieving progressively the full realisation of the right recognised in the present article. In this regard, particular account shall be taken of the needs of developing countries.

In the case of the UN declarations, member states are required to submit reports to the UN of their performance against the articles in the declarations. Again, however, without explicit national legislation, accountability is limited. There is further discussion of human rights legislation and its impacts on health visiting in Chapter 5, particularly in relation to the UNCRC. Suffice it to say at this point that the UNCRC does contain a specific article (Article 24) on the right to health of children that has relevance to health visiting and a public health role (see Box 2.2). This article sets out a comprehensive statement of the rights of children to health, taking account of wider determinants and, in particular, the right of access to healthcare. The article also makes reference to the concept of 'progressive realisation': this is an acknowledgment of governmental obligations to the UNCRC, and of the fact that the rights may be difficult to achieve on a short timescale, but it does mean that governments are required to demonstrate through their reporting to the UN that they are taking steps towards 'realisation' of the right to health (Gruskin & Tarantola, 2004). It is also clear that achievement (or otherwise) of the remaining articles of the UNCRC will have a profound impact on securing the health of children. You may wish to explore this further through Activity 2.5.

The UNCRC needs to be viewed within the context of the WHO definition of health, the UDHR (UN, 1948), and the ICESCR (UN, 1966), which all also assert rights relating to health. The UDHR is noteworthy as the first articulation of the right to health, but the ICESCR holds particular significance for public health and health visiting. The Covenant under Article 12 'recognises the right of everyone to the enjoyment of the highest attainable standard of physical and mental health' (UN, 1966) and makes specific reference to a reduction in child mortality and the healthy development of children under this article. The Covenant also places a particular emphasis on the social and economic context of people's lives and reflects upon how, in the absence of rights of freedom and protection, the infrastructure for health is lost. The UN has affirmed this with a statement that under Article 12 of the ICESCR:

States must protect this right [to health] by ensuring that everyone within their jurisdiction has access to the underlying determinants of health, such as clean water,
sanitation, food, nutrition and housing, and through a comprehensive system of
healthcare, which is available to everyone without discrimination, and economically
accessible to all.

(CESCR, 2000: para. 11)

The UN is very clear, therefore, through the ICESCR and the UNCRC, that not only
do the underlying social and economic determinants of health need to be addressed
in order to realise an attainment of health, but member states need to recognise the
unfair distribution of those determinants and that they should take steps to reduce
the impact of health inequalities, much as described in the UN's 17 sustainable development goals (UNDP, 2015b). Health visitors must recognise how this international
framework of legislation can be used to support their role as an advocate for local
children, families, and communities.

Not only is there a legislative requirement for health visitors to uphold human
rights, but it can also be argued from an ethical standpoint that health visitors have
a moral duty to promote and protect human rights as a means of securing health.
Indeed, *The Code: Professional Standards of Practice and Behaviour for Nurses
and Midwives* requires nurses, midwives, and health visitors to 'pay special attention
to promoting wellbeing, preventing ill health and meeting the changing health and
care needs of people during all life stages' (NMC, 2015: 5). This statement clearly
resonates with the role of health visitors. Furthermore, from an ethical standpoint,
health visitors need to have an understanding of how ethical health visiting practice links to a public health approach. Beauchamp & Childress (2001) identify four
principles for ethical practice: autonomy, beneficence, nonmaleficence, and justice.
Table 2.1 highlights the implications of these principles for health visitors in their
role of protecting and promoting health.

In summary, the process of defining the underlying concepts associated with public health has demonstrated clear associations with health visiting and the role of
health visitors in promoting health and reducing health inequities. This is supported
by an ethical and moral justification for promoting the health of children and their
families, based on consideration of the broad social determinants of health. It is
useful, therefore, with reference to the preceding discussion, to consider the underpinning principles of health visiting that enable an articulation of the public health
role for health visitors.

The principles of health visiting

The Acheson definition also views public health in terms of disease prevention and
health promotion. There are thus clear and direct parallels here with the role of
health visiting defined as 'The promotion of health and the prevention of ill health'
(CETHV, 1977). Such an approach clearly draws health visiting into the anticipatory
and preventive nature of public health by seeking to prevent illness and improve the
health and quality of life of whole populations of people. Health visitors undertake this
work by focusing at various times on individuals, families, groups, or communities.

Table 2.1 Principles for ethical health visiting practice.

Principle	Implication for health visiting practice
Autonomy	Supporting self-determination by building the self-esteem of clients and encouraging active participation in how they change their lives in order to improve their health
Beneficence	Supporting health improvement with individuals, families, and communities by identifying health needs, taking account of the broader social determinants of health
Nonmaleficence	Ensuring that health-visiting practice uses evidence-based approaches and is undertaken in a way that is cost-effective for disadvantaged populations. This is important for two reasons: • practice that is delivered inappropriately through outdated methods or without an evidence base may be harmful to clients • delivering care to populations with fewer needs entails time and opportunity costs for the health of those who need it the most
Justice	Ensuring that health visiting practice is delivered equitably across the population and is focused on addressing the needs of vulnerable groups and seeking to reduce the impact of health inequalities

Health visiting itself is underpinned by four principles (CETHV, 1977; Baldwin, 2012). These principles were first articulated nearly 4 decades ago by the Council for the Education and Training of Health Visitors, the regulatory body for health visiting at that time, but they have since been reaffirmed, most recently by Cowley & Frost (2006). They are said to reflect the knowledge base and process of health visiting (UKPHA, 2009), as well as providing the framework for the Nursing and Midwifery Council (NMC) SCPHN Standards (NMC, 2004):

1. The search for health needs.
2. The stimulation of an awareness of health needs.
3. The influence on policies affecting health.
4. The facilitation of health-enhancing activities.

Each of the principles is interconnected with the others, and together they form the basis for health improvement in individuals, families, and communities. They reflect a philosophy of health visiting (rather than specific activities *per se*) that focuses intervention with those identified as in greatest need, and therefore aim to reduce health inequalities. The UK Public Health Association (UKPHA, 2009) highlighted the importance of these principles for children and families – particularly the most disadvantaged, who become socially excluded and suffer comparatively poorer levels of health. The principles of health visiting are also clearly action focused, which again reflects the art of preventing disease, prolonging life, and promoting health.

A consideration of each of the principles demonstrates that they all have distinct features embedded within a public health approach.

The search for health needs

The search for health needs is viewed as an essential starting point for health improvement (South, 2015). While it forms the basis of an assessment process aimed at developing a plan to improve health, often in the form of an Health Needs Assessment (HNA), it also frames the search for health needs within a positive inter- pretation of health. HNA will be considered in more detail in Chapter 3, but suffice it to say at this point that searching for health needs broadens the horizons within which the health visitor views the people they work with and the factors they must take into account when making an assessment. The emphasis is on what needs can be fulfilled to maximise health, rather than what the health problem(s) is/are. Search- ing out need therefore goes beyond the individual client to the context within which they live their lives (e.g. their access to material resources and services, income, and employment[2]). Searching for health needs therefore aligns with a public health approach as a preventive process that takes account of the wider determinants of health.

However, it has to be acknowledged that meeting health needs will be a challeng- ing area of health visiting practice, given the increasing pressures and cuts in public- and voluntary-sector services (Bawden, 2013; CPAG, 2015). There is a risk of min- imising those health needs that the health visitor perceives may require additional assistance or referral and prioritising a focus on the client changing their individual behaviours. Given the earlier account of the client's rights to health and the duty of the health visitor to respond to those rights, health visitors need to think creatively about how they respond to unmet health needs. For example, utilising an asset-based community-development approach (South, 2015) with peer- or group-based activities can be an empowering way for clients to find solutions to their needs. Searching out health needs is therefore a challenging but important process for opening up the social determinants of health in clients' lives. This is in contrast, as Cowley & Frost (2006) point out, to other primary health care professionals, who will be framed by the presence of illness or disease and will be constrained by a focus on the health problem to be treated or rectified.

The stimulation of an awareness of health needs

The knowledge and understanding that health visitors gain from searching for health needs is a rich resource for gaining awareness of issues in need of a public health response. For example, the health visitor's awareness of the extent of domestic abuse occurring in the community, and the associated impacts on families and the community as a whole, are important pieces of information that warrant some form of action. What is less clear is whose awareness is to be stimulated. Cowley & Frost

---

[2] Material resources in this context refers to those living materials that are considered essen- tial, e.g. adequate shelter, heating, washing and cooking facilities, healthy food, and safe toys and play facilities.

(2006) suggest three different levels at which to engage in awareness-raising in order for an issue to be recognised as a priority. These can be applied to the issue of domestic abuse as follows:

1. *With individuals and communities:* Building trusting relationships and focusing on attributes and the capability to promote self-esteem in people suffering from domestic abuse, and exploring with them the unseen impact of domestic abuse on their own health and the health of their children. Such an approach can stimulate awareness of health as a positive resource.
2. *With commissioners and providers of services*: Raising awareness of the extent of domestic abuse as an often hidden and unmet need. The purpose is to give a richer understanding of the barriers and challenges that exist for health service managers and commissioners when attempting to meet key health improvement targets in local areas. For example, women experiencing domestic abuse are more likely to smoke, have an alcohol dependency, or suffer from depression. In this situation, the approach to improving health targets also means investing resources in tackling domestic abuse.
3. *With politicians and policy makers:* Raising awareness about proposed cuts in services for people experiencing domestic abuse and the subsequent impacts on individuals, society, and the economy.

Health visitors should be prepared to employ all of these levels in order to maximise the opportunities for improving the health of individuals, their families, and communities. To do so will require thinking critically and working in partnership with their service leaders and commissioners to determine the most appropriate audience with which to engage and to raise full awareness of health needs (see, for example, iHV, 2015).

The influence on policies affecting health

Influencing policy development has been perceived as the most challenging of the principles for most health visitors (Cowley & Frost, 2006; Laverack, 2015). The political nature of public health suggests that perspectives on public health and healthcare policy should be challenged to recognise the needs of the most vulnerable in society. In effect, the practitioner becomes an advocate for those with health needs, challenging and supporting policy making in order to ensure that policies have a positive health impact. Cowley & Frost (2006) suggest that this principle has three underpinning mechanisms for health visiting:

1. *Health intelligence:* A recognition of timely local population evidence, often ahead of official statistics, can be useful in determining a local policy response or service development. For example, health visitors are able to use their up-to-date knowledge of the community, through HNA and other processes (see Chapter 3), to gather qualitative information highlighting health needs.
2. *Innovation and change:* Being an active participant in change, challenging current practice, and becoming involved in new approaches (e.g. as a member of a project steering group, developing a breastfeeding policy in a local authority children's centre).

3. *Acting as a resource:* Either:
   - directly undertaking and disseminating robust research to support policy makers in identifying best practice to underpin new policies;
   - getting involved in policy development, which may include redesigning local service delivery;
   - informing or responding to policy proposals;
   - indirectly enabling community groups or pressure groups to access and interpret information on health and health services; or
   - enabling colleagues and other services to interpret the health impact of policies, in order to ensure their actions are conducive to good health (e.g. raising awareness within a local community cafe of the unhealthy nature of foods high in refined sugar or saturated fat content – and getting them to consider alternatives).

The political nature of public health and the extent to which it is dependent upon the values of those that make policy means that this is arguably one of the most important areas of health visiting practice to become involved in. It is the capacity to influence service redesign and policy making that will determine the extent to which the population will be able to maximise its health potential.

The facilitation of health enhancing activities

Milio (1986) coined the phrase 'making the healthier choice the easier choice', which became an underlying principle of the Ottawa Charter for Health Promotion, adopted in the same year (WHO, 1986; de Leeuw & Clavier, 2011; Naidoo and Wills, 2016). It suggests a focus on addressing the environment within which families and communities live as a means of achieving improvements in their health. Clearly, there are strategies that individuals can be supported to adopt in order to change their health behaviours, but to do so leaves untreated the underlying factors that may be contributing to those behaviours. Focusing on individual behaviour also places clients under substantial pressure to change their lifestyles when they may not have the capacity or resources to do so. Indeed, estimates suggest that only 10–30% of the gap in health outcomes between the most and least wealthy may be explained by differences in health-related behaviours (Lantz *et al.*, 1998). This suggests that the remaining 70–90% is determined by other factors in an individual's social environment. There is therefore a high risk of failure with the individual behaviour approach, which can stifle health enhancement.

Facilitating health focuses on multidisciplinary approaches to enabling people to actively participate in and shape their own futures. Giddens (2006: 8) highlights how the 'social contexts of people's lives are not just random assortments of events or actions; they are structured, or patterned in distinct ways'. This social patterning across populations is built on access to income and employment, cultural and community patterns and norms, adequate housing, education, and healthcare services. Tackling inequalities in health is therefore at the core of facilitating health-enhancing activity. Health inequalities will be discussed further later in the chapter, but at this point, the key issue is for health visitors not to focus solely on the health behaviours of clients but to see their role within the broader context of social determinants of health. Activity 2.6 may help you explore the principles of health visiting further.

Summary

The four principles described in this section set out the values and processes underpinning health visiting. They resonate with public health principles and form the basis for viewing the practice of health visiting in a broad context that can promote health enhancement for the most disadvantaged. The common emphasis in all four principles is on a population understanding of health and the wider determinants that impact upon people's lives. Success is best achieved, this suggests, through a process of enabling people and communities to determine how they can shape their lives to maximise their health experience by prioritising the issues that matter to them. The principles themselves have endured for over 30 years and, whatever the political landscape, they have remained as the bedrock for health visiting practice and will need to continue to do so into the foreseeable future.

The principles of health visiting are also included in the current Standards of Proficiency for Specialist Community Public Health Nurses produced by the NMC (2004). As the regulatory body for health visiting, the NMC sets the standards for entry to that part of its register that is concerned with public health nursing and provides the framework that regulates health visitors. Health visitors are not alone in this part of the register, which includes school nurses, occupational health nurses, family health nurses in Scotland, and nurses practising in a variety of settings, including sexual health and health protection. The four principles (referred to rather ambiguously as 'domains' in the NMC document) are mapped against 10 key areas developed as national occupational standards for public health practice (Skills for Health, 2004) (see Box 2.3). The purpose of the 10 areas is to identify those standards within

---

Box 2.3 Ten areas of public health practice (Skills for Health, 2004)

1. Surveillance and assessment the population's health and well being.
2. Promoting and protecting the population's health and well being.
3. Developing quality and risk management within an evaluative culture.
4. Engaging in collaborative working for health and well being.
5. Developing health programmes and services and reducing inequalities.
6. Developing and implementing policy and strategy to improve health and well being.
7. Working with and for communities to improve health and well being.
8. Providing strategic leadership for health and well being.
9. Engaging in research and development to improve health and well being.
10. Ethically managing one's self, people, and resources to improve health and well being.

which the public health workforce should practise and by which it should be measured. These ten areas were reviewed recently with nine refreshed areas making up the Public Health Skills and Knowledge Framework (PHORCaST, 2013) designed to place greater emphasis on the necessary knowledge and skills required for public health practice.

The Standards of Proficiency were developed in 2004, following the creation of the third part of the NMC register. In a controversial move, health visiting was removed from statute in 2001 upon the creation of the NMC in 2002 (UKPHA, 2009), signalling a lack of government support (Unite/CPHVA, 2009). As a profession in its own right, health visiting had been under the auspices of a regulatory body since 1962; since 2004, its status has been that of a post-registration nursing qualification. The 2014 Law Commission review of health professionals has, however, promoted renewed discussion of the regulatory position of health visitors (Cowley, 2014). As already discussed, the preventive nature of public health does not sit easily within a philosophy of healthcare that focuses on managing and caring for individuals with health problems and diseases, as is the case in nursing. The concern is that health visiting risks being increasingly diluted and constrained into a nursing rather than a public health model of delivery, and regulated within a framework that prevents people from backgrounds other than nursing and midwifery from being able to join the profession. Indeed, the Standards of Proficiency for Specialist Community Public Health Nurses (NMC, 2004) do not give a context for the underpinning theoretical framework and its association with public health. There are also gaps, particularly around public engagement and the significance of leadership, which are both important for effective public health practice.

Current policy suggests a stronger role among children and families, through improving and safeguarding health and leading, managing, and delegating programmes of work. Maintaining a public health focus through the regulatory framework in order to reduce health inequalities will clearly require an effort. Indeed, it is to the issue of health inequalities that the discussion now turns.

Health inequalities

During the 19th century, public health efforts were concentrated on addressing appalling living, sanitary, and working conditions and the impact of diseases such as cholera, smallpox, and tuberculosis (Ashton & Seymour, 1988). Improvements in the environment (including in housing, sanitation, and water supplies) during the late 19th century are said to have been the main factors associated with a reduction in deaths from infectious diseases. This became known as the environmental phase of public health (Ashton & Seymour, 1988). The origins of health visiting are said to have lain in this era (Adams, 2012; Cowley et al., 2013), and in the next phase which was concerned with maternal and child welfare.

The early 20th century saw the influence of public health measures begin to narrow in response to advances in medicine and scientific knowledge (e.g. the discovery of bacteria and viruses and the development of anaesthesia and antibiotics; Ashton &

Seymour, 1988). The result was a greater focus on treating the individual and the rise of personal health education. Indeed, as Caraher & McNab (1997) highlight, a focus for health visitors was the provision of education to poor families. The increasing emphasis on healthcare and clinical interventions, coupled with rapid technological advances in medicine, particularly after the Second World War, resulted in greater attention being paid to treating the unwell than to addressing the social conditions that prevent illness (Graham, 2007). McKinlay (cited in Graham, 2007: 101) relays a story told to him by the sociologist Irving Zola of a doctor jumping in a river to rescue drowning people, who has no time to look 'upstream' to see why they are falling in in the first place. McKinlay suggests that 'downstream' thinking relates to the delivery of medical care, while 'upstream' thinking considers the wider and prevailing set of factors that shape the experience of health.

A series of influential critiques of health policy at the latter end of the 20th century highlighted the significance of the social determinants of health (Graham, 2007) and the need for a greater emphasis on upstream thinking. Figure 2.1 shows the layers of influence that exist within the social structure and form the main determinants of health (Dahlgren & Whitehead, 1991). The innermost layer is (arguably) fixed, with age, sex, and hereditary factors being predetermined. Moving outwards, individual lifestyle behaviours, including tobacco use, diet, and exercise, also affect health, as do networks of family, friends, and others in the community. Further upstream, living and working conditions and the broader socioeconomic, cultural, and environmental context (e.g. the political landscape and governmental change, industry and business, wealth, access to services, welfare and taxation) also shape health experience. What is less evident from Figure 2.1 is that these layers interact with one another to magnify further poor health experience. For example, unemployment or low pay results in an income that prevents adequate housing arrangements from being maintained, causing family upheaval and stress. Low income also impacts on the quality of food consumed and the capacity to engage fully with social and community networks, causing and compounding stress and anxiety.

These determinants of health therefore result in variations or inequalities in health experience, with different distributions between different sectors of the population; for example, health experiences are different between men and women and across different age groups. Whitehead & Dahlgren (2006) suggest that there are three features that underpin health inequities. First, they are systematic: they do not happen randomly but show a consistent social gradient (i.e. of poor health across societies) that is heavily influenced by socioeconomic status. Essentially, the lower an individual's socioeconomic position, the worse their health (WHO, 2011). The emphasis is on the word 'gradient', as the difference is not simply between the most and least disadvantaged, but between all those in between; health statuses and levels of income are spread across the population. Hence, the steepness of the gradient is important. Second, health inequities are socially produced and therefore can be changed; as Whitehead & Dahlgren (2006: 2) highlight, 'No Law of Nature, for instance, decrees that the children of poor families should die at twice the rate as that of children born into rich families.' Third, health inequity is unjust. For example, all children should have the opportunity to be breastfed, regardless of the socioeconomic status of the parents.

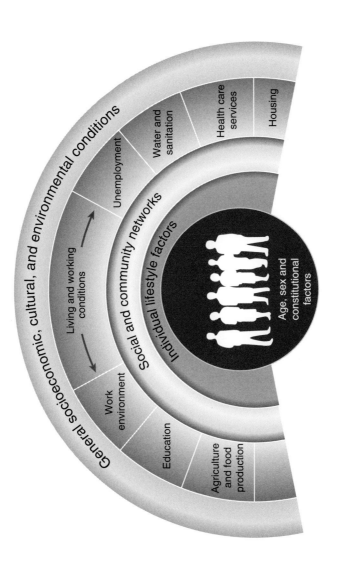

Figure 2.1 The main determinants of health. *Source*: Dahlgren & Whitehead (1991), Institute for Futures Studies, Stockholm. Reproduced with permission of Institute for Futures Studies.

On many levels, tackling health inequities is a fundamental aspect of public health and health visiting. From an ethical and human rights perspective, and as part of the duty of care, health visitors should undertake their practice with a clear focus on helping those most in need, but without losing sight of the goal of providing a universal service. This is what the Marmot Review refers to as 'proportionate universalism' (Marmot et al., 2010: 16). The purpose is to reduce the steepness of the social gradient:

> To reduce the steepness of the social gradient in health, actions must be universal, but with a scale and intensity that is proportionate to the level of disadvantage. We call this proportionate universalism. Greater intensity of action is likely to be needed for those with greater social and economic disadvantage, but focusing solely on the most disadvantaged will not reduce the health gradient, and will only tackle a small part of the problem.
>
> (Marmot et al., 2010: 10)

Recognising that socioeconomic status is a key determinant of health has led some writers to suggest pathways that provide an explanation for health inequalities (Graham, 2007). One such pathway, known as the 'lifecourse perspecitve', suggests that disadvantage starts before birth and accumulates throughout life. As the Marmot Review observes:

> From the time of birth, the individual is exposed to a wide range of experiences – social, economic, psychological and environmental … It is the accumulation of these influences, their effects and the interactions that 'cast a long shadow' over subsequent social development, behaviour, health and well-being of the individual.
>
> (Marmot et al., 2010: 40)

In other words, poor health in adulthood may have its roots in childhood disadvantage. Indeed, there is growing evidence that the circumstances in which children are conceived, born, and grow up reflect later socioeconomic inequalities in the health of adults. Work carried out by Barker (1992), known as the 'foetal origins hypothesis', suggests that impaired foetal growth during pregnancy (using low birth weight as an indicator) contributes to disease in adulthood, including cardiovascular disease and its precursors, such as diabetes, high lipid values, and high blood pressure. This indicates that maternal health should be a concern throughout pregnancy, and that maternal poverty and disadvantage can affect foetal development (Earle & O'Donnell, 2007). Indeed, disadvantaged mothers are more likely to have babies of low birth weight (Jefferis et al., 2002) and are more likely to be exposed to stress, poor diet, and alcohol, tobacco, and drug misuse during pregnancy (Marmot et al., 2010). Furthermore, Davey Smith et al. (1998) found in their prospective cohort study[3] that poor childhood circumstances increase the risk of death from stroke,

---

[3] A prospective study involves taking a cohort of subjects (e.g. a group of people born at the same time) and watching them over a long period; any outcomes (e.g. development of a disease) can then be correlated with other factors present in the subjects.

heart, and respiratory disease in later life. You may find Activity 2.7 useful at this point.

With its emphasis on childhood disadvantage, the lifecourse perspective clearly has ramifications for the role of health visitors in supporting disadvantaged families with young children. Furthermore, the lifecourse perspective gives a strong indication of the public health interventions that should be implemented, focusing on maternal nutrition, breastfeeding, and cessation of smoking. Consequently, the Marmot Review (Marmot *et al.*, 2010) frames much of its analysis through the lifecourse perspective, and not surprisingly identifies health visitors as important to any success in reducing health inequalities to disadvantaged families. The review highlights some key findings of an analysis of available material:

- People living in the poorest areas of England die 7 years earlier than those in the most affluent areas.
- The average difference in disability-free life expectancy at birth between the least and most deprived areas is 17 years; that is, people from disadvantaged areas not only die sooner than their affluent counterparts, but will also spend more of their later years with a disability.
- One in four deaths of infants under the age of 1 would be avoided if all births had the same level of risk as those among women who are least disadvantaged.
- There are higher rates of smoking and obesity amongst low-income groups and higher rates of drug use and alcohol-related admissions amongst people living in disadvantaged areas.
- There is a strong social gradient associated with the prevalence of postnatal depression.
- A child's physical, social, emotional, and cognitive development during the early years strongly influences her or his school-readiness and educational attainment:
  ○ Children with a high cognitive score at 22 months but with parents of low socioeconomic status do less well (in terms of subsequent cognitive development) than children with low initial scores but with parents of high socioeconomic status.
  ○ Children of educated or wealthy parents can score poorly in early tests but still catch up, whereas children of worse-off parents are extremely unlikely to do so.

The Marmot Review and Marmot's (2015) book, *The Health Gap*, will both be useful for the health visitor who wants to understand more about health inequalities and their impact on children, families, and communities. The Marmot Review chellenges health visitors to reflect on and consider appropriate, evidence-based responses to the public health priorities it identifies. You may find it useful to undertake Activity 2.8 here.

The Health and Social Care Bill 2012 set out arguably the most radical reforms for the NHS in its over 65-year history, with proposals for structural changes that meant commissioning of services would largely be driven by GPs in primary care. Public health was transferred to local authorities, with a ring-fenced public health budget allotting funding for specific services, including health visiting. From October 2015, health visiting has continued to be delivered through the NHS and funded through local authorities, alongside the FNP programme (see Chapter 4). The aim of this return of health visiting to its local authority roots is to foster greater levels of integration between NHS services (e.g. maternity and primary care) and local authority early years' services (e.g. children's centres) in order to deliver improvements in health outcomes for children through the Healthy Child Programme (DH, 2015).

The 2011–15 action plan for health visiting investment has resulted in a 50% increase in the workforce in England (Bennett, 2015a), while the Call to Action for Health Visiting (DH, 2011) has set out a framework for a new health visiting service. These are further explored in Chapter 3 (see Box 3.1) and Chapter 4.

Existing health visitors in England have been encouraged to refresh and develop their skills, taking lessons from the early-intervention FNP programme and other evidence-based programmes aimed at helping families with complex needs. Investment by Health Education England in educational resources through the Making the Most of Health Visiting Project has provided this increased workforce with access to resources that can help develop their knowledge from preceptorship to specialism (e.g. in one of the public health high impact areas). These resources are accessible via the eCommunity of Practice Hub on the Institute of Health Visiting website. You may find it useful to undertake Activity 2.9 at this point.

Interestingly, the Call to Action refers to work undertaken by Field (2010) and Allen & Duncan Smith (2010), with the health visitor action plan being a response to the challenges posed in these reports. Both pieces of work clearly focus on early intervention aimed at improving children's life chances; however, they look less at socioeconomic factors and social structure and more at what can be done for children and families at an individual level. Indeed, Field comments that he has 'come to view poverty as a much more subtle enemy than purely lack of money' (Field, 2010: 12), focusing on the cycle of poverty and disadvantage that occurs across the generations. From this viewpoint, and from that of other early intervention programmes such as the FNP, the behaviours and characteristics of poor parents come to be seen as the problem, and the focus of interventions is thus changes in individual behaviour. The intention is to break the alleged cycle of deprivation, much as Clarke (2006) suggests in her critique of the Sure Start initiative. However, as discussed earlier, focusing on individualistic approaches runs the risk of failing to provoke behaviour change. Additionally, psychological harm can arise among families and groups who feel powerless to respond to calls for behaviour change. The point for health visitors is that while the increased investment has been very welcome to the profession, it comes at a cost. Health visitors have to deliver a government policy that promotes individualised approaches to improving health and minimises the scope to address the broader social context. One way to counter this individualistic approach is for health visitors to consider their role in the community, which forms the first level of the four-level health visiting service structure (DH, 2011), while acknowledging that as a method of promoting health, community participation comes with its own challenges (see Chapter 3).

Recently, focus on individual behaviour change has led to an emphasis on health improvement and tackling health inequalities through approaches such as 'nudging' people to change health behaviour. 'Nudging' is a phrase coined by Thaler & Sunstein

(2008), who suggest that people are more likely to respond to instant reward than the promise of future benefit. They refer to 'libertarian paternalism' and systems of human thought that lead to instinctive or automatic responses, and base the notion of nudging on the premise that it is legitimate to influence behaviour (paternalism) to promote health, but that people should not be compelled to change their behaviour (libertarianism). Cues leading to healthy choices are 'architectured' or designed to occur in subtle ways that nudge people, through their sense of freedom, to make such choices for themselves. This might include placing healthy foods in a prominent position in a cafe or designing a building such that it is easier to take the stairs than the escalator. It also includes dispelling behaviour myths (e.g. that most people do not smoke or drink excessively) among targeted groups, in what is known as 'social norm feedback'.

Bonnell et al. (2011) argue that nudging already occurs, through social marketing techniques, peer approaches, and motivational interviewing. Marteau et al. (2011) claim nudging is 'fuzzy' and point out that while there is evidence that it works to promote unhealthy behaviours (e.g. the placement of sweets at the eye level for children at supermarket checkouts), there is little to show that it can be used to improve health, and no evidence that it is cost-effective compared to other inter-ventions. They also point to the limited effectiveness of self-regulation by the food, alcohol, and tobacco industries, which have more interest in promoting unhealthy behaviour than healthy. Public Health England (2015) has argued for a multisectoral approach to reducing sugar intake and thus addressing the obesity epidemic which has culminated in government proposals for a sugar tax to be implemented in 2018. Health visitors may also find that people from more advantaged areas are more likely to respond to nudges or cues to change health behaviours than those from disadvan-taged areas, given the increasing evidence that health inequalities can widen when using an individual-behaviour change approach (Capewell & Graham, 2010).

The concept of libertarian paternalism fits well with a conservative/liberal approach, much as does Baggott's (2011) reference earlier in the chapter to liberal ideology, which emphasises the freedom of the individual to make choices without state interference and minimises legislation and regulation. Bonnell et al. (2011) argue that public health is rarely coercive and that it seeks to influence those processes that support people's healthy choices. It is evident that the 'nudge' approach does not sit well with principles of public health that identify more with collective approaches or a willingness on the part of the state to intervene and legislate for health improvement. The health visitor must contend with government expectations that 'nudge' initiatives and early intervention approaches (through the Healthy Child Programme) will be delivered to success. The difficulty, as already discussed, is that the philosophy of health visiting does not sit easily with such individualised approaches, and that policy may limit or deny the opportunity to address socioeconomic and other factors in the social structure.

Good leadership is a fundamental aspect of public health practice. There is no doubting the complexity of the contemporary role for health visiting when engaging a public health approach in light of current policy. Herein lies the challenge for health visitors at the dawning of a new era for the profession that will require a greater readiness to integrate with other services concerned with the health, well being, and development of children. Bennett (2015b) has proposed the 4-5-6 Model of the Transformed Health Visiting Service as a way to demonstrate the contribution of health visitors to public health. Leadership in this context is centred on working with other professionals to manage the divergence within a policy agenda that focuses practice on changing health behaviour at the level of individuals (whether carried out at the individual, family, or community level) while seeking to maintain a footing in public health principles that promote a collective approach to addressing the main determinants of health. The key is to maximise all of the principles of health visiting. This will require strength, clarity of thought and vision, a willingness to build partnerships, and a recognition of human rights as the basis for advocacy, influence, and change – whether at a local or a national level.

Health visitors are currently using their leadership and management skills, through delegation and risk assessment, to lead multidisciplinary teams to deliver the Healthy Child Programme (HCP), HNA and parenting programmes, amongst other things, and to support the development of the next generation of health visitor students. As this list illustrates, and as Fanning (2013) notes, the context and requirements of leaders in the community are highly complex and challenging. Good leadership also demands a capacity to think innovatively and critically about how to respond to the needs of communities and a readiness to build partnerships and to advocate for and influence local agendas. This is particularly important given the increasing integration between local authority early years' services and NHS provision for families with young children. There will be opportunities to influence that process, but there will also be challenges (of ambiguity, ignorance, and conflict) to overcome. It is therefore important for health visitors to develop strategic and political awareness. There is also evidence, through a diverse array of leading roles, both within and without health visiting, of leaders using their health visiting principles to support change (e.g. specialists working in infant feeding, weight management, and immunisation programmes, senior leaders with a health visiting background working in public health, commissioning, procurement, and quality management).

Summary

This chapter has sought to give an understanding of the public health role of health visiting through an analysis of the context and delivery of contemporary practice. History has shown how the development of health visiting arose at a time when public health concerned itself with broader, social determinants of health. However, its development into the maternal and welfare movement resulted in an approach centred in health education and advice for most of the 20th century. The development of the principles of health visiting has given the profession a broader appreciation of the contribution that it can make to improving health and reducing health inequalities.

The concepts associated with the term 'public health' have been analysed and discussed, and a connection has been made with health visiting and its four underlying principles. An analysis of the human rights agenda and the right to health has demonstrated that solutions to tackling health inequities are interconnected with the main determinants of health, and not individual behaviour alone. Recognising the wider determinants of health highlights the importance of enabling active participation by individuals, families, and communities in shaping their own health experiences and outcomes. Almost four decades after their inception, the four principles continue to give a sound philosophical footing to health visiting practice and its contribution to reducing health inequalities.

Fortunately, the profession has a number of influential political allies who recognise the value of health visitors in supportinging children and families. Consequently, at a time of economic and social austerity, the profession finds itself at the dawning of a new era, with significant investment leading to a significant increase in the numbers of health visitors in England and to 500 new health visitors in Scotland by 2017–18. This investment comes at a cost, however, with the profession facing challenges in enacting government policy that diverges from the four principles underpinning it. The difficulties in addressing these tensions cannot be overestimated. The way forward, therefore, lies in health visitors taking a fresh approach and exploiting each of the principles to the full, with strong leadership at all levels within the profession. To do so gives the best opportunity for health visiting to be able to contribute to a more fair society and to demonstrate how it can maximise its approach to promoting health and preventing ill health.

References

Adams, C. (2012) The history of health visiting. *Nursing in Practice*, **68**. Available from: http://www.nursinginpractice.com/article/history-health-visiting (last accessed 30 March 2016).

Allen, G. & Duncan Smith, I. (2010) Early Intervention: Good Parents, Great Kids, Better Citizens. The Centre for Social Justice and The Smith Institute, London. Available from: http://www.centreforsocialjustice.org.uk/UserStorage/pdf/Pdf %20reports/EarlyInterventionFirstEdition.pdf (last accessed 30 March 2016).

Ashton, J. & Seymour, H. (1988) The New Public Health. Open University Press, Milton Keynes.

Baggott, R. (2011) Public Health: Policy and Politics, 2nd edn. Palgrave Macmillan, Basingstoke.

Baldwin, S (2012) Exploring the professional identity of health visitors. *Nursing Times*, **108**(25), 12–15.

Barker, D.J.P. (ed.) (1992) Fetal and Infant Origins of Adult Disease. BMJ Publishing, London.

Bawden, A. (2013) Charities: we've got five years left, at best. *Guardian*, 24 July 2013. Available from: http://www.theguardian.com/society/2013/jul/24/charities-voluntary-sector-five-years-existence (last accessed 30 March 2016).

Beaglehole, R. & Bonita, R. (1997) Public Health at the Crossroads. Cambridge University Press, Cambridge.

Beauchamp, T. & Childress, J. (2001) Principles of Biomedical Ethics, 5th edn. Oxford University Press, Oxford.

Bennett, V. (2015a) Transforming health visiting: thank you to the profession, partners and parents. Public Health England blog. Available from: https://vivbennett.blog.gov .uk/2015/03/23/transforming-health-visiting-open-letter-thanks/ (last accessed 30 March 2016).

Bennett, V. (2015b) The 4-5-6 Model of the Transformed Health Visiting Service. Public Health England blog. Available from: https://vivbennett.blog.gov.uk/2015/03/05/ the-4-5-6-model/ (last accessed 30 March 2016).

Blair, M., Stewart-Brown, S., Waterston, T. & Crowther, R. (2010) Child Public Health, 2nd edn. Oxford University Press, Oxford.

Bonnell, C., McKee, M., Fletcher, A., Wilkinson, P. & Haines, A. (2011) One nudge forward, two steps back. *British Medical Journal*, **342**, d401.

Capewell, S. & Graham, H. (2010) Will cardiovascular disease prevention widen health inequalities? *PLoS Medicine*, **7**(8), e1000320.

Caraher, M. & McNab, M. (1997) Using lessons from health visiting's past to inform the public health role. *Health Visitor*, **70**, 380–4.

CESCR (2000) Substantive Issues Arising in the Implementation of the International Covenant on Economic, Social and Cultural Rights: General Comment No. 14. Committee on Economic, Social and Cultural Rights, New York. Available from: http://data.unaids.org/publications/external-documents/ecosoc_cescr-gc14_en.pdf (last accessed 30 March 2016).

CETHV (1977) An Investigation into the Principles of Health Visiting. Council for the Education and Training of Health Visitors, London.

Clarke, K. (2006) Childhood, parenting and early intervention: a critical examination of the SureStart national programme. *Critical Social Policy*, **26**(4), 699–721.

Conservative Party (2014) Protecting Human Rights in the UK: The Conservatives' Proposals for Changing Britain's Human Rights Laws. The Conservative Party, London.

Council of Europe (1950) Convention for the Protection of Human Rights and Fundamental Freedoms (Amended, 2010). Council of Europe. Available from: http://conventions.coe.int/treaty/en/Treaties/Html/005.htm (last accessed 30 March 2016).

Cowley, S. (2014) Position Paper on Health Visitor Regulation. Available from: http://ihv.org.uk/wp-content/uploads/2015/08/Law-Comission-Position-statement-on-HV-regulation-final-20-05-14.pdf (last accessed 30 March 2016).

Cowley, S. & Frost, M. (2006) The Principles of Health Visiting: Opening the Door to Public Health Practice in the 21st Century. Community Practitioners' and Health Visitors' Association, London.

Cowley, S., Whittaker, K., Grigulis, A., Malone, M., Danetto, S., Wood, H., Morrow, E. & Maben, J. (2013) Why Health Visiting? A Review of the Literature about Key Health Visitor Interventions, Processes and Outcomes for Children and Families. National Nursing Research Unit, King's College London, London. Available from: https://www.kcl.ac.uk/nursing/research/nnru/publications/Reports/Why-Health-Visiting-NNRU-report-12-02-2013.pdf (last accessed 30 March 2016).

CPAG (2015) Welfare Reform and Work Bill 2015. Child Poverty Action Group, London. Available from: http://www.cpag.org.uk/content/welfare-reform-and-work-bill-2015 (last accessed 30 March 2016).

Craig, P.M. (2000) The nursing contribution to public health. In: Nursing for Public Health. Population-Based Care (eds P.M. Craig & G.M. Lindsay). Churchill Livingstone, London.

Dahl, B.M. & Clancy, A. (2015) Meanings of knowledge and identity in public health nursing in a time of transition: interpretations of public health nurses narratives. *Scandinavian Journal of Caring Sciences*, **29**, 679–87. Available from: http://onlinelibrary.wiley.com/doi/10.1111/scs.12196/epdf (last accessed 30 March 2016).

Dahlgren, G. & Whitehead, M. (1991) Policies and Strategies to Promote Social Equity in Health. Institute for Futures Studies, Stockholm.

Davey Smith, G., Hart, C., Blane, D., Gillis, C. & Hawthorne, V. (1997) Lifetime socioeconomic position and mortality: prospective observational study. *British Medical Journal*, **314**, 547.

Davey Smith, G., Hart, C., Blane, D. & Hole, D. (1998) Adverse socioeconomic conditions in childhood and cause specific adult mortality: prospective observational study. *British Medical Journal*, **316**, 1631.

Dawson, A. (ed.) (2011) Public Health Ethics: Key Concepts and Issues in Policy and Practice. Cambridge University Press, Cambridge.

de Leeuw, E. & Clavier, C. (2011) Healthy public in all policies. Health Promotion International, **26**(S2): ii237–44. Available from: http://heapro.oxfordjournals.org/content/26/suppl_2/ii237.full.pdf (last accessed 30 March 2016).

DH (1988) Public Health in England: the Report of the Committee of Inquiry into the Future Development of the Public Health Function. Department of Health, London.

DH (1999) Saving Lives: Our Healthier Nation. The Stationery Office, London.

DH (2003) Liberating the Public Health Talents of Community Practitioners and Health Visitors. Department of Health, London.

DH (2007) The Government Response to Facing the Future: a Review of the Role of Health Visitors. Department of Health, London. Available from: http://webarchive.nationalarchives.gov.uk/20071204130045/http://dh.gov.uk/prod_consum_dh/idcplg?IdcService=SS_GET_PAGE&siteId=en&ssTargetNodeId=566&ssDocName=DH_080007 (last accessed 30 March 2016).

DH (2009) Healthy Child Programme: Pregnancy and the First Five Years of Life. Department of Health, London. Available from: https://www.gov.uk/government/uploads/system/uploads/attachment_data/file/167998/Health_Child_Programme.pdf (last accessed 30 March 2016).

DH (2010) Healthy Lives, Healthy People: Our Strategy for Public Health in England. Stationery Office, London. Available from: https://www.gov.uk/government/publications/healthy-lives-healthy-people-our-strategy-for-public-health-in-england (last accessed 30 March 2016).

DH (2011) Health Visitor Implementation Plan 2011–15: Call to Action. Department of Health, London. Available from: https://www.gov.uk/government/publications/health-visitor-implementation-plan-2011-to-2015 (last accessed 30 March 2016).

DH (2015) Transfer of 0–5 Children's Public Health Commissioning to Local Authorities: Overview 2: Health Visiting and Family Nurse Partnership Services. Department of Health, Stationery Office, London. Available from: https://www.gov.uk/government/uploads/system/uploads/attachment_data/file/407645/overview2-health-visit.pdf (last accessed 30 March 2016).

DH/DCSF (2009) Healthy Lives, Brighter Futures – The Strategy for Children and Young People's Health. Department of Health and Department for Children, Schools and Families, Stationery Office, London. Available from: http://webarchive.nationalarchives.gov.uk/+/www.dh.gov.uk/en/publicationsandstatistics/publications/publicationspolicyandguidance/DH_094400 (last accessed 30 March 2016).

Earle, S. (2007) Exploring health. In: Theory and Research in Promoting Public Health (eds S. Earle, C.E. Lloyd, M. Sidell & S. Spurr). Sage, London.

Earle, S. & O'Donnell, T. (2007) The factors that influence health. In: Theory and Research in Promoting Public Health (eds S. Earle, C.E. Lloyd, M. Sidell & S. Spurr). Sage, London.

Faculty of Public Health (2010) What is Public Health? Available from: http://www.fph.org.uk/what_is_public_health (last accessed 30 March 2016).

Fanning, A. (2013) Leadership: measuring the effectiveness of care delivery. In: Community and Public Health Nursing, 5th edn (eds D. Sines, S. Aldridge-Bent, A. Fanning, P. Farrelly, K. Potter & J. Wright). Wiley-Blackwell, Chichester. Ch. 14, pp. 241–56.

Field, F. (2010) The Foundation Years: Preventing Poor Children from Becoming Poor Adults. Cabinet Office, London. Available from: http://www.frankfield.com/campaigns/poverty-and-life-changes.aspx (last accessed 30 March 2016).

Fromer, M.J. (1981) Ethical Issues in Healthcare. CV Mosby, St Louis.

Giddens, A. (2006) Sociology, 5th edn. Polity Press, Cambridge.

Glass, N. (1999) Sure Start: The development of an early intervention programme for young children in the United Kingdom. *Children and Society*, **13**, 257–64.

Graham, H. (2007) Unequal Lives. Open University Press, Maidenhead.

Gruskin, S. & Tarantola, D. (2004) Health and human rights. In: Oxford Textbook of Public Health, 4th edn (eds R. Detels, J. McEwen, R. Beaglehole & H. Tanaka). Oxford University Press, Oxford.

HM Government (2006) Reaching Out: An Action Plan on Social Exclusion. Cabinet Office, Social Exclusion Task Force, London. Available from: http://webarchive .nationalarchives.gov.uk/20070402091623/cabinetoffice.gov.uk/social_exclusion_ task_force/publications/reaching_out/ (last accessed 30 March 2016).

Home Office (1998) Supporting Families: A Consultation Document. Stationery Office, London.

HSC (2009) Health Inequalities: Third Report of Session 2008–09. Health Select Committee, House of Commons, London. Available from: http://www.publications .parliament.uk/pa/cm200809/cmselect/cmhealth/286/286.pdf (last accessed 30 March 2016).

iHV (2015) Understanding Local Government. Professional Guidance. Institute of Health Visiting. Available from: http://ihv.org.uk/wp-content/uploads/2015/06/PB_Local-Government_V3-WEB.pdf (last accessed 30 March 2016).

Jefferis, B.J.M.H., Power, C. & Hertzman, C. (2002) Birth weight, childhood socioeconomic environment, and cognitive development in the 1958 British birth cohort study. *British Medical Journal*, **325**, 305.

Lansley, A. (2010) Health Committee – Minutes of Evidence Responsibilities of the Secretary of State for Health. Question 38. Available from: http://www.publications .parliament.uk/pa/cm201011/cmselect/cmhealth/380/10072004.htm (last accessed 30 March 2016).

Lantz, P.M., House, J.S., Lepkowski, J.M., Williams, D.R., Mero, R.P. & Chen, J. (1998) Socio-economic factors, health behaviours and mortality. *Journal of the American Medical Association*, **279**(21), 1703–8.

Laverack, G. (2015) Public Health: Power, Empowerment and Professional Practice, 3rd edn. Palgrave Macmillan, Basingstoke.

Marmot, M. (2015) The Health Gap: The Challenge of an Unequal World. Bloomsbury Publishing, London.

Marmot, M., Atkinson, T., Bell, J., Black, C., Broadfoot, P., Cumberlege, J., Diamond, I., Gilmore, I., Ham, C., Meacher, M. & Mulgan, G. (2010) Fair Society, Healthy Lives: The Marmot Review. Marmot Review Team, University College, London. Available from: http://www.instituteofhealthequity.org/projects/fair-society-healthy-lives-the-marmot-review (last accessed 30 March 2016).

Marteau, T.M., Ogilvie, D., Roland, M., Suhrcke, M. & Kelly, M.P. (2011) Judging nudging: can nudging improve population health? *British Medical Journal*, **342**, d228.

Milio, N. (1986) Promoting Health through Public Policy. Canadian Public Health Association, Ottawa.

Naidoo, J. & Wills, J. (2009) Foundations for Health Promotion, 3rd edn. Bailliere Tindall Elsevier, Edinburgh.

Naidoo, J. and Wills, J. (2016) Foundations for Health Promotion. 4th edn. Bailliere Tindall Elsevier, Edinburgh.

NHSE (2014) 2015–16 National Health Visiting Core Service Specification. NHS England, London. Available from: http://www.england.nhs.uk/wp-content/uploads/2014/12/ hv-serv-spec-dec14-fin.pdf (last accessed 30 March 2016).

NMC (2004) Standards of Proficiency for Specialist Community Public Health Nurses. Nursing and Midwifery Council, London.

NMC (2015) The Code: Professional Standards of Practice and Behaviour for Nurses and Midwives. Nursing and Midwifery Council, London.

Orme, J., Powell, J., Taylor, P. & Grey, M. (2007) Mapping public health. In: Public Health for the 21st Century: New Perspectives on Policy, Participation and Practice (eds J. Orme, J. Powell, P. Taylor & M. Grey), 2nd edn. Open University Press, Maidenhead.

PHORCaST (2013) Public Health Skills and Knowledge Framework Refresh Final Report. PHORCaST, London. Available from: http://www.phorcast.org.uk/page.php?page_id=313 (last accessed 30 March 2016).

Public Health England (2015) Sugar Reduction: The Evidence for Action. Public Health England, London. Available from: https://www.gov.uk/government/uploads/system/uploads/attachment_data/file/470179/Sugar_reduction_The_evidence_for_action.pdf (last accessed 30 March 2016).

RCN (2012) Going Upstream: Nursing's Contribution to Public Health. Prevent, Promote and Protect. Royal College of Nursing, London. Available from: https://www2.rcn.org.uk/__data/assets/pdf_file/0007/433699/004203.pdf (last accessed 30 March 2016).

Ryan, W. (1976) Blaming the Victim. Vintage, New York.

Sirkin, S., Iacopeno, V., Grodin, M.A. & Danieli, Y. (2005) The role of health professionals in protecting and promoting human rights. In: Perspectives on Health and Human Rights (eds S. Gruskin, M.A. Grodin, S.P. Marks & G.J. Annas). Routledge, Abingdon.

Skills for Health (2004) National Occupational Standards for the Practice of Public Health Guide. Skills for Health, Bristol.

SmithBattle, L., Diekemper, M. & Leander, S. (2004) Moving upstream: becoming a public health nurse, Part 2. Public Health Nursing, 21(2), 95–102.

South, J. (2015) A Guide to Community-Centred Approaches for Health and Well-Being. Full Report. Public Health England, London. Available from: https://www.gov.uk/government/uploads/system/uploads/attachment_data/file/417515/A_guide_to_community-centred_approaches_for_health_and_wellbeing__full_report_.pdf (last accessed 30 March 2016).

Symonds, A. (1991) Angels and interfering busy bodies: the social construction of two occupations. Sociology of Health and Illness, 13, 249–64.

Thaler, R.H. & Sunstein, C.R. (2008) Nudge: Improving Decisions about Health, Wealth, and Happiness. Yale University Press, London.

UKPHA (2009) Health Visiting Matters: Re-establishing Health Visiting. UK Public Health Association, London. Available from: http://www.ukpha.org.uk/media/14945/health%20visiting %20matters%20final%20report.pdf (last accessed 30 March 2016).

UN (1948) United Nations Universal Declaration on Human Rights. United Nations, New York. Available from: http://www.un.org/en/universal-declaration-human-rights/index.html (last accessed 30 March 2016).

UN (1966) United Nations International Covenant on Economic, Social and Cultural Rights. United Nations, New York. Available from: http://www.un-documents.net/icescr.htm (last accessed 30 March 2016).

UN (2000) United Nations Millennium Declaration. United Nations, New York. Available from: http://www.un.org/millennium/declaration/ares552e.htm (last accessed 30 March 2016).

UNDG (2013) A Million Voices: The World We Want – A Sustainable Future with Dignity for All. United Nations Development Group, New York. Available from: http://www.undp.org/content/undp/en/home/librarypage/mdg/a-million-voices--the-world-we-want/ (last accessed 30 March 2016).

UNDP (2015a) Building the Post-2015 Development Agenda. United Nations Development Programme, New York. Available from: http://www.undp.org/content/undp/en/home/librarypage/mdg/building-the-post-2015-development-agenda/ (last accessed 30 March 2016).

UNDP (2015b) Sustainable Development Goal. Available from: http://www.undp.org/content/undp/en/home/mdgoverview/post-2015-development-agenda.html (last accessed 30 March 2016).

UNICEF (1989) The United Nations Convention on the Rights of the Child. United Nations International Children's Emergency Fund. Available from: http://www.unicef.org.uk/UNICEFs-Work/UN-Convention/ (last accessed 30 March 2016).

UNICEF (2009) The State of the World's Children 2009 Report. United Nations International Children's Emergency Fund. Available from: http://www.unicef.org/sowc09/ (last accessed 30 March 2016).

UNICEF (2015) Progress for Children: Beyond Averages: Learning From the MDGS. United Nations International Children's Emergency Fund. Available from: http://www.unicef.org/publications/index_82231.html# (last accessed 30 March 2016).

Unite (2009) Fall in Health Visitor Numbers is 'A National Scandal', Nursing Commission Told. Press Release.

Unite/CPHVA (2009) Regulatory Issues and the Future Legal Status of the Health Visitor Title and Profession. Unite/Community Practitioners' and Health Visitors' Association, London.

Verweij, M. & Dawson, A. (2009) The meaning of 'public' in 'public health'. In: Ethics, Prevention, and Public Health (eds A. Dawson and M. Verweij). Oxford University Press, Oxford.

Whitehead, M. & Dahlgren, G. (2006) Concepts and Principles for Tackling Social Inequities in Health: Levelling Up, Part 1. World Health Organization, Regional Office, Copenhagen. Available from: http://www.euro.who.int/en/health-topics/health-determinants/social-determinants/publications/2007/concepts-and-principles-for-tackling-social-inequalities-in-health (last accessed 30 March 2016).

WHO (1946) Constitution of the World Health Organization. New York, 22 July, 1946. World Health Organization, Geneva.

WHO (1986) Ottawa Charter for Health Promotion. World Health Organization, Geneva.

WHO (2011) Social Determinants of Health: Key Concepts. Commission on Social Determinants of Health, World Health Organization, Geneva. Available from: http://www.who.int/social_determinants/thecommission/finalreport/key_concepts/en/index.html (last accessed 30 March 2016).

Activities

Activity 2.1

Populations

What distinct populations might health visitors work with?

Activity 2.2

Health promotion

What do you consider are your underpinning values for health promotion?

Activity 2.3

Defining 'public health'

- How would you define public health?
- Have a discussion with your colleagues from other professional groups or agencies and ask them how they would define public health.
- Reflect on the value of this activity. Why might gaining different views be helpful?

Activity 2.4

Perspectives on public health

Consider the range of ideological perspectives outlined by Baggott (2011). Interpret and apply these ideologies to addressing the needs of children and families.

Activity 2.5

Relevance of the UNCRC to public health

Given that 'promoting and protecting human rights can be the most effective means to securing health', what relevance do each of the articles of the UNCRC (http://www.unicef.org/crc/files/Rights_overview.pdf) have for public health?

Activity 2.6

Reflection on the principles of health visiting

1. The search for health needs.
2. The stimulation of an awareness of health needs.
3. The influence on policies affecting health.
4. The facilitation of health-enhancing activities.

Think critically about the extent to which the principles of health visiting are embedded in local practice. What are the strengths, weaknesses, opportunities, and threats to fulfilling the principles in practice? How can you respond to these?

Activity 2.7

Reflection on experiences in childhood

Take some time to think of your own childhood experiences. How have they influenced your opportunities in life so far? How have they have impacted upon your health?

Activity 2.8

Tackling health inequalities

Familiarise yourself with any local strategies that contribute to tackling health inequalities. What added value can your public health role offer to these strategies?

Activity 2.9

Six High-Impact Areas

Familiarise yourself with the six high-impact areas on the eCommunity of Practice section of the iHV website (https://cophv.evidence-hub.net/ui/pages/login.php?ref=https%3A%2F%2Fcophv.evidence-hub.net%2F). Reflect on how your practice can adapt and develop in response to these.

3

The Community Dimension

Rosamund M. Bryar

City University London, London, UK

Introduction

Health visitors are fundamentally community public health workers – they work in communities, they work with communities, and they are part of communities. In 2004, the Nursing and Midwifery Council (NMC) opened the Specialist Community Public Health Nursing (SCPHN) Register, emphasising in its title and in the qualification both the *community* and the *public health* role of the practitioners – including health visitors – on that register. In Chapter 2, the case was made that in undertaking community work, health visitors are essentially working with individuals who are part of a community to address the health of that community (that community's public health) at the level of individual behaviour change. Draper *et al.* (2010) cite O'Dwyer *et al.*'s (2007) systematic review of area-based interventions and comment that the differentiation between these two approaches to working with communities is not often acknowledged:

> The distinction between community-based interventions (programmes that are based in communities, but focus on achieving change in individuals) and community-level interventions (programmes that seek to achieve change in a whole community via participation and other community wide changes) is also rarely made.
>
> (Draper *et al.*, 2010: 1104)

Hogg *et al.* (2013) discuss the tension in health visiting between the individual-level and community-level approaches to public health in a study of the views of parents and health visitors about parents' need for support in parenting. This distinction is further demonstrated in the model or 'family of community-centred approaches' (South, 2015a: 4) in guidance from Public Health England, which includes roles that develop individuals ('volunteer and peer roles') and processes that 'strengthen communities', including community development and social network approaches.

Health Visiting: Preparation for Practice, Fourth Edition.
Edited by Karen A. Luker, Gretl A. McHugh and Rosamund M. Bryar.
© 2017 John Wiley & Sons, Ltd. Published 2017 by John Wiley & Sons, Ltd.

Health visitors, in putting into practice the principles of health visiting (Cowley & Frost, 2006), are seeking through such work to influence community-level health (through both community-based and community-level interventions), wider public health policies, and the main determinants of health (Dahlgren & Whitehead, 1991; Morgan & Cragg, 2013).

In working with and in communities, health visitors are responding to the identification within the Declaration of Alma-Ata (Health for All by the Year 2000) (WHO/UNICEF, 1978), reiterated in *Primary Health Care – Now More Than Ever* (WHO, 2008) and in the Primary Health Care Performance Initiative (www.phcperformanceinitiative.org), of the importance of communities to the health of individuals, populations, and countries. The Health for All declaration identifies that communities should be involved in the development, provision, and monitoring of health services and sees health care as contributing to overall community development. This focus was reinforced in the primary health care reforms proposed by the World Health Organization (WHO) in 2008, which sought to move health systems towards health for all through making services more people-centred, promoting and protecting the health of the public, and improving health equity: 'reforms that secure healthier communities, by integrating public health actions with primary care and by pursuing healthy public policies across sectors ...' (WHO, 2008: xvi).

This focus on the development and involvement of communities was reinforced in 2015 by the adoption by the UN General Assembly of 17 sustainable development goals, to be achieved by 2030, which are concerned with five Ps: people, planet, prosperity, peace, and partnership. The UN is one form of community, bringing together 193 of the 196 countries in the world, and the 'world' community focus is evident in the resolution which records the adoption of the goals:

> All countries and all stakeholders, acting in collaborative partnership, will implement this plan. We are resolved to free the human race from the tyranny of poverty and want and to heal and secure our planet. We are determined to take the bold and transformative steps which are urgently needed to shift the world onto a sustainable and resilient path. As we embark on this collective journey, we pledge that no one will be left behind.
>
> (UN, 2015: 1)

The launch of these sustainable development goals was accompanied by the launch of the Primary Health Care Performance Initiative (phcperformanceinitiative .org), which identifies the value of interventions in communities through actions in primary health care, including, for example, improving equity in health and supporting people to become active decision makers with regard to their health – which is fundamental both to the sustainable development goals and to public health.

Lang & Rayner (2012: 4) support the need for the multisectoral approach evident in the UN and WHO documents: 'Today public health requires multilevel action, coordinated across not just the state but private spheres, commerce and civil society.' In the UK, the National Health Service (NHS) Five Year Forward View (NHS England, 2014a: 4) emphasises the need for integrated working and the importance of prevention and public health, proposing that 'the future health of millions of children, the sustainability of the NHS, and the economic prosperity of Britain now depend on a

radical upgrade in prevention and public health' (emphasis in original). Health visitors as front-line public health workers working with local communities are in a prime position to contribute to this urgent agenda.

The aim of this chapter is to examine the role of health visitors in communities, the value of community-level activities, and the skills needed to undertake this type of work. The focus will be on working with groups or populations within communities, while acknowledging that this may often be achieved through engagement with individuals. Many of the skills health visitors make use of in working with individuals, such as health promotion theories (Stockdale *et al.*, 2011; Cragg *et al.*, 2013), motivational interviewing (Miller & Rollnick, 2012), and nudge methods (see Chapter 2), are also utilised in working with communities.

Public health and communities

Chapter 2 provided a definition of public health and found it to be concerned with *improvement* in the health of populations: 'through *action* with populations that take account of the wider social determinants of health' (p. 60). The wider social determinants of health (Dahlgren & Whitehead, 1991; Morgan & Cragg, 2013) provide one of the many frameworks for considering public health practice. In this chapter, the underpinning approach taken is that of ecological public health proposed by Rayner & Lang (2012). This framework recognises the complex interrelationships between human beings and the world which impact on human (and world) health. Rachel Carson's (1962) famous *Silent Spring*, in which she discusses the impact of pesticides on the food chain, leading to the death of birds and the 'silent spring', illustrates this ecological approach to considering public health. Rayner & Lang (2012) identify four dimensions of existence which interrelate and contribute to prevention and public health:

- 'the *material*, which refers to the physical and energetic infrastructure of existence;
- the *biological*, which refers to the bio-physiological processes and elements, not just 'blood and bodies' but all that grows;
- the *cultural*, which refers to the importance of how people think and to the formation of collective consciousness;
- the *social*, by which we mean interactions between people, and their mutual engagement in collectivities, in the form of institutions through which societies operate.'

Rayner & Lang (2012: 315)

These four dimensions provide a focus for action by individuals, governments, communities, and public health practitioners, which Rayner & Lang (2012: 320–1) illustrate through an application to the obesity epidemic. Taking just the material dimension, local authorities can use planning laws to build physical activity into people's lives (e.g. by developing cycle paths); governments can pass laws which link food producers' profits to the production of healthier food ranges; and the public can seek to live more healthily by demanding increased access to public space and making use of play spaces for children in streets and parks (e.g. through schemes such as Play Streets) (Gill, 2015; Play England, 2015).

The ecological public health approach is based on the interaction between human health and the health of the environment – both local and global. The model also suggests, therefore, that the responsibility for improving the health of the public is multidimensional:

> The complexity and multiple interactions which Ecological Public Health assumes mean that no one or few institutions, bodies or professions can resolve public health problems on their own. Public health is inevitably about teams, about the collective of actors, not the intrinsic superiority of one profession.
>
> (Rayner & Lang, 2012: 314)

This framework emphasises the need for collective action to improve individual health and the health of communities. This is recognised as one of the key messages of Public Health England:

> local government and the NHS, together with the third sector, have vital roles to play in building confident and connected communities as part of efforts to improve health and reduce health inequalities
>
> (South, 2015a: 3)

Health visitors, with their unique access to all of the families within a community, therefore have a key role to play as part of the team of health and social care practitioners working with the community to improve health. In England, this role has been specified as occurring at the community level within the 2011 service model of health visiting (DH, 2011), but as illustrated in Box 3.1, health visitors need to make use of their community-work skills at all four levels of provision. Working with local communities, they can help to develop the community's skills and knowledge to address local health issues. Working with professional communities, such as midwives and social workers, in providing universal and universal plus services, they need to know and understand local services and have relationships with people within those services in order to make appropriate referrals.

Box 3.1 The new health visiting service: a partnership approach

- **Community:** Interactions at community level – **building capacity** and **using that capacity to improve health outcomes**; leading the Healthy Child Programme.
- **Universal:** Universal services for all families – **working with** midwives, **building strong relationships** in pregnancy and early weeks, and planning future contacts with families; leading the Healthy Child Programme for families with children under the age of 5.

- **Universal plus:** Additional services that any family may need some of the time, including providing care packages for maternal mental health, providing **parenting support**, and helping with baby/toddler sleep problems (where the health visitor **may provide, delegate, or refer**); **intervening early** to prevent problems developing or worsening.
- **Universal partnership plus:** Additional services for vulnerable families requiring **ongoing support** for a range of special needs (e.g. families at **social disadvantage**, families with a child with a disability, teenage mothers, and adults with mental health or substance misuse problems).

Making sure the appropriate health visiting services form part of the high-intensity multiagency services for families where there are safeguarding and child protection concerns.

(Adapted from: DH, 2011: 10)

Defining 'community'

The idea of community is central to the provision of health care, to public health, and to the description of social life in general, but there are very many different interpretations of what it denotes. Community is one of the traditional concepts in sociology, and Delanty (2003) argues that:

> The idea of community, which perhaps explains its enduring appeal, is related to the search for belonging in the insecure conditions of modernity. The popularity of community today can be seen as a response to the crisis in solidarity and belonging that has been exacerbated and at the same time induced by globalization.
>
> Delanty (2003: 1–2)

Activity 3.1 will help you explore your understanding of 'community'.

'Community' is a complex term, as captured in the definition used by the National Institute for Health and Care Excellence (NICE):

> A community is defined as a group of people who have common characteristics. Communities can be defined by location, race, ethnicity, age, occupation, a shared interest (such as using the same service) or affinity (such as religion and faith) or other common bonds. A community can also be defined as a group of individuals living within the same geographical location (such as a hostel, a street, a ward, town or region).
>
> (NICE, 2008: 38)

The word 'community' originates from the Latin *communis*, which can mean 'affable', 'collective', 'common', 'open', 'public', 'social', and 'universal' (www.wordhippo .com). In attempting to analyse the word further, Tonnies (published 1887; cited in

Harris, 2001) contrasted the concepts of *Gemeinschaft and Gesellschaft. Gemeinschaft* is described as the most basic form of human grouping, characterized by rich and satisfying relationships. *Gesellschaft*, on the other hand, describes those relationships which are essentially superficial and impersonal. The quality of relationships within a community is identified as a defining characteristic in a discussion of the term on the Resilience website (www.resilience.org), where the following definition is proposed: 'A community is a network of social and economic relationships and the places where those relationships interact'. This definition, in using the word 'places' rather than a defined geographical location as a characteristic of a community, allows for other types of locations of interaction, such as digital locations and Internet communities (e.g. Facebook, WhatsApp, the Health Visiting Community of Practice Evidence Hub). As McNaught (2009: 167) comments, 'What gives the notion of community its strengths is the self-perception and awareness of its members that they are a "community".'

Communities and theories about communities are not static (Crow, 2002). The changes that can occur in one community over time are made very clear by the case of the East End of London. In 1957, Young & Willmott (2007) published a classic study entitled *Family and Kinship in East London*, which showed the value of the strong relationships in that community in supporting its resilience. Almost 50 years on, a new study of the area, revealingly entitled *The New East End: Kinship, Race and Conflict* (Dench et al., 2006), found that the community had changed radically and that tensions between different groups characterised relationships in the area.

The various meanings and confusions surrounding the concept of 'community' occur because the word is used in both descriptive and evaluative terms. Just think of the many ways we use it: we talk of community nursing, community spirit, community policing, the European Community, community education, and so on. In addition, it often not only describes a range of features in social life but puts these features in a favourable perspective. As Hawtin & Percy-Smith (2007: 39) note, definitions of community 'are almost always positive, evoking feelings of warmth and closeness.' Unlike many other terms relating to social organization, such as 'state' or 'society', the term 'community' is seldom used in an unfavourable sense. However, as discussed in Chapter 2, considerable disparities and inequalities exist between and within communities, which have the potential to undermine a local community or wider society. Health inequalities, social disturbance (e.g. riots), and rapid changes in population composition suggest that the work of community building has the potential to impact on community health, social cohesion, and community capacity (Lawrence, 2008; Community Development Foundation, 2014).Health visitors work with a range of different communities, whether defined by location (e.g. a neighbourhood), by interest (e.g. new mothers), or by ethnicity (e.g. a Turkish women's group), and interface with others, such as those on the Internet (e.g. Netmums: www.netmums.com). From the preceding discussion, it can be seen that communities play a central part in people's lives, and it is therefore important to ask what impact they have on the health of individuals, families, and on the communities themselves.

Impact of communities on health

The experience of community has a significant impact on well being, physical and mental health, and inequalities in health. South (2015b: 32) summarises the evidence on the impact of community-centred approaches on health, identifying improvements in health literacy, increased social capital, increased civic engagement by community members, and – at the organisational level – outcomes including increased uptake of preventive services. Health visitors' work with local communities or neighbourhoods – including understanding, intervening in, and measuring the well being and health of these communities – contributes to the wider public health in an area.

If we focus on the neighbourhood, the usual workplace for health visitors, the Young Foundation suggests:

> Neighbourhoods are ultra-local communities of place. Most people feel they intuitively understand what they mean, in the shape of neighbourly interactions, mutual support, gathering places and a friendly, attractive environment – or a 'bad neighbourhood', danger, anti-social interaction, exclusiveness, isolation and dereliction.
> (Young Foundation, 2010: 9)

The Young Foundation (2010: 11) also mentions the rule of thumb of planners of new towns that 'the overall size of a neighbourhood should be dictated by "the maximum walking distance for a woman with a pram"'. The neighbourhood – or a group of neighbourhoods – forms the usual area of practice of the health visitor and health visiting team, although in many rural areas neighbourhoods may be spread over a large area.

The Young Foundation (2010) suggests that our understanding of neighbourhoods has three aspects (see Figure 3.1): the administrative wards or geographic boundaries of an area; our personal identification and mental map of our neighbourhood;

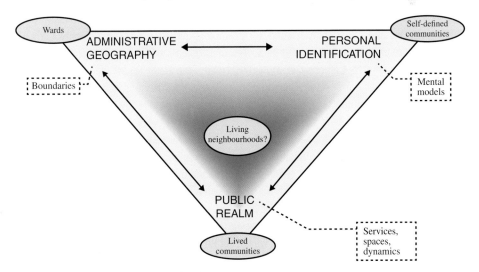

Figure 3.1 Elements of neighbourhoods.
Source: The Young Foundation (2010). Reproduced with permission of the Young Foundation.

and the public realm, including open spaces, services, schools, and community centres. The interaction of these three aspects provides a description and understanding of the experience of a neighbourhood. From a health visiting point of view, it also indicates the role that local public services, such as health visiting, play in the experience of the community and raises questions concerning joint working between different public services to support a positive neighbourhood experience.

An individual's experience of their neighbourhood includes feelings of mutual support and their relationships within the community, which help them cope with and enhance their health and the health of their families. These subjective elements go to make up what Moos (Kloos *et al.*, 2012) terms the 'social climate', which affects the quality of life of individuals and of the community. The social climate in a particular setting results from the interplay of three elements: relationships and the support experienced by community members; personal development and the extent to which individuals are supported to grow and develop skills in a particular environment; and system maintenance and change, in which emphasis is put on maintenance of order and behaviour in the setting. Moos (1976) suggests that environments have unique personalities, just as people do: some are supportive, some competitive. This approach, using the environmental-social, rather than the environmental-physical, emphasises impressionistic elements of description, which are, however, measurable using various measurement scales, including the Family Environment Scale (Moos, 2002), used recently in a study of the German application of the Family Nurse Partnership (FNP) model (Sierau *et al.*, 2015).

Historically, planners and policy makers have relied on objective measures of a community. They have measured such things as housing and unemployment, because it is argued that such factors influence people's lives. These types of measure are useful because they enable comparisons to be made between areas and groups and can be a guide to changing socioeconomic conditions. The question, however, remains as to the meaning of these statistics and their relationship to the subjective experience. We can, for example, measure the housing density, but what does that tell us about the pleasures or problems of living in a particular estate? According to Campbell *et al.* (1976), who were early researchers in the field of quality-of-life measures, the use of social indicators alone is not sufficient: in order to know the quality of life experiences, one must go directly to the individual for a description of what their life is like. In a review of quality-of-life measures, Bowling (2014) discusses these wider measures (with reference to Campbell *et al.*'s (1976) work), which take into account people's perceptions of the quality of their lives and the factors which matter to them and influence their feelings of well being. Krupat & Guild (1980) identified in their early research a number of factors which they suggest could be used to capture the social climate of a city or community. These factors can be seen now to inform the work being undertaken by the Office for National Statistics (ONS) to measure national well being: 'We must measure what matters – the key elements of national well-being. We want to develop measures based on what people tell us matters most' (ONS, 2015). Six factors which are meaningful to people and by which social climate can be described emerge in Krupat & Guild (1980)'s work:

1. *Warmth and closeness:* This first and most important factor contains items reflecting general feelings of security and support which an environment may provide, such as a relaxed atmosphere, a sense of intimacy, a safe, healthy, and peaceful place, and friendly people.

2. *Activity and entertainment:* This factor contains items such as activity, entertainment, diverse selection, dense population, and an atmosphere of culture. Density is seen as being related to the opportunity for activity and entertainment, and reflects positive aspects of urban life, rather than the isolation and anonymity that are often described.

3. *Alienation and isolation:* This factor contains items such as apathy, dirty surroundings, loneliness, distrust, confusion, and violence. It predominantly includes items referring to the characteristics of people, but it also refers to the physical condition of the environment, which is seen as something which fosters – or is a result of – a breakdown in interpersonal solidarity.

4. *Good life:* This factor contains items such as intellectual people, affluent people, liberal people, prestigious places, the valuing of old ways, and people who are interesting because they are not locals. It again refers to the characteristics of the people, and it may be seen as elitist. Different values will be important in different communities. Included here is the recognition of spatial mobility and innovation.

5. *Privacy:* This factor includes items such as gossip, intrusion, ignorance, and pettiness. It refers to a dimension of life involving privacy and carries a strong negative connotation, with the inclusion of items noting pettiness and ignorance on the part of people.

6. *Uncaring:* This factor includes items such as snobby people, a depressing environment, and insensitive people. It represents the uncaring aspects of social climate and includes aspects of people's behaviour and feelings about the overall social life.

It can be seen that the elements of the social climate of a community relate to the material, biological, cultural, and social framework discussed earlier (Rayner & Lang, 2012). These factors suggest areas which need to be addressed in developing the infrastructure of new communities. Current approaches to new developments aim to bring together those involved with the design of new houses and the physical environment of communities with members of the community and public health practitioners to build more healthy communities (Ross & Chang, 2012; House, 2015).

The level of support in a neighbourhood indicates the networks and relationships or social capital present there, which interact to reinforce a salutogenic approach to health and well being. Such relationships and networks enable people to manage and deal with the challenges in their lives, leading to the question – of great relevance to health visitors working with communities – posed by Antonovsky (1996):

> What can be done in this 'community' – factory, geographic community, age or ethnic or gender group, chronic or even acute hospital population, those who suffer from a particular disability, etc. – to strengthen the sense of comprehensibility, manageability and meaningfulness of the persons who constitute it?
>
> (Antonovsky, 1996: 16)

One response to this question can be seen in the launch of the Big Society by Prime Minister David Cameron in 2010, which aimed to 'give power back to the people, to involve us all in creating a fairer society' (Civil Exchange, 2015: 4). The Coalition Government's and the present Conservative Government's policies can be seen to be promoting the three key areas underpinning the notion of the Big Society: community empowerment, opening up public services, and social action. In relation to health visiting, the increase in the number of health visitors achieved under the Coalition Government (2010–May 2015), which now, arguably, enables health visitors to fulfil the community level of the Health Visitor Service Model (NHS England, 2014b), has the potential to contribute to both building community capacity (BCC) and community empowerment, and promoting the health of communities. The University of Kansas Group for Community Health and Development, as part of its role as a WHO Collaborating Centre, has produced a free Community Tool Box (University of Kansas, 2015) to support work to build healthy communities and contribute to social change, which health visitors should find very useful in working towards delivering the community element of health visiting practice.

Well-being extends the idea of social climate (Krupat & Guild, 1980) and has been described by Layard & Dunne (2009) (cited by Roberts et al., 2009) as resulting from the interaction of seven factors:

1. family relationships;
2. financial situation;
3. work;
4. community and friends;
5. health;
6. personal freedom;
7. personal values.

Individual, subjective well-being is therefore impacted by a person's health and feelings of being healthy. Mguni & Bacon (2010) define an individual's feeling of well-being as a combination of subjective well-being and community well-being:

> The focus of our work has been on individual 'subjective well-being', how people experience the quality of their lives, alongside community well-being – the extent to which local services and infrastructure has the capacity to support or reduce well-being. We see this as the most fundamental test of any area: does it provide its citizens with a good life?
>
> (Mguni & Bacon, 2010: 11)

These authors illustrate the relationship between community well-being and an individual's sense of well-being and health in a circular diagram (see Figure 3.2). When we consider the elements of this figure in relation to the discussion of the model of the main determinants of health (Dahlgren & Whitehead, 1991) in Chapter 2 (Figure 2.1), we can see how the experiences of individuals of, for example, poor access to quality education and thus a lack of job opportunities, interact to form a community with a reduced sense of wellness, a poorer sense of social capital (Gilchrist, 2007), and a greater need for inclusion in the Big Society (Mulgan, 2010).

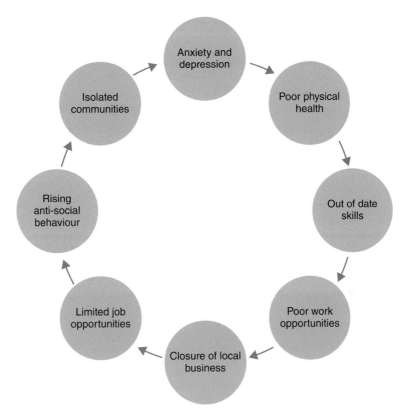

Figure 3.2 How local environments can interact with individual characteristics in harmful ways.
Source: Mguni & Bacon (2010). Reproduced with permission of the Young Foundation.

Communities living close together can have widely different health experiences. The iconic map of the London Underground system provides a graphic representation of the different levels of community health within one small geographic area. As shown in Figure 3.3, communities located along the Jubilee Line from affluent Westminster in the centre of London to the more deprived Canning Town experience a loss of 1 year in life expectancy for each stop you move further east.

Evidence of the impact of the different factors on health and the identification of the needs of a local community enable us to identify where interventions (e.g. through children's centres, parents' sense of well-being, social networks, and relationships) have the potential to change communities, people's experience of their neighbourhood, wellness, and health:

> Even when families live in poor housing with inadequate income and experience unemployment and multiple deprivations, finding ways to enhance adult well-being can have positive repercussions on the whole family, giving all its members a better chance of constructing a different kind of future.
>
> (Roberts *et al.*, 2009: 13)

Differences in Life Expectancy within a small area in London

Travelling east from Westminster, each tube stop represents nearly one year of life expectancy lost

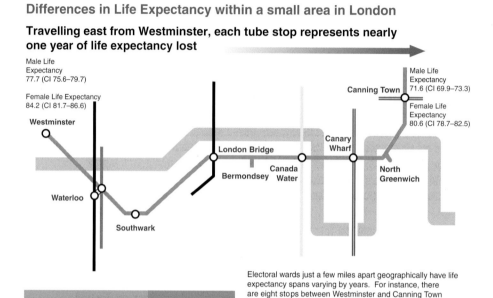

Male Life Expectancy
77.7 (CI 75.6–79.7)

Female Life Expectancy
84.2 (CI 81.7–86.6)

Westminster

Male Life Expectancy
71.6 (CI 69.9–73.3)

Canning Town

Female Life Expectancy
80.6 (CI 78.7–82.5)

Canary Wharf

London Bridge

Waterloo

Canada Water
Bermondsey

North Greenwich

Southwark

Electoral wards just a few miles apart geographically have life expectancy spans varying by years. For instance, there are eight stops between Westminster and Canning Town on the Jubilee Line – so as one travels east, each stop, on average, marks nearly a year of shortened lifespan.[1]

London Underground   Jubilee Line

[1] Source: Analysis by London Health Observatory using Office for National Statistics data. Diagram produced by Department of Health

Figure 3.3 Differences in life expectancy: taking the Jubilee Line route to health inequalities. Source: London Health Observatory (2007). Analysis by London Health Observatory using ONS data. Diagram produced by Department of Health. Available from: http://www.lho.org.uk/viewResource .aspx?id=12381 (last accessed 30 March 2016).

As long ago as 1971, Tudor Hart put forward the concept of the inverse care law: the availability of good medical (and nursing) care tends to vary inversely with the need for it in a given population (Tudor Hart, 1971; Watt, 2002). That is, people with greater health care needs have less access to good health care provision. One way to address this imbalance is through a reorientation of health care to an approach that is people-centred, includes a focus on health needs and enduring personal relationships, is comprehensive and continuous, takes responsibility for the health of the whole community across the life span, has responsibility for tackling the determinants of ill health, and integrates public health with primary care provision (Starfield 1996; WHO, 2008; Bryar *et al.*, 2012), and in which 'People are partners in managing their own health and that of their community' (WHO, 2008: 43). Public health practitioners, as part of health systems, therefore have a role to play in improving the health of communities. The next section will consider the role of the health visitor in this regard.

The role of health visitors in working with communities

There is a long history of community and public health work in health visiting. Since the establishment of health visiting in 1862, there has been an ongoing tension for health visitors and health visiting services between working at the community or public health level and working with individuals and families on a one-to-one basis (see Chapter 2). Craig (1995: 5), in *A Different Role: Health Visiting in a Community Project*, refers to both aspects in a description of the work of the first health visitor employed in Glasgow, who worked with the city's first woman doctor in the early 20th century 'to supervise the Milk Depot Scheme and undertake infant consultation sessions'. The tension between a public health/community focus and a focus on individuals is also reflected in public health policy: measures such as the ban on smoking in public places (Bauld, 2011) are aimed at changing the exposure of whole populations to tobacco smoke, while strategies such as Change4Life (http://www.nhs.uk/Change4Life/Pages/change-for-life.aspx) are aimed at changing individuals' health behaviours to improve both their own health and that of the whole population.

The public health role has long been included in courses for student health visitors. One of the functions of the health visitor identified in 1967 was in the 'Recognition and identification of need and mobilization of appropriate resources' (Council for the Education and Training of Health Visitors, 1967; cited in Robinson & Elkan, 1996: 4). Robinson & Elkan comment that 'The formalization of group and population-based health needs assessment (HNA) by nurses working in community settings can be traced from 1965, when a new syllabus of training for health visitors was introduced' (Council for the Education and Training of Health Visitors 1965; cited in Robinson & Elkan, 1996: 4). The increasing emphasis on the community role of the health visitor at this time is illustrated in the earlier editions of the present volume (Luker & Orr, 1992; Orr, 1992) and evident in the principles of health visiting first defined in 1977 (see Chapter 2, p. 63).

In the 1970s to 1980s, there was a resurgence of interest in the community role of health visitors, as Drennan (1988) notes in *Health Visitors and Groups: Politics and Practice*:

> While envisaging a role that responds to present-day society, health visitors have come to look increasingly to group and community work methods of practice, with their emphasis on consumer-expressed definitions of need. Health visitors are not alone in this change of emphasis. Increasingly, the philosophies of the provision of health care are now embracing the notion of partnership between the professional and individual and community at large. More emphasis has been given to client or community perceptions and definitions of need, participation in planning and active involvement in the provision and evaluation of care.
>
> (Drennan, 1998: 8)

As previously discussed, the philosophy of partnership identified by Drennan almost 30 years ago has been given a new impetus in the NHS Five Year Forward View (NHS England, 2014b). Examples of this type of work are provided by the Stockport Model of Health Visiting (Swann & Brocklehurst, 2004), which enabled and required health visitors to engage with the public health elements of the role; the multifaceted public health/community development activities in Glasgow (Craig, 1995; Craig & Lindsay, 2000); the community-development approach used in work in a community health house set up on a council estate in the Welsh Valleys (Bryar

& Fisk, 1994); and, more recently, the community projects initiated as part of the BCC developments (Pearson, 2013; McInnis *et al.*, 2015), which form part of the delivery of the community level of the Health Visiting Service Model (NHS England, 2014a).

During the 1990s and into the 21st century, the focus of health visiting work reverted to one on individuals away from work at the community/public health level. This reorientation resulted from a number of changes, including the NHS focus on targets, the influence of evidence-based documents (which raised questions concerning the efficacy of some of the screening work undertaken by health visitors; Hall & Elliman, 2006), and changes in the regulation of health visitors. The development of Sure Start/children's centres from the late 1990s further reduced the need for health visitors to lead or provide group- and community-level initiatives. The closure of the health visiting register by the NMC in 2002, which led to a reduction in the number of health visitors, further contributed to the decline. Given these pressures, managers of health visiting services required health visitors to prioritise work with individuals at the expense of community-focussed work. This dichotomy in provision has been perceived as a tension for many health visitors (Craig & Lindsay, 2000). Cameron & Christie (2007) interviewed health visitors in 2003, and one of the respondents, looking back over the previous 10 years of her practice (to 1993) in various parts of the UK, describes the lack of focus on community/public health work:

> My early experience of health visiting was mainly crisis visiting and coping with a very large 0–5 caseload, with lots of problems and public health was a very small component of the work and only in relation to core under 5 work. I can't remember doing any groups or development work.
>
> (Cameron & Christie, 2007: 84)

At the same time, work on setting competency standards for the wider public health workforce was taking place, supported by public health organisations including the Community Practitioners and Health Visitors Association (CPHVA). This resulted in the publication of a framework identifying the 10 key areas of public health practice – with associated competencies – that could be applied to all public health practitioners (see Chapter 2, Box 2.3). Activity 3.2 will help you explore the use of one of these elements of public health practice in your work with a community. This framework was applied to the education of SCPHNs, including health visitors, in the *Standards of Proficiency for Specialist Community Public Health Nurses* (NMC, 2004), which aligns the standards of proficiency for the 10 areas of public health practice to the four principles of health visiting (termed 'domains of practice' in the document). All 25 NMC standards, which guide learning at university and in practice, can be seen to relate to the development by health visitors of skills in promoting the health of communities. Table 3.1 provides examples of standards in relation to each of the domains of practice (principles of health visiting) and its associated principle (area of public health practice). (As noted in Chapter 2, the use of the terms 'principle' and 'domains' in the NMC document is both ambiguous and confusing.)

Table 3.1 Selected NMC standards of proficiency for health visiting that relate to working with communities.

Principle	Domain: Search for health needs
Surveillance and assessment of the population's health and well-being	• Collect and structure data and information on the health and well-being of a defined population • Develop and sustain relationships with groups and individuals with the aim of improving health and social well-being
Principle	**Domain: Stimulation of awareness of health needs**
Working with, and for, communities to improve health and well-being	• Communicate with individuals, groups, and communities about promoting their health and well-being • Raise awareness about the actions that groups and individuals can take to improve their health and social well-being
Principle	**Domain: Influence on policies affecting health**
Developing health programmes and services and reducing inequalities	• Work with others to plan, implement, and evaluate programmes and projects to improve health and well-being • Identify and evaluate service provision and support networks for individuals, families and groups in the local area
Principle	**Domain: Facilitation of health-enhancing activities**
Promoting and protecting the population's health and well-being	• Work in partnership with others to prevent the occurrence of needs and risks related to health and well-being • Work in partnership with others to protect the public's health and well-being from specific risks

Since the publication of the NMC standards in 2004, there have been several refinements of the public health framework. The first, the *Public Health Skills and Career Framework* (Public Health Resource Unit/Skills for Health, 2008), refined the 10 areas of public health practice into four core areas and, in addition, identified five defined areas of practice. In 2013, a further review refined the four core areas of practice and five defined areas (Public Health Online Resource for Careers, Skills and Training, 2013). The four core areas of practice for all public health practitioners are central to the work of health visitors and to working with communities (see Box 3.2).

> ### Box 3.2   Core areas of public health
>
> - Surveillance and assessment of the population's health and well-being.
> - Assessment of the evidence of the effectiveness of interventions, programmes, and services to improve population health and well-being.
> - Policy and strategy development and implementation for population health and well-being.
> - Leadership and collaborative working for population health and well-being.

However, as identified by Cameron & Christie (2007), the low priority that has been given to public health/community skills in recent years has led to many health visitors feeling daunted by the prospect of re-engaging in community-level work, as required by the health visiting service model (DH, 2011) and the commissioning framework in England (NHS England, 2014a), which identifies the remit of the health visiting service as:

> Leading, with local partners, in developing, empowering and sustaining families and communities' resilience to support the health and well-being of their 0–5 year olds by working with local communities and agencies to improve family and community capacity and champion health promotion and the reduction of health inequalities.
>
> (NHS England, 2014a: 12 para. 5.1)

This anxiety was recognised in the roll out of the Health Visitor Implementation Plan 2011–15 (DH, 2011) and led to the commissioning of the BCC module from a team headed by Professor Pauline Pearson of the University of Northumbria. This module provides a combination of online and work-based facilitation support for health visitors, allowing them to reinvigorate or develop new skills in community work by undertaking a community capacity-building project in their area of practice. It is available as an open access module on the e-Learning for Healthcare website (http://www.e-lfh.org.uk/programmes/building-community-capacity/). Through redevelopment of these skills, enabling health visitors to better connect with communities, it is anticipated that health outcomes for children and their families will be improved (Lynch et al., 2010; NICE, 2008). The BCC module is discussed further on p. 110. If health visitors are going to fulfil their role in working with communities and contributing to local Joint Strategic Needs Assessments (JSNAs) they need skills in learning about and working with communities. The next section discusses a range of ways in which they can develop such skills.

Gaining an understanding of the health of your local community

There are a range of approaches to gaining a picture of the health of your local community or neighbourhood. Knowing the local community is fundamental to working in an area, as Gilchrist (2007) notes:

> Learning about other people's cultures and histories is an important aspect of networking, enabling people to empathize with perspectives that are different from their own and to operate appropriately in different settings.
>
> (Gilchrist, 2007: 146)

This section outlines three approaches which help move from a general understanding of the needs of your community to a more detailed picture of the needs of a particular section of that community:

- windshield survey;
- public health walk;
- health needs assessment.

Windshield survey

The first activity a health visitor should undertake in a new area is to 'walk the patch' or drive around the area, undertaking a 'windshield survey' or 'walking survey'. The purpose of this is to gain information on the obvious characteristics of the area and so identify potential strengths and challenges (Brown & Collins, 2015). Hunt (2013: 142) provides an outline assessment tool for collecting information on the people, places, and social systems evident in the community by making use of 'the five senses and powers of observation'. Questions to ask while undertaking the survey include: Who are the people in the streets, parks, shops, and community centres? How are they dressed and what are they doing? What are the boundaries of the neighbourhood or area? What types of building are there, and how old are they? What condition are the houses in? Are there any open spaces, and if so, what are these used for? What types of shop are there? How many fast food outlets are there? What services are available? What health services are available? Is there a library, and if so, what types of health information does it provide? Are there any schools, religious buildings, or cinemas? (Hunt 2013: 142–3).

These questions suggest the need to consider carefully the main purpose of the survey, the area it will include, at what time of day to do it, and what the information gained will be used for – as discussed by Rabinowtiz (2015) in the University of Kansas Community Tool Box. Doing a windshield survey at different times of day or on different days will yield different information (e.g. a park might be used by older people on a health walk, younger people playing football, or pet owners exercising their dogs). Rabinowitiz (Rabinowtiz, 2015) provides detailed guidance on undertaking these surveys and the need to consider personal safety, but also suggests participation in community activities – go on the buses, shop in the shops, eat in the cafes, perhaps even walk around with a pram and experience the community from the perspective of a new mother.

Public health walk

A windshield survey may identify evidence of public health issues, such as local reservoirs linked to water supply, buildings which were once local hospitals, old

Table 3.2 A public health walk in Tower Hamlets, London.

Evidence in the community	Relevance
The (former) Women's Library (now part of London Metropolitan University)	Previously the local wash house
Tall Georgian houses with large windows on the top floor	Homes of the Huguenot weavers, providing light for their work – evidence of immigration
A mosque	Previously a synagogue – evidence of immigration
Signs on a building indicating a soup kitchen for Jewish immigrants	Immigration; poverty; community support

industrial waste indicating possible health risks or unemployment, the use made of parks, the number of fast food outlets in the area, children's centres, and the number of people in a shopping centre during the day. Identification of these elements can help in understanding the health issues impacting on the current population, as well as some of the attitudes of local people to health care provision.

Once these public health aspects have been identified, they can be examined in more depth through an exploration of the history of the area, examining the local public health reports, reading novels and other books about the area, and talking to local practitioners and residents. This exploration will provide information of help in understanding the relevance and impact of the different public health features identified, which can then be woven together to form a walk tracing the public health history of the area. In East London, one such walk has been developed by the lecturer and historian John Eversley, which provides an introduction for student health visitors to the public health history of part of the borough of Tower Hamlets. Some of the elements included in this walk are shown in Table 3.2. Activity 3.3 will help you construct your own public health walk.

Health needs assessment

An HNA involves the collection and analysis of information of relevance to the health of a particular population. The Health Development Agency (HDA) defines HNA as:

> a systematic method for reviewing the health issues facing a population, leading to agreed priorities and resource allocation that will improve health and reduce inequalities.
>
> (HDA, 2004a: 3)

HNA is therefore vital in terms of the commissioning of services and of supporting the direction of the activities of a particular health visiting team. This definition is expanded by the HDA to identify the key elements of HNA:

> HNA is an approach that reviews systematically the health issues facing a given population. The starting point in HNA is a defined **population**. Health issues selected as priorities will usually be those that can help reduce **health inequalities**. The **primary outputs** are a **set of recommendations, an action strategy** based on the evidence gathered about that population, and the **identification of effective and acceptable interventions**. These should be used to **influence policies and service delivery** in order to **improve health outcomes** (highlight added, apart from 'population'; bold in original)
>
> (HDA, 2004b: 5)

It can be seen from this description that HNA involves the identification of a need, plans to address that need, and evaluation of the impact of the interventions put in place to meet the need. Hooper & Longworth (2002: 9) state that there are three underpinning principles to HNA: improvement, integration, and involvement.

1. *Improvement* of health and inequalities by making changes that improve the most significant conditions or factors affecting health ...
2. *Integration* of this improvement in health into the planning processes ...
3. *Involvement* of:
   - people who know about the health issues in a community
   - people who care about those issues
   - people who can make changes happen.

These definitions focus on the identification of needs. Stewart *et al.* (2009: 133) stress the importance of identifying health assets alongside needs: 'The purpose of health needs assessment (HNA) is to identify the health assets and needs of a given population to inform decisions about service delivery to improve health and reduce health inequalities'.

Understanding need

Before examining the process of HNA, it is important to consider our understanding of need. Stewart *et al.* (2009) discuss a number of approaches, including Maslow's hierarchy of needs (Maslow, 1954). Maslow identifies need from the perspective of the individual, ranging from the fulfilment of basic physiological needs through to self-actualisation (the individual's fulfilment of their own potential). This approach may be contrasted with that of Bradshaw (1972, 1994), who categorises need from 'the perspective of the person or organisation identifying the need' (Stewart *et al.*, 2009: 136). Although Bradshaw first proposed his taxonomy many years ago, Scriven (2010) notes that it is still of great use in distinguishing levels of need. Bradshaw's fourfold classification is based on the derivation of the criteria adopted to recognize need, be they diagnostic or prescriptive. He identifies four types of need:

1. normative needs;
2. felt needs;
3. expressed needs;
4. comparative needs.

Normative needs

Normative needs are defined in accordance with some agreed standard. A desirable standard is laid down by an expert or professional and is compared with a standard which already exists. If an individual or group falls short of the desirable standard, they are identified as being in need. A normative definition of need is by no means absolute. It may not correspond with other definitions, and, of course, different experts may have conflicting standards. It is relatively easy to lay down standards for housing – where, for example, inside plumbing and electricity may be accepted as two standards of adequate housing – but it is more difficult to set standards in less tangible areas such as health without becoming involved in making value judgments. Thus, normative definitions of need may differ according to the value judgments of different experts. Furthermore, the idea of normative need demonstrates a particular view of service delivery, in that it places the expert or professional at the centre of needs assessment.

Felt needs

A felt need is a need expressed by an individual or community. It is termed a 'want'. Felt need alone may be an incomplete measure because it is limited by the perceptions and knowledge of the individual or community, who may express a desire for a service without needing it, fail to recognize their own need, or assume that no acceptable solution exists.

Expressed needs

Expressed need, or 'demand', is a felt need turned into action. Under this definition, total need is defined as 'those people who demand a service'. Commercial weight-management classes provide an example of a response by industry to an expressed need (Scriven, 2010). Expressed need alone is an unsatisfactory measure, however, because some people will not turn felt need into demand or, again, will not recognize their own need. Waiting lists are an insufficient measure of unmet need, for example, as some people will be pre-symptomatic. Other forms of information are also needed; for example, any self-help groups in an area or any demand for well women clinics or parenting information for fathers may be seen as examples of expressed need.

Comparative needs

Comparative needs are the imputed needs of an individual or group not in receipt of services but similar in relevant characteristics to others receiving such services. For example, if a person receives a service because they have particular characteristics and another person with those characteristics is not receiving that service, then we can say that the second person has a comparative need. Note, however, that provision may not correspond with need: even if area A is receiving more resources than area B, area A may still be in need.

Using the Bradshaw taxonomy, we can consider the interrelations between these four definitions of need. For example, taking the example of fluoridation of water supplies, this need was accepted by public health experts (i.e. was a normative need) long before it was felt, demanded, or supplied. The application of Bradshaw's taxonomy raises many issues for practice, not the least of which is the lack of clarity about what health visitors should determine to be a normative need and what criteria we should use in comparing provision in our area with what is available in other parts of the district or country. As Naidoo & Wills (2016: 273) conclude, 'needs are not objective and observable entities to which we must just match our interventions. The concept of need is a relative one, and is influenced by values and attitudes and by other agendas.' Such other agendas will, of course, also include access to resources and finance that can support services aimed at meeting the identified needs of the community. The process of HNA, in partnership with community members and public health colleagues, and with reference to evidence such as that provided by Marmot *et al.* (2010), is one way of seeking to address these dilemmas.

Steps to undertaking HNA

The HDA (which was joined with the National Institute for Clinical Excellence, forming the National Institute for Health and Clinical Excellence in 2005, now the National Institute for Health and Care Excellence (NICE)) has produced a guide (HDA, 2004a) and workbook (Hooper & Longworth, 2002) to support people in undertaking HNAs. A five-step process is provided in Table 3.3, and Activity 3.4 will help you to use these steps in undertaking an HNA in your locality.

An HNA may be undertaken by a range of different people, but involvement across different services and disciplines will enable collection and sharing of a wide range of information and will ensure that those participating are ready to be involved in the planning and implementation of change. Hooper & Longworth (2002) suggest that some or all of the following might be involved in an HNA: members of the community affected by the issue; community leaders; religious leaders; shop owners; teachers and social workers; police, probation, and community safety officers; GPs and members of the primary care team; local authority staff and elected members; service commissioners; and members of community organisations (e.g. allotment associations). They also suggest that the following questions will be helpful in deciding who should be involved in the HNA:

- Who *knows* about the issue?
- Who *cares* about the issue?
- Who can *make change happen related* to the issue?

(Hooper & Longworth, 2002: 29)

An HNA may therefore be undertaken by such a cross-community team, or else a health visiting team may undertake an HNA of an area of its practice population to help plan the types of service it will provide and engage with members of the wider community as part of this. An HNA can cover a whole population (e.g. a neighbourhood) or be focused on a particular part (e.g. families with children over the age of 2). Such groups may or may not identify themselves as a community (refer back to Figure 3.1 in thinking about communities of interest). Once the focus of the HNA has been decided, the team undertaking it must develop a realistic time plan.

A major part of an HNA is the collection of information of relevance to the health needs of the population under study. This information will be both quantitative

Table 3.3 Steps in undertaking a health needs assessment (HNA).

Steps	Activities
Step 1: Getting started	What population? What are you trying to achieve? Who needs to be involved? What resources are required? What are the risks?
Step 2: Identifying health priorities	Population profiling Gathering data Perceptions of needs Identifying and assessing health conditions and determinant factors
Step 3: Assessing a health priority for action	Choosing health conditions and determinant factors with the most significant size and severity impact Determine effective and acceptable interventions and actions
Step 4: Planning for change	Clarifying aims of intervention Action planning Monitoring and evaluation strategy Risk-management strategy
Step 5: Moving on/review	Learning from the project Measuring the impact Choosing the next priority

Source: HDA (2004a: 2).

and qualitative. It will involve accessing information from local, national, and international sources and undertaking local forms of qualitative data collection, which might include interviews, focus groups, and observation of the use of services or spaces. Sources of information are shown in Table 3.4, while methods of identifying information with the local community are shown in Table 3.5 (other sources are provided in Chapter 7).

The information collected through these various methods may then be used to identify the extent of a health need in a particular population, the attitudes of people to that need, and the ability of the population to respond to the need. The health profiles on the Association of Public Health Observatories website will make a good starting point for identifying the health priorities in your area. Table 3.6 provides information from the health profiles of two contrasting areas of England, demonstrating the different focuses of health visiting intervention between them. Activity 3.5 will help you explore the information in the health profile relevant to your area.

Table 3.4 Examples of sources of quantitative information on the health of a population.

SourceTypes of information	
The local public health report (e.g. https://www.croydon.gov.uk/sites/default/files/articles/downloads/Annual%20Public%20Health%20Report%20for%202015.pdf)	Local health needs and current priorities
The local commissioning plan (e.g. https://www.northsomersetccg.nhs.uk/media/medialibrary/2014/07/North_Somerset_CCG_Five_Year_Strategic_Plan.pdf)	Plan of action across local organisations to meet health and social needs
Association of Public Health Observatories, www.apho.org.uk	• Health profiles • Health impact assessment reports • Marmot indicators for local authorities in England • APHO Tools Directory and Guide to Key Data Sources

UK National Statistics, www.gov.uk/government/statistics	• Census information
	• Theme areas, including:
	  ○ children, education, and skills
	  ○ health and social care
	  ○ people and places

NHS Evidence, www.evidence.nhs.uk	• Clinical and nonclinical evidence • Local, regional, national, and international evidence • Government policy Used to support high-quality health care
NICE, www.nice.org.uk	• Clinical and cost-effectiveness guidance • Appraisals of evidence • Tools to support implementation of evidence into practice
Child and Maternal Health Observatory, www.chimat.org.uk	• Child health profiles • Information relating to the health of children and young people and to maternal health • Tools to support needs assessment

(Continued)

Table 3.4 (Continued)

SourceTypes of information	
Birth cohort studies – Centre for Longitudinal Studies, www.cls.ioe .ac.uk	• Evidence of the impact of determinants of health on the development and progress of children
PEGASUS (Professional Education for Genetic Assessment and Screening), http://cpd.screening.nhs .uk/pegasus	• Antenatal and newborn screening statistics for local areas • Educational resources for health practitioners
Marmot Review, http://www .instituteofhealthequity.org	• Marmot Report (2010) • Updated inequalities data • Evidence of initiatives to address inequalities in health
Joseph Rowntree Foundation, http:// www.jrf.org.uk	• Social policy research concerned with poverty, inequalities, community development, and empowerment
World Health Organisation, www.who.int	• World health statistics • World guidelines • Annual world health report
Public Health England, http://www .gov.uk/government/organisations/ public-health-england	• Statistics • Guidance • Current public health issues
Public Health Wales, http://www .wales.nhs.uk/sitesplus/888/home	• Data and statistics • Guidance • Current public health issues

Organisations use a range of other approaches to identify needs, and the reports and strategies produced by local authorities and others as part of these processes provide valuable information about health needs in different areas. A health impact assessment: 'enables the identification, prediction and evaluation of likely changes to health, both now and in the future, as a consequence of a policy programme or plan.' (Naidoo & Wills, 2016: 187). It may be used to measure the impact of both health-related policies and of other strategies which are not directly related to health but have consequences for it (Lock, 2000) (see Table 3.6). Health equity audits are another way in which the health of populations can be assessed, usually by organisations such as health trusts or local authorities. Health equity is different to health inequality but may contribute to it: 'health equity describes *differences in opportunity* for different population groups which result in different life chances,

Table 3.5 Examples of sources of qualitative information on the health of a population.

Methods of gathering local information
Observation of the use of facilities and services in the local community
Interviews with users of facilities and services
Interviews with key informants (e.g. informal group leaders, shopkeepers, religious leaders)
Public meetings and forums
Focus groups
Using local media, including radio phone-ins
Reviewing local newspaper content
Using Internet sites (e.g. a local community site, Facebook or Twitter groups)
Community health panels and citizens' juries
Research techniques, including structured observation, rapid appraisal, and ethnographic studies

Source: Naidoo & Wills (2009: 264).

Table 3.6 Comparison of health profile information.

Kingston-upon-Hull Health profile information, June 2015	Surrey Health profile information, June 2015
The health of people in Hull is generally worse than the average for England	The health of people in Surrey is generally better than the England average
Life expectancy is 12.1 years lower for men and 8.2 years lower for women in the most deprived areas compared to the least deprived	Levels of deprivation are low and life expectancy is higher than average
Early deaths from cancer, heart disease, and stroke and deaths from smoking are all worse than the England average	Obesity in children (age 6) is below the England average
In Hull, *breastfeeding initiation, smoking at time of delivery and teenage pregnancy are all worse than the England averages.* However, the percentage of obese children (age 6) is close to the England average	For all but 2 of the 32 indicators (*road traffic accidents and malignant melanoma*), health in Surrey is better than the England average

Source: http://www.apho.org.uk/default.aspx?QN=HP_FINDSEARCH2012 (last accessed 30 March 2016).

access to health services ...', which can lead to health inequalities (Hamer *et al.*, 2003: 11). Hamer *et al.* (2003: 11) describe a health equity audit as focusing on '*how fairly resources are distributed in relation to the health needs of different groups. (This may include resources such as services, facilities, and the determinants of health like employment and education.)*'

Local authorities and local health commissioners were required under the Local Government and Public Involvement in Health Act 2007 to undertake a JSNA to identify the health and well-being needs of their local population and draw up plans to address them (DH, 2007). The Health and Social Care Act 2012 revised the requirement for the production of local JSNAs and associated Joint Health and Wellbeing Strategies (JHWSs) through health and wellbeing boards, led by the local authority and the local clinical commissioning groups (DH, 2013; NICE, 2014). JHWSs provide the means to address the needs identified through the JSNA process and guide commissioning of services. In England, the commissioning of services is led by clinical commissioning groups, which produce commissioning plans stating how local services will respond to identified needs (http://www.wellards.co.uk/papers/courses/diplomas_comms2014_TIER2/what_are_comm_plans2.html). Health visitors have responsibilities identified in the Health Visiting Service Specification (NHS England, 2014b) to contribute to the development of the JSNA and to the delivery of JHWSs. In relation to their role at the community level, they should be:

> Providing and developing intelligence about communities' assets in partnership with communities to support the health and well-being of 0–5 year olds, to inform the Joint Strategic Needs Assessment (JSNA)
>
> (NHS England, 2014b: 13, 5.7.1)

Once evidence of the extent of health needs has been compiled, the HNA process moves on to the development of interventions and the creation of an action plan to address the health needs in the local commissioning plans (see Table 3.4). Discussion of the utilisation and evaluation of the BCC approach by health visitors will help demonstrate how health visitors and health visiting services can develop and implement these skills.

Building community capacity

As previously discussed, recognition of the need to refresh and extend health visitors' skills in working with communities led to the commissioning by the Department of Health of the BCC module developed by the University of Northumbria (Pearson, 2013). Some universities have also developed their own modules and learning resources (e.g. Sheffield Hallam University), while others have incorporated the e-learning module into their SCPHN programmes (e.g. University of West of England). A wide range of resources are now available to support health visitors in working with communities. Some have been specifically written for health visitors, including *Building Community Capacity (BCC): An Introductory Toolkit for Health Visitors* (Kenyon, 2015), while others are aimed at a wider audience, such as the guidance produced by the Scottish Community Development Centre for Learning Connections (2007) and the online Community Tool Box (University of Kansas, 2015) produced by the Work Group for Community Health and Development, University of Kansas, a WHO Collaborating Centre, as a worldwide free resource (see Box 3.3).

Box 3.3   Community Tool Box resources, University of Kansas (http://ctb.ku.edu/en)

Overview An overview of the Community Tool Box and frameworks for guiding, supporting and evaluating the work of community and system change.

Community assessment Information about how to assess community needs and resources, get issues on the public agenda, and choose relevant strategies.

Communications to promote interest and participation Communications that promote interest and encourage involvement.

Developing a strategic plan and organizational structure Information about developing a strategic plan and organizational structure, recruiting and training staff and volunteers, and providing technical assistance.

Leadership and management Information about the core functions of leadership, management, and group facilitation.

Analyzing community problems and designing and adapting community interventions Information about analyzing community problems to design, choose, and adapt interventions for different cultures and communities.

Implementing promising community interventions Information on illustrative interventions using various strategies for change.

Cultural competence and spirituality in community building Information on understanding culture and diversity, how to strengthen multicultural collaboration, and spirituality and community building.

Organizing for effective advocacy Information on advocacy principles, advocacy research, providing education, direct action campaigns, media advocacy, and responding to opposition.

Evaluating community programs and initiatives Information on developing a plan for evaluation, evaluation methods, and using evaluation to understand and improve the initiative.

Maintaining quality and rewarding accomplishments Information on achieving and maintaining quality performance, public reporting, providing incentives, and honoring colleagues and community champions.

Generating, managing, and sustaining financial resources Information on writing grants, preparing an annual budget, and planning for financial sustainability.

Social marketing and institutionalization of the initiative Information on conducting a social marketing effort (promoting awareness, interest, and behavior change), and planning for long-term sustainability.

The authors of the guidance produced by the Scottish Community Development Centre for Learning Connections (2007) make the important point that community capacity building is not the same as community development or community engagement, both of which may be longer-term outcomes of community capacity building. This organisation makes use of the following definition of community capacity building:

> Activities, resources and support that strengthen the skills, abilities and confidence of people and community groups to take effective action and leading roles in the development of communities.
>
> (Skinner, 2006; cited in Scottish Community Development Centre for Learning Connections, 2007: 3)

It emphasises the need to take a strengths-based approach to community capacity building and makes the point that 'Community capacity building should be complemented by parallel work to enhance the skills of public bodies in their partnerships and programmes with communities.' (Scottish Community Development Centre for Learning Connections, 2007: 3). The work on BCC in health visiting can be seen as responding to this skills deficit and as a first step in the process of health visitors' full engagement with communities.

The BCC module (available from http://www.e-lfh.org.uk/programmes/building-community-capacity/learning-zone/) is an open-access online module which aims to 'help you to refresh and extend your knowledge and skills in relation to particular aspects of building community capacity and enabling people to identify and address their health needs' (University of Northumbria, 2013). Resources and master classes are available online and include material on policy issues, service improvement, community development, and behavioural approaches. Those following the module are asked to complete the online work and undertake a community engagement project within 6 months. There is the option to gain masters level credits for the module. Organisational support and access to a workplace advisor are required to facilitate the translation of learning to practice and completion of the community project. The impact of the module in developing community initiatives has been reported through a number of publications and conferences. In Dorset, projects have been reported relating to provision of information on when to attend A&E with a child, strengthening the parent role as the primary educator, and working with parents to better manage their family finances, amongst others (Dorset Healthcare NHS, 2013). A report on a number of projects in the East of England (Health Education East of England, 2014) highlights the role that health visitors can play in identifying needs and working with others to establish projects (e.g. to address social isolation amongst parents). This report shows that some projects become embedded in a community, with group members taking on the task of running them, but that in other cases additional resources or engagement with the wider health and social care system are needed in order for the project to succeed. In the North West of England, a large number of projects have been initiated by health visitors and student health visitors who have undertaken the BCC module, including projects supporting parents to develop parenting skills, to participate in exercise, and to provide peer support. A presentation at a conference in Manchester in 2015 on projects undertaken in the North West of England showed that successful achievement is dependent on a range of factors, which Pearson (2013) identified from a review of BCC projects. Support from local organisational leaders, involvement of the local Higher Education Institution (HEI), alignment to the local JSNA, and team working were all found to contribute to success, while high workload and lack of access to resources had a negative impact. Pearson (2013: 708) concludes her review by asking, 'where or for whom is this building capacity, and what difference is it making to health and well-being in the local community?' McInnis *et al.* (2015: 22), in a review of the uptake of the BCC module in the North West of England, provide a useful flow diagram, which in part responds to Pearson's questions. This diagram indicates that undertaking the BCC module is the first step in helping health visitors work more effectively with communities. With the additional skills they acquire, they can identify local needs, develop joint initiatives, and ultimately act as a resource to a community or community group that is implementing initiatives. The impact on community health of these initiatives will become evident further down the line. The authors of the report identify a range of recommendations and emphasise the need for managerial support to enable staff to access BCC education and put their new skills into practice: 'Organisations should ensure clear communication strategies are in place to enable accurate information sharing about BCC opportunities, planning and growth and to embed community capacity as a service priority' (McInnis *et al.*, 2015: 27). The value of BCC, the Introductory Toolkit (Kenyon, 2015), and other resources is that they help health visitors develop those skills needed to deliver at the community level, as Kenyon (2015: 4) notes: 'Building Community Capacity is not an "add on" activity that can be carried out when time permits, rather it is part of the core programme as it has the potential to reduce health inequalities and promote sustainable health and well-being.' South (2015b: 36) reinforces the view that developing community health is a process which starts with identification of community strengths and needs, and goes on to make use of community-centred approaches in order to increase equity, community control, voice, and connectedness and so achieve individual health and well being, strong connected communities, and vibrant civil societies. These aims are ambitious, and building the capacity of health visitors to engage with communities is a step towards achieving them.

Using health promotion models to support community working

There are a range of health promotion models that may be applicable to work with communities (Tones & Tilford, 2001; Cragg *et al.*, 2013; Naidoo & Wills, 2016). Health promotion is concerned with change in populations and communities. Skovdal (2013) outlines four concepts which underpin it: critical consciousness, derived from the work of Freire (1973); community participation; social capital; and health assets. The focus in the present chapter has been on supporting community participation, enabling the development of social capital and health assets through awareness raising amongst health visitors and the communities with which they work. Beattie's

(2003) model has a particular focus on community development as one aspect of the collective focus of an intervention. It describes health promotion interventions as being top-down or bottom-up and as focusing on the community or on the individual. Where the focus is on the community and a bottom-up approach is taken, community development activity will be supported. Naidoo & Wills (2009) identify the characteristics of community development based on Beattie's model as follows:

- To *enfranchise* or *emancipate* groups or communities so they recognize what they have in common and how social factors influence their lives
- Practitioner is the role of 'advocate'
- Radical political ideology
- Activities include community development and action

(Naidoo & Wills, 2016: 84, Fig. 5.2)

The health visitor using this model is working in partnership with community members, supporting them, acting as an advocate on their behalf, and facilitating their empowerment. Working with communities in these ways helps identify needs that are important to people, as opposed to needs identified by policy makers (normative needs). For example, a qualitative interview study of residents in parts of London found that they expressed great concern about dog fouling in their neighbourhoods and that this concern was related to their feelings of social and environmental neglect (Derges *et al.*, 2012). The researchers suggest that the issue of 'dog poo' cannot be addressed simply through environmental clean up but that it acts as a metaphor for a wider discontent, which might better be addressed through community engagement activities.

An important part of the process of working with communities is strengthening networks and the relationships between networks to enhance social capital. Gilchrist (2007) discusses the literature demonstrating the importance of networks in providing support for health improvement and the resilience of a community:

> While the physiological mechanisms for this resilience are unclear, it is probable that social networks provide a variety of forms of support and affirmation, including practical advice around health matters.
>
> (Gilchrist, 2007: 142)

The work of the health visitor interfaces with very many people and organisations, and this gives her or him the ability to provide a means of bridging and strengthening informal networks, as well as professional and statutory network links. In her PhD study, Joly (2009; Joly *et al.*, 2011) demonstrates the existence of multiple overlapping and separate networks concerned with the care of people who are homeless. The mapping of networks provides a means to locate gaps and communication problems between organisations working with the same community, and thus a means of resolving these issues.

Identification of networks and work to strengthen networks is essentially concerned with taking a strength-based/assets approach to practice. One such approach is that of appreciative inquiry, which is based on the 4-D model: discovery (the best of what is or has been), dreaming (what might be), designing (what should be), and destiny (what will be) (Reed, 2007; Radford, 2009). Using an appreciative inquiry approach requires participants to identify what has worked in the past and to draw on that experience to design solutions that address current needs. Whittaker *et al.* (2013) used appreciative inquiry as part of a study of recruitment and retention in health visiting, asking participants to bring to workshops an example of when they felt happiest working as a health visitor. The discussions identified the key motivator to be 'making a difference to children and families' (Whittaker *et al.*, 2013: 54), and this can be used to design strategies that might support health visitors to experience this positive aspect of work more often, thus facilitating recruitment and retention.

Another approach to the identification of strengths and challenges is participatory appraisal (PA), which makes use of visual and other tools. Pearson (2003) comments that PA focuses on community-level health and is an ideal approach for community-based practitioners, such as health visitors:

> PA takes a whole community approach to development rather than focusing on individuals, or individual groups of people in isolation. This has the effect of looking for rich, deep and broad community explanations for issues that would be missed if a narrower approach were used. Community practitioners who know and are part of communities are well placed to be involved in PA as facilitators, participants and users.
>
> (Pearson, 2003: 176)

Participatory Appraisal enables participation by people whose voices may not usually be heard. For example, in using PA in a rural community in Mexico, the voices of children and women were captured in the various activities used to collect information about community needs (Torres & Carte, 2013). Participatory approaches are essentially about trying to address the power differentials between those with power (e.g. governments, organisations, professions) and those without (e.g. marginalised communities, individuals experiencing abuse) (Laverack, 2015). As Green *et al.* (2014) note, community members should be involved in designing the tools used to collect information, and the range of tools that can be used – from social mapping to photography – is only limited by the imagination of those involved in the process.

The approaches discussed in this section may be helpful in engaging communities – particularly those that have long been disenfranchised. The term 'participation' has many different meanings, and efforts to engage people to participate may be met with both enthusiasm and resistance. Arnstein (1969) was the first to outline a ladder of the different levels of community participation:

8 citizen control;
7 delegated power;
6 partnership;
5 placation;
4 consultation;
3 informing;
2 therapy;
1 manipulation.

(Naidoo & Wills, 2009: 16)

This ladder helps to demonstrate the limits of the transfer of power at the different levels of participation, and Arnstein:

ranks the different degrees of citizen participation starting at the lowest rung of manipulation and ascending upwards to the highest level of participation, citizen control in which power is directly transferred from government to people

(Draper *et al.*, 2010: 1103)

The application of this ladder to work with communities or to the health visitor's experience in her or his team or work setting assists in the identification of barriers to the development of participant engagement in activities. As will be apparent, participation is a complicated concept, and the process of encouraging participation may be used by organisations to achieve different ends. The title of a book by Cooke & Kothari (2001), *Participation: The New Tyranny?*, suggests the complexity of this process and the need to appreciate the power dynamics and purposes behind community participation activities (Powell & Geoghegan, 2004). South (2015b) suggests that understanding where power lies and the purpose of participation is helpful for both practitioners and communities in managing expectations of the involvement process.

Another challenge in working with communities is how to measure both the process and the outcomes of community-based work (see Chapter 7). Rifkin (2014) concludes in an updated literature review that community participation should be viewed as a process factor supporting the implementation of initiatives to achieve service outcomes, such as improved birth outcomes. To gain an understanding of the level of participation of communities in health initiatives, Rifkin (1985) developed a measurement approach which examines participation on a continuum from narrow to wide (Draper *et al.*, 2010). Five features which impact on participation by community members were identified from a systematic review: needs assessment, leadership, organisation, resource allocation, and management. These are represented in Figure 3.4. By linking the scores for the five areas, a spidergram is produced showing the strength or weakness of each feature in a particular project (see Figure 3.5). This approach has been widely used in community health projects, some of which modify the elements that form the spidergram (e.g. in community-based child survival programmes in low-income countries (Draper *et al.*, 2010) or in a health planning project in Ghana (Baatiema *et al.*, 2013)).

Summary

This chapter has considered some of the issues that need to be addressed by the health visitor and the health visiting team when working at the community level to support and enhance the experience of community health. Health has been considered in the context of ecological public health, highlighting the connections between material, biological, cultural, and social factors. Following an exploration of the meaning of community and the impact of community on health, we considered the role of the health visitor and the skills and competencies needed to deliver health visiting at the

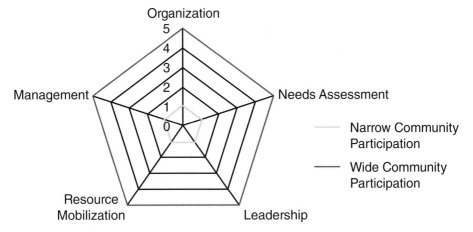

Figure 3.4 Spidergram measuring community participation.
Source: Baatiema *et al.* (2013).

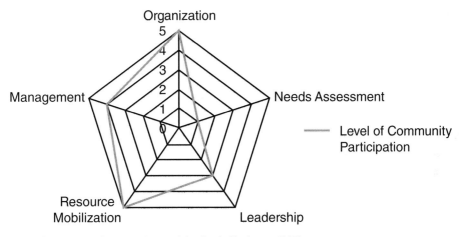

Figure 3.5 Level of community participation in Nachanta CHPS.
Source: Baatiema *et al.* (2013).

community level. Working with a community requires the health visitor to develop an in-depth knowledge of the strengths and needs of that community. This may be achieved in a variety of ways, including by working one-to-one and making use of current knowledge and skills. At the level of the community, three approaches to developing such knowledge were outlined: the windshield survey, public health walk, and HNA. Following this, BCC resources were discussed. Building health visitors' knowledge of working with communities and with partners in community building in public health, such as local authorities and third sector-organisations, was identified as the first step in the process of health visitors working with local communities as communities, as opposed to working with individual community members as individuals. Working with communities to improve health and community resilience is a long-term process that will require both knowledgeable health visitors and a radical rebalancing of health care towards prevention and the promotion of health.

References

Antonovsky, A. (1996) The salutogenic model as a theory to guide health promotion. *Health Promotion International*, **11**(1), 11–18.

Arnstein, S. (1969) A ladder of citizen participation. *American Institute of Planners Journal*, **35**(4), 216–24.

Baatiema, L. Skovdal, S., Rifkin, S. & Campbell, C. (2013) Assessing participation in a community-based health planning and service programme in Ghana. *BMC Health Services Research*, **13**, 233–46. Available from: http://bmchealthservres.biomedcentral .com/articles/10.1186/1472-6963-13-233 (last accessed 30 March 2016).

Bauld, L. (2011) The Impact of Smokefree Legislation in England: Evidence Review, March 2011. Department of Health, London.

Beattie, A. (2003 [1991]) Knowledge and control in health promotion: a test case for social policy and social theory. In: The Sociology of the Health Service (eds J. Gabe, M. Calnan & M. Bury). Routledge, London. Ch. **7**, pp. 162–202.

Bowling, A. (2014) Quality of Life: Measures and Meanings in Social Care Research. Methods Review 16. NIHR School for Social Care Research, London School of Economics and Political Science, London.

Bradshaw, J. (1972) The concept of social need. *New Society*, **30**, 640–3.

Bradshaw, J. (1994) The conceptualisation and measurement of need – a social policy perspective. In: Researching the People's Health (eds. J. Popay & G. Williams). Routledge, London. Ch. 3, pp. 45–57.

Brown, J. & Collins, G. (2015) Embedding simulated practice: health of the community experience. *Primary Health Care*, **25**(6), 26–9.

Bryar, R. & Fisk, L. (1994) Setting up a community health house. *Community Practitioner*, **67**(6), 203–5.

Bryar, R., Kendall, S., & Mogotlane, S.M. (2012) Reforming Primary Health: A Nursing Perspective Contributing to Health Care Reform, Issues and Challenges. ICHRN, Geneva. Available from: http://www.icchnr.org/documents/PHCNursing.pdf (last accessed 30 March 2016).

Cameron, S. & Christie, G. (2007) Exploring health visitors' perceptions of the public health nursing role. *Primary Health Care Research and Development*, **8**(1), 80–90.

Campbell, A., Converse, P. & Rodgers, W. (1976) The Quality of American Life: Perceptions, Evaluations and Satisfaction. Russell Sage Foundation, New York.

Carson, R. (1962) Silent Spring. Houghton Mifflin, New York.

Civil Exchange (2015) Whose Society? The Final Big Society Audit. Civil Exchange, London. Available from: http://www.civilexchange.org.uk/wp-content/uploads/2015/ 01/Whose-Society_The-Final-Big-Society-Audit_final.pdf (last accessed 30 March 2016).

Community Development Foundation (2014) *Tailor-Made: How Community Groups Improve People's Lives*. Available from: http://www.cdf.org.uk/wp-content/uploads/ 2014/10/Tailor-made-How-Community-Groups-Improve-Peoples-Lives.pdf (last accessed 30 March 2016).

Cooke, B. & Kothari, U. (2001) Participation: The New Tyranny? Zed Books, London.

Council for the Education and Training of Health Visitors (1965) Syllabus Examination for Health Visitors in the United Kingdom. Council for the Education and Training of Health Visitors, London.

Council for the Education and Training of Health Visitors (1967) The Function of the Health Visitor. Council for the Education and Training of Health Visitors, London.

Cowley, S. & Frost, M. (2006) The Principles of Health Visiting: Opening the Door to Public Health Practice in the 21st Century. Community Practitioners' and Health Visitors' Association, London.

Cragg, L., Davies, M. & Macdowell, W. (eds) (2013) Health Promotion Theory, 2nd edn. Open University Press, McGraw-Hill Education, Maidenhead.

Craig, P. (1995) A Different Role: Health Visiting in a Community Project. Glasgow City Health Project, Glasgow.

Craig, P.M. & Lindsay, G.M. (eds) (2000) Nursing for Public Health: Population-Based Care. Churchill Livingstone, London.

Crow, G. (2002) Community studies: fifty years of theorization. *Sociological Research Online*, **7**(3), 1–13. Available from: http://www.socresonline.org.uk/7/3/crow.html (last accessed 30 March 2016).

Dahlgren, G. & Whitehead, M. (1991) Policies and Strategies to Promote Social Equity in Health. Institute for Future Studies, Stockholm.

Delanty, G. (2003) Community. Routledge, London.

Dench, G., Gavron, K. & Young, M. (2006) The New East End: Kinship, Race and Conflict. The Young Foundation, London.

Derges, J., Lynch, R., Clow, A., Petticrew, M. & Draper, A. (2012) Complaints about dog faeces as a symbolic representation of incivility in London: a qualitative study. *Critical Public Health*, **22**(4), 419–25.

DH (2007) Guidance on Joint Strategic Needs Assessment. Department of Health, London.

DH (2011) The Health Visitor Implementation Plan 2011–15. A Call to Action. Department of Health, London.

DH (2013) Statutory Guidance on Joint Strategic Needs Assessments and Joint Health and Well-Being Strategies. Department of Health, London.

Dorset Healthcare NHS Trust (2013) Building Community Capacity Projects. Dorset Healthcare NHS Trust, Poole. Available from: http://www.dorsethealthcare.nhs.uk/WS-Dorset-HealthCare/Downloads/Health%20Visiting%20Related%20Links/BCC%20A4%20leaflet%20-2013.pdf (last accessed 30 March 2016).

Draper, A.K., Hewitt, G. & Rifkin, S. (2010) Chasing the dragon: developing indicators for assessment of community participation in health programmes. *Social Science & Medicine*, **71**(6), 1102–9.

Drennan, V. (ed) (1988) Health Visitors and Groups: Politics and Practice. Heinemann Professional Publishing, Oxford.

Freire, P. (1973) Education for Critical Consciousness. Seabury Press, New York.

Gilchrist, A. (2007) Community development and networking for health. In: Public Health for the 21st Century, 2nd edn. (eds J. Orme, J. Powell, P. Taylor & M. Greys). Open University Press McGraw-Hill Education, Maidenhead. Ch. **8**, pp. 135–52.

Gill, T. (2015) Hackney Play Streets Evaluation Report. Hackney Play Association, London. Available from: http://www.hackney.gov.uk/Assets/Documents/play-streets-evaluation-report.pdf (last accessed 30 March 2016).

Green, J., Tones, K., Cross, R. & Woodall, J. (2014) Health Promotion: Planning and Strategies, 3rd edn. SAGE, London.

Hall, D.M.B. & Elliman, D. (2006) Health for All Children, 4th revised edn. Oxford University Press, Oxford.

Hamer, J., Jacobson, B., Flowers, J. & Johnstone, F. (2003) Health Equity Audit Made Simple: A Briefing for Primary Care Trusts and Local Strategic Partnerships. Working Document January 2003. NICE, London.

Harris, J. (ed) (2001) Tonnies: Community and Civil Society. Cambridge University Press, Cambridge.

Hawtin, M. & Percy-Smith, J. (2007) Community Profiling: A Practical Guide, 2nd edn. Open University Press, McGraw-Hill Education, Maidenhead.

HDA (2004a) Health Needs Assessment: A Practical Guide. Health Development Agency, National Institute for Health and Care Excellence, London. Available from: https://www.urbanreproductivehealth.org/sites/mle/files/Health_Needs_Assessment_A_Practical_Guide.pdf (last accessed 30 March 2016).

HDA (2004b) Clarifying Health Impact Assessment, Integrated Impact Assessment and Health Needs Assessment. Health Development Agency, National Institute for Health and Care Excellence, London. Available from: https://www.google.com/url?sa=t&rct=j&q=&esrc=s&source=web&cd=1&cad=rja&uact=8&ved=0ahUKEwiu64rk1cXLAhXM7CYKHXI1DhIQFggiMAA&url=http%3A%2F%2Fwww.apho.org.uk%2Fresource%2Fview.aspx%3FRID%3D44782&usg=AFQjCNH-RmvoqeCPxk0VaXmrd2e3WuMAkQ (last accessed 30 March 2016).

Health Education East of England (2014) Building Community Capacity Health Visiting Case Studies. Health Education East of England, Cambridge. Available from: https://heeoe.hee.nhs.uk/sites/default/files/1410863281_rrnz_bcc_booklet_-_july_14_-_final.pdf (last accessed 30 March 2016).

Hogg, R., Ritchie, D., de Kok, B., Wood, C. & Huby, G. (2013) Parenting support for families with young children – a public health, user-focused study undertaken in a semi-rural area in Scotland. Journal of Clinical Nursing, 22(7–8), 1140–50.

Hooper, J. & Longworth, P. (2002) Health Needs Assessment Workbook. Health Development Agency, National Institute for Health and Care Excellence, London.

House, A. (2015) The TCPA New Communities Group: Ambitious Councils Working Together to Deliver Large-Scale New Communities. Town and Planning Association, London.

Hunt, R. (2013) Introduction to Community-Based Nursing, 5th edn. Walters Kluwer, Lippincott Williams and Wilkins, Philadelphia.

Joly, L.M.A. (2009) A Mixed Method Study to Explore Interagency Working to Support the Health of People who are Homeless. Unpublished PhD thesis. University College London, London.

Joly, L., Goodman, C., Froggett, K. & Drennan, V. (2011) Interagency working to support the health of people who are homeless. Social Policy and Society, 10(4), 523–36.

Kenyon, L. (2015) Building Community Capacity (BCC): An Introductory Toolkit for Health Visitors. Institute of Health Visiting, London. Available from: http://ihv.org.uk/wp-content/uploads/2015/10/iHV_BCC-Toolkit.pdf (last accessed 30 March 2016).

Kloos, B., Hill, J., Thomas, E., Wandersman, A., Elias, M. & Dalton, J. (2012) Community Psychology: Linking Individuals and Communities, 3rd edn. Wadsworth CENGAGE Learning, Belmont.

Krupat E. & Guild W. (1980) Defining the city: the use of objective and subjective measures for community description. Journal of Social Issues, 36(3), 9–28.

Lang, T. & Rayner, G. (2012) Ecological public health: the 21st century's big idea? British Medical Journal, 345, e5466.

Laverack, G. (2015) Public Health: Power, Empowerment and Professional Practice, 3rd edn. Macmillan Education Palgrave, Basingstoke.

Lawrence, A. (2008) Better Together: A Guide for People in the Health Service on How You Can Help to Build More Cohesive Communities. Available from: http://resources.cohesioninstitute.org.uk/Publications/Documents/Document/DownloadDocumentsFile.aspx?recordId=5&file=PDFversion (last accessed 30 March 2016).

Layard, R. & Dunne, J. (2009) A Good Childhood Inquiry: Searching for Values in a Competitive Age. Penguin, London.

Lock, K. (2000) Health impact assessment. *British Medical Journal*, **320**, 1395–8.

Luker, K. & Orr, J. (eds) (1992) Health Visiting: Towards Community Health Nursing. Blackwell Science, Oxford.

Lynch, J.W., Law, C., Brinkman, S., Chittleborough, C. & Sawyer, M (2010) Inequalities in child health development: some challenges for effective implementation. *Social Science & Medicine*, **71**(4), 1244–8.

Marmot, M., Atkinson, T., Bell, J., Black, C., Broadfoot, P., Cumberlege, J., Diamond, I., Gilmore, I., Ham, C., Meacher, M. & Mulgan, G. (2010) Fair Society, Healthy Lives: The Marmot Review. Marmot Review Team, University College, London. Available from: http://www.instituteofhealthequity.org/projects/fair-society-healthy-lives-the-marmot-review (last accessed 30 March 2016).

Maslow, A. (1954) Motivation and Personality. Harper, New York.

McInnis, E., Nettleton, R., Whittaker, K. & Kenyon, L. (2015) Building Community Capacity: A Perspective on Practice. Institute of Health Visiting, London.

McNaught, A. (2009) Leadership in community development. In: Professional Practice in Public Health (eds J. Stewart & Y. Cornish). Reflect Press, Exeter. Ch. **12**, pp. 165–76.

Mguni, N. & Bacon, N. (2010) Taking the Temperature of Local Communities: The Well-Being and Resilience Measure (WARM). The Young Foundation, London.

Miller W.R. & Rollnick, S. (2012) Motivational Interviewing. Helping People Change, 3rd edn. Guilford Press, New York.

Moos, R.H. (1976) The Human Context: Environmental Determinants of Behaviour. John Wiley, New York.

Moos, R.H. (2002) The mystery of human context and coping: an unravelling of clues. *American Journal of Community Psychology*, **30**(1), 67–88.

Morgan, A. & Cragg, L. (2013) The determinants of health. In: Health Promotion Theory, 2nd edn (eds L. Cragg, M. Davies & W. Macdowell). Open University Press, McGraw-Hill Education, Maidenhead. Ch. 7, pp. 98–113.

Mulgan, G. (2010) Investing in Social Growth: Can the Big Society be More than a Slogan? The Young Foundation, London.

Naidoo, J. & Wills, J. (2009) Foundations for Health Promotion. 3rd edn. Bailliere Tindall Elsevier, Edinburgh.

Naidoo, J. & Wills, J. (2016) Foundations for Health Promotion, 4th edn. Bailliere Tindall Elsevier, Edinburgh, elsevierhealth.com.

NHS England (2014a) Five Year Forward View. NHS England, London. Available from: https://www.england.nhs.uk/wp-content/uploads/2014/10/5yfv-web.pdf (last accessed 30 March 2016).

NHS England (2014b) 2015–16 National Health Visiting Core Service Specification. NHS England, London. Available from: http://www.england.nhs.uk/wp-content/uploads/2014/12/hv-serv-spec-dec14-fin.pdf (last accessed 30 March 2016).

NICE (2008) Community Engagement. NICE Public Health Guidance No 9. National Institute for Health and Care Excellence, London. Available from: http://www.apho.org.uk/resource/view.aspx?RID=85472 (last accessed 30 March 2016).

NICE (2014) Community Engagement to Improve Health. NICE Local Government Briefings. National Institute for Health and Care Excellence, London. Available from: http://www.nice.org.uk/advice/lgb16/resources/community-engagement-to-improve-health-60521149786309 (last accessed 30 March 2016).

NMC (2004) Standards of Proficiency for Specialist Community Public Health Nurses. Nursing and Midwifery Council, London.

O'Dwyer, L.A., Baum, F., Kavanagh, A. & Macdougall, C. (2007) Do area-based interventions to reduce health inequalities work? A systematic review of the evidence. *Critical Public Health*, **17**(4), 317–35.

ONS (2015) Measuring National Well-Being. Available from: http://www.ons.gov.uk/ons/guide-method/user-guidance/well-being/index.html (last accessed 30 March 2016).

Orr, J. (1992) The community dimension. In: Health Visiting: Towards Community Health Nursing (eds K. Luker & J. Orr). Blackwell Science, Oxford. Ch. 2, pp. 43–72.

Pearson, L. (2003) Capturing client voices for community development using participatory appraisal. In: Practice Development in Community Nursing: Principles and Processes (eds R.M. Bryar & J.M. Griffiths). Arnold, London. Ch. 9, pp. 175–93.

Pearson, P. (2013) Working with communities to improve health: the Building Community Capacity programme. *Journal of Health Visiting*, **1**(12), 704–9.

Play England (2015) Street Play Briefing for Public Health Professionals. Play England. Available from: http://www.playengland.net/wp-content/uploads/2015/10/Play-England-Street-Play-Briefing-for-Public-Health-Professionals.pdf (last accessed 30 March 2016).

Powell, F. & Geoghegan, M. (2004) The Politics of Community Development: Reclaiming Civil Society or Reinventing Governance? A. & A. Farmar, Dublin.

Public Health Online Resource for Careers, Skills and Training (2013) *Public Health Skills and Knowledge Framework*. Available from: http://www.phorcast.org.uk/page.php?page_id=44 (last accessed 30 March 2016).

Public Health Resource Unit/Skills for Health (2008) *Public Health Skills and Career Framework: Multidisciplinary/Multi-Agency/Multi-Professional*. Available from: http://www.publichealthcoursesguide.nhs.uk/PDF/NESC_Public_Health_Report_Web_April_20090608.pdf (last accessed 30 March 2016).

Rabinowtiz, P. (2015) Section 21. Windshield and walking surveys. In: Chapter 3. Assessing Community Needs and Resources. The Community Tool Box. Work Group for Community Health and Development, University of Kansas. Available from: http://ctb.ku.edu/en/table-of-contents/assessment/assessing-community-needs-and-resources/windshield-walking-surveys/main (last accessed 30 March 2016).

Radford, A. (2009) Reflections on AI and their implications for sustaining AI as a way of life. Available from: www.aradford.co.uk (last accessed 30 March 2016).

Rayner, G. & Lang, T. (2012) Ecological Public Health: Reshaping the Conditions for Good Health. Routledge, Abingdon.

Reed, J. (2007) Appreciative Inquiry – Research for Change. Sage, London.

Rifkin, S.B. (1985) Health Planning and Community Participation: Case Studies in South-East Asia. Croom Helm, Beckenham.

Rifkin, S.B. (2014) Examining the links between community participation and health outcomes: a review of the literature. Health Policy and Planning, **29**, ii98–106.

Robinson, J. & Elkan, R. (1996) Health Needs Assessment: Theory and Practice. Churchill Livingstone, Edinburgh.

Roberts, Y., Brophy, M. & Bacon, N. (2009) Parenting and Well-Being: Knitting Families Together. The Young Foundation, London.

Ross, A. & Chang, M. (2012) Reuniting Health with Planning – Healthier Homes, Healthier Communities. Town and Country Planning Association, London.

Scriven, A. (2010) Promoting Health: A Practical Guide. Balliere Tindall Elsevier, Edinburgh.

Scottish Community Development Centre for Learning Connections. (2007) Building Community Capacity: Resources for Community Learning & Development Practice. A Guide. The Scottish Government, Edinburgh. Available from: http://www.scdc.org.uk/media/resources/what-we-do/building-comm-cap/building_community_capacity_resource_for_cld.pdf (last accessed 30 March 2016).

Sierau, S., Dahne, V., Brand, T., Kutz, V., von Klitzing, K. & Jungmann, T. (2015) Effects of home visitation on maternal competencies, family environment, and child development: a randomized controlled trial. *Prevention Science*, **17**(1), 40–51.

Skinner, S. (2006) Strengthening Communities: a Guide to Capacity Building for Communities and the Public Sector. Community Development Foundation, London.

Skovdal, M. (2013) Using theory to guide change at the community level. In: Health Promotion Theory, 2nd edn (eds L. Cragg, M. Davies & W. Macdowell). Open University Press, McGraw-Hill Education, Maidenhead. Ch. 6, 79–97.

South, J. (2015a) A Guide to Community-Centred Approaches for Health and Well-Being. Briefing. Public Health England, London. Available from: https://www.gov.uk/government/uploads/system/uploads/attachment_data/file/402889/A_guide_to_community-centred_approaches_for_health_and_wellbeing__briefi___.pdf (last accessed 30 March 2016).

South, J. (2015b) A Guide to Community-Centred Approaches for Health and Well-Being. Full Report. Public Health England, London. Available from: https://www.gov.uk/government/uploads/system/uploads/attachment_data/file/417515/A_guide_to_community-centred_approaches_for_health_and_wellbeing__full_report_.pdf (last accessed 30 March 2016).

Starfield, B. (1996) Public health and primary care: a framework for proposed linkages. American Journal of Public Health, 86(10), 1365–9.

Stewart, J., Cornish, Y. & Patel, S. (2009) Health needs assessment. In: Professional Practice in Public Health (eds J. Stewart & Y. Cornish). Reflect Press, Exeter. Ch. 10, pp. 133–47.

Stockdale, J., Sinclair, M., Kernohan, G. & Keller, J. (2011) Understanding motivational theory and the psychology of breastfeeding. In: Theory for Midwifery Practice, 2nd edn (eds. R. Bryar & M. Sinclair). Palgrave Macmillan, Basingstoke. Ch. 4, pp. 92–112.

Swann, B. & Brocklehurst, N. (2004) Three in one: the Stockport model of health visiting. Community Practitioner, 77(7), 251–6.

Tones, K. & Tilford, S. (2001) Health Promotion: Effectiveness, Efficiency and Equity, 3rd edn. Nelson Thornes, Cheltenham.

Torres, R.M. & Carte, L. (2014) Community participatory appraisal in migration research: connecting neoliberalism, rural restructuring and mobility. Transactions of the Institute of British Geographers, 39, 140–54.

Tudor Hart, J. (1971) The inverse care law. The Lancet, i, 405–12.

UN (2015) Sustainable development goals. Available from: https://sustainabledevelopment.un.org/?menu=1300 (last accessed 30 March 2016).

University of Kansas (2015) Community Tool Box. University of Kansas, Kansas. Available from: http://ctb.ku.edu/en (last accessed 30 March 2016).

University of Northumbria (2013) Building Community Capacity module. Available from: http://www.e-lfh.org.uk/programmes/building-community-capacity/ (last accessed 30 March 2016).

Watt, G. (2002) The inverse care law today. The Lancet, 360(9328), 252–4.

Whittaker, K., Griguils, A., Hughes, J., Cowley, S., Morrow, E., Nicholson, C., Malone, M. & Maben, J. (2013) Start and Stay: The Recruitment and Retention of Health Visitors. National Nursing Research Unit, King's College London, London.

WHO/UNICEF (1978) Declaration of Alma-Ata. World Health Organization, Geneva. Available from: http://www.who.int/publications/almaata_declaration_en.pdf (last accessed 30 March 2016).

WHO (2008) Primary Health Care: Now More than Ever. World Health Organization, Geneva.

Young Foundation (2010) How can Neighbourhoods be Understood and Defined? The Young Foundation, London.

Young, M. & Willmott, P. (2007 [1957]) Family and Kinship in East London. Penguin Modern Classics, London.

Activities

Activity 3.1

Your definition of community and your communities

Write down your definition of community and discuss it with a colleague. Do you share the same understanding? What are the differences in your definitions?

Think about the different communities that you belong to. Write down all of these communities and group them under relevant headings.

Activity 3.2

Public health practice

Consider the 10 areas of public health practice listed in Table 3.7 and identify an example from your practice with a community which illustrates your application of one or more of them.

Table 3.7 Areas of public health practice.

Area	Example(s) from your practice
Surveillance and assessment of the population's health and wellbeing	
Promoting and protecting the population's health and wellbeing	
Developing quality and risk management within an evaluative culture	
Collaborative working for health and wellbeing	
Developing health programmes and services and reducing inequalities	
Policy and strategy development and implementation to improve health and well being	
Working with and for communities to improve health and wellbeing	
Strategic leadership for health and wellbeing	
Research and development to improve health and wellbeing	
Ethically managing self, people and resources to improve health and wellbeing	

Activity 3.3

Developing a public health walk

Explore your local area on foot, talk to local health visitors and public health colleagues, consult the local librarian and library services, and talk to local residents to identify the historical and contemporary public health issues in your area. Construct a walk to illustrate the impact of these issues. Invite colleagues and local residents to participate in and develop the walk.

Activity 3.4

Undertaking a health needs assessment

Identify a neighbourhood in which you are working and use the HDA five-step model (HDA, 2004a) to undertake an HNA of it. In doing this, identify a health need and develop an implementation plan and evaluation process to address it (Table 3.8).

Table 3.8 Blank health needs assessment (HNA) form.

Steps	Activities	Your neighbourhood
Step 1: Getting started	What population? What are you trying to achieve? Who needs to be involved? What resources are required? What are the risks?	
Step 2: Identifying health priorities	Population profiling Gathering data Perceptions of needs Identifying and assessing health conditions and determinant factors	
Step 3: Assessing a health priority for action	Choosing health conditions and determinant factors with the most significant size and severity impact Determine effective and acceptable interventions and actions	

(Continued)

Activity 3.4: *(Continued)*

Table 3.8 *(Continued)*

Steps	Activities	Your neighbourhood
Step 4: Planning for change	Clarifying aims of intervention Action planning Monitoring and evaluation strategy Risk-management strategy	
Step 5: Moving on/review	Learning from the project Measuring the impact Choosing the next priority	

Activity 3.5

Accessing health profile information

Access the health profile for your area on the APHO website (www.apho.org .uk) and compare it with a contrasting area in another part of Britain. What are the key priorities for health visiting that you can identify from this information? How does the comparison affect your assessment of health issues in your area?

4

Approaches to Supporting Families

Karen I. Chalmers
The University of Manchester, Manchester, UK

Karen A. Whittaker
University of Central Lancashire, Preston, UK

Introduction

Health visitors are well positioned to contribute to the public health system and improve the health of the nation (DH & Public Health England, 2015). Improving the social determinants of health is critical if health inequalities are to be reduced across social groups (Marmot *et al.*, 2010). The Department for Work and Pensions (DWP) social justice team estimates that the gap in educational attainment for disadvantaged children aged 4 is 9%, and that it escalates throughout childhood (HM Government, 2013). Disadvantages include having no parent in the family in work, living in poverty or overcrowded housing, having no parent with educational qualifications, having a mother with mental health problems, and living in a family with low income. The impact of poverty is seen in the 35-fold increase in the number of people relying on emergency food provided by the UK-wide network of Trussell Trust Foodbanks (Perry *et al.*, 2014). Research funded by the Economic Social Research Council (ESRC) and published by Poverty and Social Exclusion UK (2013) reports that over 3.5 million adults are unable to feed themselves properly and that over half a million children (4%) live in food-insecure households. Worryingly, children who regularly experience hunger are likely to have poorer health and thus increased vulnerability (Ke & Ford-Jones, 2015). Additionally, there is increasing evidence of the impact of the home environment on the neurological development and physical and psychosocial health of infants and young children, and these impacts can have a long-lasting effect on children's health and development. Building resilience and well being in young children across the social gradient is critical to improving the health of the population (Marmot *et al.*, 2010). Supporting families with young children is seen as an important approach to improving the social determinants of a population.

Health Visiting: Preparation for Practice, Fourth Edition.
Edited by Karen A. Luker, Gretl A. McHugh and Rosamund M. Bryar.
© 2017 John Wiley & Sons, Ltd. Published 2017 by John Wiley & Sons, Ltd.

Furthermore, nurse-led home visiting programmes modelled to some extent on UK health visiting are promoted (e.g. by UNICEF, working with Eastern European countries (Whittaker & Bowne, 2014)) as a viable mechanism for improving early child development and thereby later health.

Supporting families to improve health and prevent ill health, particularly families with young children, has been the cornerstone of health visiting practice since the inception of the service. This chapter explores approaches and programmes in which health visitors support families with young children with the goal of improving family health. The specific objectives of the chapter are to:

- Assess some models of intervention in family life and their application to health visiting practice.
- Explore the role of policies influencing health visitors' work in supporting families.
- Examine programmes to support families with young children.
- Examine the role of the health visitor–client relationship in providing supportive care to young families.
- Reflect on the challenges when planning services for and working with families.

Models of intervention in family life

The 'family' is viewed as an important institution in our society, not only for individual welfare but for society as a whole. The family is used as a symbol in all discussions of social life and social welfare, and it is seen as a necessary function of the state that it intervene in family life through the provision of services and benefits and by controlling behaviours through policies and laws (e.g. the use of infant and child car seats). Health visitors are, more than most other health workers, involved in visiting families in their homes, and they provide a unique service by working with families across all social classes and during periods of family transition and crisis. To work with families in this way gives health visitors considerable experience of family life and the tensions which are a normal part of living, placing them in a privileged position to monitor social and economic policies affecting health. Working with individuals and families in this personal and important sphere of their lives is a also a great responsibility. The notion of intervening in family life to assess need is a complex one, and it has within it tensions based on the relationships between the state and the family. On the one hand, the family is seen as being a private and personal unit, especially when there are no children and the dominant values of society are being upheld. On the other hand, due to the importance of the family, particularly in relation to the well being of children, intervention is seen by many as a legitimate action of the state. Governments recognise the need to develop policies on many fronts in order to increase the life chances of children living in poverty, including policies to support child rearing, improve nutrition, and help parents access work (HM Government, 2014a).

The state often first intervenes in the family when a woman becomes pregnant and almost always when the child is born. Pregnancy and childbirth result in the private family being scrutinised by professionals. Doctors often legitimise when a woman is pregnant and decide on the availability of abortion, if that is requested. The medical profession tends also to control contraception, at least in part. Social workers, and more recently health visitors, have a major role in deciding if children are being adequately cared for and when, or if, they should be taken into care, and parents may perceive that they have to 'measure up' to professionals' expectations. The focus on child-rearing skills objectifies parenting as caring labour and hides the fact that it has a gendered status and is largely undertaken by women in the family. Also, it is women who usually find themselves on the interface with social and health services, particularly if they are caring for children or aged or disabled family members (Carers UK, 2014). Of concern is the substantial number of children and young people in England who find themselves in caring roles and the damaging impact this has on education and life chances (The Children's Society, 2013). Campaigning by charity groups has facilitated increased recognition of the social costs imposed on carers, and increasingly carers' needs are being identified by governments (e.g. DH, 2014; HM Government, 2014b), although the impacts of this remain to be seen.

Three models relevant to health visiting practice in families with young children

Historically, the focus of health visitors' work was on families, specifically families with infants and pre-school children. Although individuals, social groups, and 'the community' were also cited in health visitor texts and position statements, in practice, the dominant focus was usually children and women in the mothering role. In England, the current service vision introduced by the Health Visitor Implementation Plan 2011–15 (DH, 2011b), updated as The Plan (DH, 2013), reintroduces health visitors' wider public health roles, although there remains a dominant emphasis on working to support young families.

Articulating the theoretical underpinnings of practice may assist practitioners in clarifying what actually or potentially influences their day-to-day work. This section outlines three models or approaches to health visitors' work in supporting young families: the child-centred model, the family-centred model and the ecological model. These models have not been generated strictly from empirical research, although there is some research which supports how health visitors work with young families (see later). Rather, they have been synthesised from the health visitor literature.

The child-centred model

This model has been the dominant model of health visiting practice for many years. Within it, the proper focus of services is seen to be the well being of the young child, with other family members – especially fathers – playing secondary roles. Health visitors work primarily with mothers in their homes and clinics, with the goal of promoting the healthy development of children. They have contact at designated times to carry out development assessments (as advocated by the Healthy Child Programme (HCP) (DH, 2009; Public Health England, 2015)), and provide health teaching and support. All families receive the home visiting service; the universality of the service is seen as eliminating the stigma of professionally perceived needs or problems, permitting intervention 'upstream' (Marmot et al., 2010: 155) to prevent health and behavioural problems (primary prevention) or to detect these problems early, before they become entrenched (secondary prevention).

Health visitors have no statutory right of access to the home, but negotiate their entry based on the universality of the service ('everyone receives it'). Because the focus is on the child, the well being of other family members is perceived to be secondary or is minimally considered. There is currently strong research evidence of the importance of prenatal and early childhood development, including neuro-logical development, as a determinant of health and health equalities (Center on the Developing Child at Harvard University, 2010). Interventions to promote healthy child development are critical. While health teaching to parents related to child develop-ment remains important, the means to promote healthy child development are also now seen as entailing a wider focus than just the child within the family.

The family-centred model

The family-centred model also recognises the importance of children's health; how-ever, the means of securing enhanced child health is viewed within a holistic 'fam-ily lens'. This approach has the satisfactory health and functioning of the family as its main aim. It tends to be concerned with resolving difficulties and conflicts within the family and thus improving the overall functioning and well being of the family as a whole, as well as those of its members. The underpinnings of this model are influenced by family theories, primarily family systems theory, but also structural-functioning theory and family development theory (Wright & Leahy, 2013). These theories were developed in social science disciplines and adapted by some applied disciplines, such as clinical psychology and specialty fields within social work. Aspects of them are now taught in nursing and health visiting courses. For example, genograms of families (see Figure 4.1) are used as a pictorial means of viewing the family holistically (McGoldrick et al., 2008), particularly when con-sidering safeguarding practice issues (Calder et al., 2012). To build on informa-tion provided by a genogram and so understand parents' wider personal social

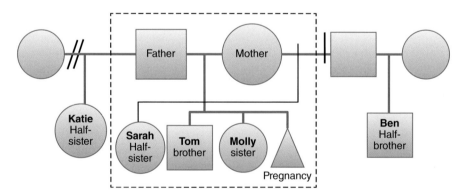

Figure 4.1 Family genogram. The dotted lines denote the current family arrangement. The scenario is a mother (separated) living with her current partner and three children: Sarah (from her previous husband), Tom, and Molly. She is expecting her fourth child. Her current partner was previously married and is now divorced with one child, Katie, who lives with her mother. Sarah has a half-brother, Ben, as her father is in a new relationship.

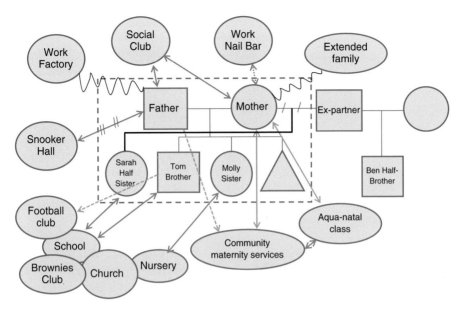

Figure 4.2   Family eco-map of the same family as shown in Figure 4.1.

networks, an eco-map can be created (Whittaker, 2014). This extended visual map (see Figure 4.2) illustrates community resources and connections within the reach of families. As in the genogram, both the quantity and quality of relationships can be depicted (Feeley & Gottlieb, 2000). Activity 4.1 provides further information about the symbols used, as well as the opportunity to create your own genogram and eco-map. Creating these visuals with a family can be a useful means of highlighting the circumstances surrounding them. Within safeguarding contexts, professional practice has been criticised for concentrating focus on the parents and giving insufficient attention to the circumstances surrounding the child (Munro, 2011). Thus, genograms and eco-maps are included in child protection resource packs, such as that produced on behalf of the Scottish Government (Calder *et al.*, 2012), as tools for detailing the child's situation and thereby keeping their needs in mind whilst working with adult carers.

It is important, though, that theories developed and applied by other disciplines are not 'imported' into health visiting without careful consideration of the practice context. These theories may assist health visitors to view families holistically, expand their 'lens' of practice from 'child' to 'family', and direct them to view the influences on the child's health from a broader perspective.

Ecological model

This model has its origins in Bronfenbrenner's (1979) 'person in context' framework. This is an integrated framework which recognises the interrelationship and interdependence of all aspects and levels in society. For example, the young child can be viewed as nestled within a family, which is viewed within the neighbourhood and community and the larger sociopolitical and cultural environments. The model outlines four distinct levels: the microsystem, mesosystem, exosystem, and macrosystem.

Viewing children's health through this approach acknowledges the various immediate and more distant environments as major impacts on children's health and development. It also provides additional 'targets' for legitimate health visitor interventions. This might involve meeting with extended family members and parents to discuss the child's health needs (i.e. mesosystem) or developing groups to support young families in the community (i.e. exosystem) or influencing governments to implement child health promotive policies (macrosystem).

This model recognises the transitions of families and communities and helps to provide a means of viewing today's families within the context of the many influences on their lives. For example, it would direct the health visitor to recognise the diversity of family units (e.g. sole parent, same-sex parents, adoptive families) and assess the strengths, resources, and stressors coming from the different systems which influence individual and family health.

This model also resonates with the Health Visitor Plan for England (DH, 2013) which supports health visitor fulfilment of public health roles with families in the context of their community through building community capacity (BCC) activities. The ecological feature of recognising the person-in-situation is understood as a key feature of health visiting (Cowley et al., 2014), and thus the model is advocated as a promising approach for the health visiting service. However, further research is needed to test directly the utility of the framework in practice (Bryans et al., 2009: 564). Bronfenbrenner's (1979) ecological model is also one of the theoretical underpinnings of the Family Nurse Partnership (FNP) and Maternal Early Childhood Sustained Home Visiting (MECSH) programmes (see 'Current Home Visiting Programmes', later in the chapter).

Application of the models in practice

Although these models are presented separately, there is little empirical evidence that, in actual practice, health visitors in the past or at present function solely within one conceptual perspective. Health visitors' practice with young families is also influenced by many other factors, such as the numbers of other health visitors in the community and other available resources. One of the most important factors is the policy initiative under which the service is offered. For example, policies might direct health visitors' service provision to all under-5s or to a targeted group of young children who are deemed to be at particular risk for poor health and development. (The influence of policy on health practice is outlined in more detail in the next section and in Chapter 2.)

Understanding of how practice is actually delivered is gleaned from empirical research. Research studies that gather information through observation and interviews with health visitors and clients are particularly helpful. For example, Cowley et al.'s (2014) narrative review of published literature on health visiting practice identified interventions which may contribute to positive outcomes in families and outlined the 'conceptual orientation' underpinning health visitors' practice, which may contribute to benefits. Across studies, health visiting practice was found to emphasise key principles such as valuing the person, a strengths- and solution-based approach to practice, and viewing the client within his/her wider environment The review also noted that in delivering a service underpinned by these principles, health visitors appear to engage in three core activities when making contact with families: home visiting, relationship formation, and continual needs assessment.

By operating within conceptual models, health visitors place more or less emphasis on particular aspects of their work. For example, in an early study of health visiting practice in the North of England, health visitors were interviewed about aspects of their practice (Chalmers, 1992a). At that time, all health visitors in the study were carrying out universal home visiting to families with children from the early postnatal period to age 5. Although the focus of the study was not directly on how health visitors worked with fathers, this could be seen from the analysis of their descriptions of practice. The particular approach that the health visitors used was influenced by their conceptualisation of men/fathers as important (or not) in promoting the family's health, including the health of young children, and also by factors in the actual client–health visitor situation which enhanced or restricted their work with the fathers. There was considerable variation in the approach to promoting the health of the children and in involvement with the fathers in these households. Some health visitors, for example, did not appear to conceptualise men as particularly important in their work with the families, but did seek them out (i.e. worked with them) when they assessed the mother to be incompetent in some way in the mothering role. Some health visitors were clearly working from a child-centred model, while others were more family-focused.

In a study on health visiting practice in central Scotland, carried out in 2003–04 (Bryans et al., 2009), the actions of the health visitors in their day-to-day work with families were analysed from an ecological perspective. This study used a mixed-method design, involving audio-recorded interviews with health visitors and clients, observations of health visitor–client interactions during home visits, and a review of documents and workshops with health visitor participants. The findings illustrated considerable work by the health visitors at the micro-, meso-, and exosystem levels. The researchers articulated that Bronfenbrenner's (1979) framework captured how health visitors worked with individuals and families in a culturally sensitive, person-focused, and context-specific way (Bryans et al., 2009: 571). Thus, research on actual practice can help to uncover what 'informal' models may be influencing health visiting practice, regardless of the policies operating at the time.

Policies

As already noted, health visitors' practice with young families is highly influenced by government policies. Governments attempt to direct social change by various policy instruments, including programmes to benefit specific groups, such as children. It is governments which develop, implement, revise, and retire polices. In addition, other nongovernmental organisations, such as professional associations, unions, and voluntary associations, attempt to influence government policies by lobbying, making presentations at government committee meetings, and producing position statements or other reports on topics of interest to their agendas.

Health visiting is increasingly seen at the forefront of government plans to deal with health inequalities and improve public health (Department of Health, Social Services and Public Safety (Northern Ireland), 2010; NHS Scotland, 2011; Public Health England, 2015). Several government policies over the past few decades have been directed at supporting families and improving children's health. A notable early publication was *Supporting Families* by the Home Office (1998), which introduced the Sure Start programme.

The Green Paper, *Every Child Matters* (HM Government, 2003), proposed the development of a national Common Assessment Framework (CAF) (see Chapter 5), which is now widely used across England (Collins & McCray, 2012). Research examining its impact indicates that the CAF is a useful means of assessing families' needs and delivering services. Parents and carers generally report satisfaction with the CAF related to support in assessing their needs and emphasise the importance of the lead professional (Holmes *et al.*, 2012).

The *Every Child Matters* report was followed by the *National Service Framework for Children, Young People and Maternity Services* report (DH, 2004) and set out the framework for delivering requirements of the Children Act 2004. An outcome of this report was the initiation of the Child Health Promotion Programme (DH, 2008), now the HCP (DH, 2009), aimed at providing preventative services tailored to the individual needs of children and families. Of note is that a body of research evidence was also published to support the HCP (Barlow *et al.*, 2008), which has since been updated and published by Public Health England (2015).

Health visitors are the identified leads for the HCP. Since its publication in 2009, health and social care services have undergone immense change, as political influences have shifted with changing governments. Similarly, in Scotland, the health visitor is the named person for the 0–5 age group and is understood to be the key provider of universal services in the early years as part of the Getting it Right for Every Child (GIRFEC) programme (NHS Scotland, 2011).

In England, the Health Visitor Implementation Plan (DH, 2013) supported an unprecedented expansion in the size of the health visitor workforce to enable comprehensive and targeted delivery of the HCP, and set out a new model for service delivery. Described as the 'family offer' (DH, 2011a), this model informed – by principles of proportionate universalism (Marmot *et al.*, 2010) – ensures universal provision to all parents, with additional, targeted help for those with more complex needs.

Health visiting services in England are now based on the Health Visitor Implementation Plan 'family offer' (DH, 2013) and are detailed in the NHS England (2014) health visiting service specification as operating on four levels: the community, universal, universal plus, and universal partnership plus. The community level recognises the importance of strengthening the community and ensuring the availability of community resources. The universal level includes services available to all families with young children, such as breastfeeding guidance, health and development assessments for infants and children, support for parents, and access to a range of community services/resources. Universal plus level services provide additional support and a rapid response when specific expert help is needed (e.g. to assist with postnatal depression, a sleepless baby, or weaning, or to answer any concerns about parenting). Universal partnership plus is designed for families that need support from a range of services working together to deal with complex issues over time (e.g. services from Sure Start children's centres, other community services (including charities), and, where appropriate, the FNP programme (NHS England, 2014)). By ensuring a range of services based on need and connections with community capacity, the England service model takes a public health approach to improving the health of young families.

The transformed health visiting service that has resulted now includes mandated times at which the health visitor will have contact with families during the child's early years. These are the antenatal visit, the new birth visit, 6–8 weeks, 12 months, and 2 to 2.5 years (DH & Public Health England, 2015). The DH (2013) health visiting implementation plan also outlines six high-impact areas (areas of focus for health visitors' work): transition to parenthood and the early weeks; maternal mental health (perinatal depression); breastfeeding (initiation and duration), healthy weight, healthy nutrition, and physical activity; managing minor illness and reducing hospital attendance and admission; health, well being, and development of the child age 2–2.5 years (integrated review); and support to be 'ready for school' (https://www.gov.uk/government/publications/commissioning-of-public-health-services-for-children). These initiatives are sometimes referred to as the 4-5-6 Plan (4 levels, 5 contacts, 6 impact areas). It is important to note that the work emanating from the DH (2013) health visiting implementation plan addresses policies in England only. In Scotland, there have been similar developments, although on a smaller scale, with the Scottish Health Secretary announcing in 2014 that there would be an expansion of the health visitor workforce of 500 people by 2018. It is anticipated that this will support the GIRFEC approach and allow fulfilment of the named-person role for the 0–5 age group, now required following the Children and Young People (Scotland) Act 2014 (Scottish Government, 2014). Other policy initiatives focus on meeting certain health indices for various groups in the population. For example, the policy Reducing Obesity and Healthy Eating (DH & Ellison, 2013) addresses, among other issues, the growing problem of obesity in children: the UK government aims to achieve a sustained downward trend in the levels of excess weight in children by 2020, from the estimated 28% of children between the ages of 2 and 15 who are overweight or obese today. To assist commissioners and practitioners in working towards this goal, Public Health England (2014) has published an electronic Children and Young People's Health Benchmarking Tool, which provides health outcomes data for different communities, highlighting key statistics that can be used to support discussions and planning, http://fingertips.phe.org.uk/profile/cyphof.

Clearly, from this brief review of current policy documents, the well being of children is an increasing government concern, and health visitors are seen as contributing to the support of families with young children. Regardless of the approach or the programme which directly structures health visitors' work, health visiting is situated within broader policy, social, and community contexts. These influences may provide additional supports with which to assist families. Whittaker (2014) outlines the influences on and facilities for parenting education and details the multiple sources of support – formal, semi-formal, and informal – which health visitors may draw upon in order to assist families. In the following sections, the evidence for family support programmes is explored.

The contemporary policies influencing health visiting practice remain consistent with the Council of Education and Training of Health Visitors' (CETHV's) original principles, which addressed searching for health needs, stimulating an awareness of health needs, influencing policies that affect health needs, and facilitating health-enhancing activities (CETHV, 1977).

Evidence for interventions to support families

Over the years, several home visiting and other child health programmes have been developed to address the needs of families with young children. Most of the interventions are home visiting programmes or group programmes specifically developed for work with young families. Other interventions focus more on an 'approach' to practice with parents, rather than a specific programme. For example, the Family Partnership Approach, based on a 'parent advisor' model, developed by Davis et al. (2002) and evaluated through a European programme of research (Puura et al., 2005) and a UK randomised controlled trial (RCT) (Barlow et al., 2007a), aims to equip health visitors to invest in strengthening the practitioner–parent relationship using a structured helping process. Training in this approach is used for health visitors working with the MECSH programme (discussed later) and the HENRY childhood obesity preventive programme (Brown et al., 2013). Another example is the Solihull Approach (www.solihullapproachparenting.com), now used widely across the UK. Preparation in the Solihull Approach enables health visitors to work with a model for enhancing parent–child relationships that draws on psychoanalytic, child development, and behaviourist theories. Support for parents can be offered in group and one-to-one situations, helping them learn to understand their child and apply principles of containment, reciprocity, and behaviour management to support emotional development throughout the child's life (Douglas, 2010). This approach can sensitise health visitors to the importance of promoting emotional well being in infants and children, regardless of the programme focus in their work setting. Although widely adopted, with favourable parent and practitioner feedback, evidence for the outcomes resulting from the Solihuill Approach has only been generated using small-scale evaluations (Douglas & Brennan, 2004; Johnson & Wilson, 2012; Brown, 2014).

These interventions and approaches build on a long tradition of child health services delivered by health visitors (in the UK) and public health nurses (in the USA, Canada, and other countries). With the growing number of well-designed longitudinal studies, there is increasing evidence – primarily from North America – that home visiting programmes contribute to several improved outcomes in mothers and children. Many of these studies have been critiqued and reported in a number of systematic reviews and meta-analyses (e.g. Elkan et al., 2000; Bull et al., 2004; Public Health England, 2015). While the focus of the programmes and the variables used to assess outcomes may vary, all of the studies are designed to gather evidence as to 'what works' in supporting young families. From reviews, the evidence suggests that home visiting programmes are associated with improved parenting, improvements in some child behaviours, improved cognitive development (particularly in some subgroups, such as low-birth-weight or premature infants), reductions in accidental child injuries, and improved detection and management of postnatal depression. Other studies have also shown prevention of postnatal depression in women receiving health visitor intervention (Brugha *et al.*, 2011) and short-term improvement in the emotional and behavioural adjustment of young children (Barlow *et al.*, 2010), although longer-term benefits are not known.

A recent extensive review of the literature on health visiting interventions and outcomes by Cowley *et al.* (2013a) concluded that there was specific benefit for families and children in the prevention, identification, and treatment of postnatal depression and in the provision of parenting support by specialist health visitors or through structured home visiting/early intervention programmes (Cowley *et al.*, 2013a: 20). Christie & Bunting (2011) also showed increased service satisfaction and reduced reliance on emergency care, although these benefits were not found in some groups (e.g. low-risk mothers parenting young infants). The strongest evidence for the benefit of health visitor support to families is found in studies in which health visitors have received additional training and education on the delivery of specific interventions (Puura *et al.*, 2005; Cowley *et al.*, 2013a).

Despite the promising findings from evaluation studies and reviews, the variation in their design, sample characteristics, data collection periods, and many other factors makes it difficult to 'tease out' the critical features of the home visiting programme that are contributing to their outcomes. In an earlier meta-analysis of 60 home visiting programmes, no one characteristic was found to be a significant influence across outcomes (Sweet & Applebaum, 2004). However, while programmes and approaches may vary, there are several key elements in most, including the provision of support for parenting, parental education (informal or formal), and the transmission of practical skills.

Characteristics of services and programmes to support families with young children

Programmes and approaches to support young families can vary in many important characteristics. Some questions that need to be considered when examining and evaluating programmes are outlined in Box 4.1. Whilst this list is not exhaustive, it may assist you in thinking about the number of factors which will influence the development, implementation, and evaluation of programmes to support families. Use this list to complete Activity 4.2.

Box 4.1   Questions to consider when assessing child health programmes

- Is the programme/approach delivered by a generalist health visitor or a health visitor specifically prepared for a programme/approach (specialist role)?
- Is the service offered to all infants/children (universal) or to a particular group (targeted)?
- If the latter, what criteria are used to identify the target group?

(Continued)

Box 4.1 (Continued)

- Is the programme designed to enrol women during the prenatal or post-natal period or during either time period?
- What are the conceptual underpinnings of the programme, if known (e.g. strengths-based, learning theory, support based on interpersonal/therapeutic relationships between parent and nurse, etc.)?
- Who delivers the programme: the professional (health visitor or public health nurse) or an assistant (a home visitor, community 'mothers', etc.)?
- What is the programme's age cut off for the child (2 years, school enrolment, etc.)?
- What services does the family receive and how often does it receive them?
- What services does the family receive (if any) once it completes the programme?

The following sections examine several programmes delivered in the UK and the evidence available to evaluate their outcomes. Similarities and differences in the conceptual underpinnings of programmes are identified, where possible, as are how the programmes were operationalised or put into actual practice. Also outlined are the key elements of the programmes and what variables or criteria were used to evaluate them. Where possible, information is provided on the programmes' evaluated findings, with additional recommendations for changes or future development.

Early home visiting programmes

First Parent Health Visiting Programme

Home visiting is now recognised globally as an important public health approach for supporting and nurturing care giving practices that buffer the effects of toxic stress and associated threats to infant development (Garner, 2013). The first and major structured home visiting programme in the UK was the Child Development Programme (also called the First Parent Health Visiting Programme), which originated at Bristol University under the leadership of Professor Walter Barker and was supported by the Bernard Van Leer Foundation at The Hague (Barker, 1984; Barker & Anderson, 1988). This was a large-scale programme intervention and evaluation project, which focused on altering the human environment surrounding the child during the earliest years of life and on supporting parents to make positive changes.

The First Parent health visitor visited antenatally and postnatally at monthly intervals (or more frequently, if necessary, in the early months), by appointment. The home visits focused on seven fields of child development: language, social development, cognitive development, pre-school educational development, nutrition, health, and general development. The health visitors' work was specialised in that they did not engage in other health visiting duties. The programme stressed the importance of working in partnership with parents, recognising their expertise. Health visitors acted as guides rather than authorities on child care, providing help to enable parents to seek their own solutions to child-rearing challenges.

The programme was evaluated during 1986–92 (retrospective data on 2113 families) and 1993–98 (prospective data from 459 families) as part of the National Health Service (NHS) provision (Emond et al., 2002: 150). Evidence of outcomes when children were aged 1 and 2 years was disappointing, indicating few differences between intervention and comparison mothers and children; the only clear outcome was an improvement in breastfeeding rates in the first parent group. However, the programme was delivered simultaneously with universal home visiting to all new infants and children: it was possible that generic health visitors adapted their practice when working alongside First Parent visitors, thereby masking any potential differences between the services.

Despite the evaluation outcomes, this remains a seminal programme on health visiting. The concepts introduced – targeting the disadvantaged child, structured home visiting, an emphasis on positive parenting and parents as experts, respectful relationships between the health visitor and parent, and the importance of support – are the cornerstones of most home visiting programmes which followed.

Community Mothers Programme (CMP)

As part of the development of the First Parent Programme, the concept of a 'Community Mothers' Programme (CMP) was developed in Dublin in 1983 in response to limitations in resource provision for high-needs families. Community mothers visit families with first and (sometimes) second children monthly. Women are selected on the basis of being experienced and competent mothers with the ability to empathise with and empower others. The mothers are volunteers, although they are given nominal expenses for each visit. The emphasis is on support, encouragement, and guidance, rather than direct advice. The programme is run in the Republic of Ireland by the Health Service Executive (Molloy, 2008).

Evaluations indicate some successes likely attributable to the CMP. Mothers and children had improved diets, and improvements were seen in children's receipt of primary immunisations and exposure to play and learning opportunities. Mothers were also reported to have reduced experiences of tiredness and depressive feelings (Johnson et al., 1993). What is more, follow-up research indicated that these child and maternal benefits were sustained 7 years later (Johnson et al., 2000), confirming that nonprofessionals can deliver a health promotion programme on child development effectively.

Modified versions of the CMP were initiated in some other communities in the UK. For example, the Essex-based charity Parents 1st (www.parents1st.org.uk) has developed community parent volunteers, and in Lanarkshire, Scotland there is a CMP specifically to support breastfeeding (www.nhslanarkshire.org.uk). It is also worth noting that the extensive Home Start programme operating across the UK and in other nations (www.home-start.org.uk) works with 16 000 volunteers to provide support in the home for 32 000 families with additional needs. First established in the 1970s in Leicestershire, Home Start has undergone several evaluations, offering mixed evidence for the value of family support provided by volunteers (McAuley *et al.*, 2004; Barnes *et al.*, 2006; Hermanns *et al.*, 2013). Collectively, the evidence suggests that whilst cost-effective outcomes are hard to demonstrate, families perceive personal benefits from volunteer family support, and thus further research is warranted (Hermanns *et al.*, 2013). Whilst there is evidence from other jurisdictions that substituting paraprofessionals for professional public health nurses in home visiting programmes results in less positive outcomes for children (Olds *et al.*, 2007), the role of volunteers as an additional support was not studied. It is evident that the question remains as to the use of replacements for health visitors when families have additional needs.

Current home visiting programmes

Family Nurse Partnership (FNP) Programme

Background

The US Model

The FNP programme (sometimes referred to as the Nurse Family Partnership Programme) is supported by a National Unit commissioned jointly by licence holders the Department of Health and Public Health England. The national unit supports local organisations to implement this model of intensive, nurse-led home visiting for vulnerable, first-time, young parents in the UK. The concept was developed in 1977 by psychologist David Olds, who worked with nurses to test the idea of home visiting with disadvantaged mothers who had at least one of the following risk factors: being a teenager, being unmarried, or being of low socioeconomic status (Olds *et al.*, 1986).

The intent of the programme is to provide support to the new mother as she learns to parent her infant, often in a very stressful environment. The nurses receive extensive training for the role, including in building therapeutic relationships. Nurses work with approximately 25 families during hour-long visits, beginning prior to the 29th week of pregnancy. Visits take place every 2 weeks. The mother's participation in the programme is voluntary. The focus of the visits is on six domains: personal health, environmental health, friends and family, the maternal role, use of health care and human services, and 'maternal life course development' (which encompasses planning for future pregnancies, education, and employment) (Dawley *et al.*, 2007).

Evidence from three large randomised trials carried out with participants in three participating cities in the USA (Elmira, NY, Memphis, TN, and Denver, CO) have shown that the programme provides significant and consistent improvements in the health and well being of the most disadvantaged children and their families in both the short and the long term. Benefits include: improved school readiness; better prenatal health; improvement in women's antenatal health; fewer subsequent pregnancies; greater interval between births; reductions of between 50 and 70% in child injuries, neglect, and abuse; increases in employment; increases in the father's involvement; reductions in welfare dependency; and reduced substance use initiation (Kitzman *et al.*, 1997; Olds *et al.*, 1997, 1998, 2007). More recent follow-up of the children, some to the age of 19 years, continues to find physical, emotional, and social benefits, including improved behavioural and language functioning (Olds *et al.*, 2013); reductions in the number of girls entering the criminal justice system (Eckenrode *et al.*, 2010); reduced mortality among mothers; and reduced preventable-cause mortality in first-born children living in highly disadvantaged settings (Olds *et al.*, 2014).

The UK FNP Programme

The FNP programme was introduced in England in September 2006 as part of the government's Social Exclusion Action Plan (Cabinet Office, n.d.). Initially, it was piloted at 10 sites in England; now there is extensive coverage, with FNP offered in more than 130 local authority areas as of March 2015 (FNP National Unit, 2015a).

FNP nurses (mainly health visitors with additional training, known as 'family nurses') visit parents from early pregnancy until the child is 24 months old, building a close, supportive relationship with the whole family and guiding mothers to adopt healthier lifestyles, improve their parenting skills, and become self-sufficient (FNP National Unit, 2015a). Families are referred to the FNP through Midwifery Services and other partner agencies, such as Leaving Care, Teenage Pregnancy Services, and general practitioners (GPs). The enrolment criteria are: age 19 and under at the point of conception; first-time mother; gestation 14–28 weeks; and not newly delivered (i.e. must be pregnant) (FNP National Unit, 2015a).

The programme is voluntary, and each highly trained family nurse works with up to 25 mothers, providing intensive support through home visiting, whilst liaising closely with other community health and local authority services. The family nurses work exclusively on the FNP programme and are all registered with the Nursing and Midwifery Council (NMC). They work in teams of up to eight, led by FNP supervisors.

Characteristics

While the FNP Programme is modelled after the US programme, it has been customised to the UK context. The programme entails weekly or fortnightly structured home visits. It is theoretically driven based on ecological (Bronfenbrenner, 1979), attachment (Bowlby, 1969), and self-efficacy (Bandura, 1977) theories. Ecological theory stresses social context and interactions among individuals and the environments in which they are situated (see earlier). Attachment theory highlights the importance of the mother–infant relationship, while self-efficacy theory focuses on the importance of individuals' beliefs in achieving and directing behaviours. Self-efficacy in the parent role is encouraged by the strengths-based focus (i.e. focus on the parents' strengths, not their limitations) (FNP National Unit, 2015b).

The curriculum is specific and detailed, with a plan for the number, timing, and content of the visits. There is ongoing supervision of the practitioner, and detailed records are kept. The core of the programme is the formation of a strong, therapeutic, empathetic relationship with the mother (FNP National Unit, 2015a).

The home visits, delivered during pregnancy, infancy, and toddlerhood, focus on five domains, with specific times allotted to address each one (Ball *et al.*, 2012):

- personal health (35–40%);
- environmental health (5–7%);

- life course development (10–15%);
- maternal role (23–25%);
- family and friends (10–15%).

Evaluation and outcomes

Initial evaluations

The initial evaluation focused on the feasibility of the programme (prenatal and post-partum periods). It was important to know whether the programme, adapted from another jurisdiction (the USA), could be implemented in England; that is, could participants be recruited and retained in the programme and could the home visitors deliver the programme as outlined? The findings indicated that the programme was acceptable to the first-time mothers, as well as the fathers who participated. Participating practitioners valued the programme, although they found the work to be demanding. Some study sites found it challenging to meet recruitment and retention targets, and the number of visits to women was just over half (53%) of the targeted number. The evaluation was helpful in identifying best practice and barriers to working effectively with families, including how to strengthen the delivery of the service (Barnes *et al.*, 2008; Ball *et al.*, 2012).

Two follow-up evaluation studies addressed the implementation of the FNP Programme in 10 pilot sites in England. The first focused on the infancy phase (birth to 12 months; second-year evaluation) (Barnes *et al.*, 2009) and the second on the toddler age group (12–24 months; third-year evaluation) (Barnes *et al.*, 2011). The former aimed to uncover how the programme could be delivered with consistency and fidelity to the original programme model (i.e. that of David Olds) and how well the programme was meeting its stated objectives. Overall, the findings were positive, with most clients receiving at least half of the expected visits in infancy, retention rates on target (Ball *et al.*, 2012) and the programme being well received by families, family nurses, and supervisors (Barnes *et al.*, 2009; Ball *et al.*, 2012). The third-year evaluation (families followed until the child was 24 months – the usual programme leaving time) continued to find similar positive results, suggesting that the programme goals were being met. Some selective findings include general satisfaction with the programme among parents, a low attrition rate during the toddler period (7%) (Barnes *et al.*, 2011; Ball *et al.*, 2012), continued involvement of many fathers in the home visits, positive attitudes and interactions between mothers and their toddlers, and, for many mothers, a move to taking up education or paid work (Barnes *et al.*, 2011; DH, 2011a: 10).

These initial studies were formative evaluations, providing information and support for refinement of the delivery of the programme in order to maximise benefits. The next step was to design and implement a major evaluation of the outcomes of the FNP programme.

Evaluation of outcomes

Although the initial three evaluations were positive, the Department of Health in England commissioned a further evaluation to generate evidence about the benefits and costs of the FNP. Using an RCT, the researchers compared the initial (short-term) outcomes of the programme with those of standard services (study referred to as the Building Blocks Trial). The study was carried out in 18 primary care trusts/local authority sites across England. Over 12 months from June 2009, 1645 pregnant first-time mothers were recruited, with half randomised to receive routine care from maternity services plus FNP and the other half to receive routine care from maternity and child health services. Participants were followed up until their child's second birthday (Robling *et al.*, 2015).

Data were collected at the time of enrolment (baseline) and then via telephone interviews at 34–36 weeks prenatal and at 6 and 18 months following the birth. A face-to-face interview was carried out at 2 years after the birth. The study outcomes addressed (i) pregnancy and birth, (ii) the health and well being of the child, and (iii) the life course and economic self-sufficiency of the mother. Short-term primary outcomes (at 2 years) indicate few differences in pregnancy and birth outcomes. Tobacco use among mothers later in pregnancy was similar in both groups. There were no differences in birth weights, rates of a second pregnancy within 2 years, or children's emergency room visits or hospital admissions (Robling *et al.*, 2015). Assessments of secondary outcomes suggest some small positive benefits to children's cognitive development (as reported by mothers) and increased social support for mothers and mothers' intention to breastfeed. On most other criteria, though, there were few or no differences (Robling *et al.*, 2015).

In addition to client outcomes, the economic costs – including unit costs and cost-effectiveness (Owen-Jones *et al.*, 2013) – were assessed. The additional cost for enrolment in the programme was £1993 per mother. In view of the absence of evidence indicating programme cost-effectiveness, the study's lead researcher was unable to recommend its continuation (Robling *et al.*, 2015).

The findings from this major study will, undoubtedly, receive considerable scrutiny from policy makers, and their decisions will have a major impact on health visitors' work with young families in the future.

Flying Start – Wales

Background
Flying Start is an initiative of the Welsh Assembly Government, introduced in 2007 (National Assembly for Wales, 2014), one component of which is the Flying Start Health Visiting Core Programme, which focuses on partnership with parents and other professionals to provide support to families from the antenatal period through school age. The long-term aim of the initiative is to reduce income inequality by increasing the skill base of the population. It is an area-based programme, geographically targeted to some of the most disadvantaged areas of Wales, and is universally available to families with children from birth to age 4 in those areas.

Characteristics
Services are directed to families with children under 4 years old. They include enhanced health visiting, parenting support, support for early language development (primarily in the form of Language and Play programmes), and free, high-quality, part-time childcare for 2- to 3-year-old children (Government of Wales, 2013: 5). All mothers receive a detailed assessment in the antenatal period, and a detailed care plan is developed. The intensity of the follow-up is based on the level of need that

is identified (low, medium, or high). The goal is to provide all families with the level of care they need, reflecting the notion of progressive universalism (see earlier).

Evaluation and outcomes

A series of national evaluation reports for Flying Start are published on the Welsh government websites. These evaluations address a number of child and parental health impact criteria and suggest that the Flying Start programme is having an impact on parents' uptake of community services, satisfaction with services, and perceptions of support, which may translate, in the future, to enhanced parenting and improvement in children's well being. However, no statistically significant differences are found between Flying Start children and those not in the programme on measures of child cognitive and language skills, social and emotional development, and independence/self-regulation, although the possibility has been raised that the Flying Start children may have begun with lower cognitive and language skills than the comparison children (Government of Wales, 2013: 8).

The Triple-P (Positive Parenting Programme)

Background

The Triple-P (Positive Parenting Programme) is a prevention and treatment programme targeting children from birth to 16 years of age. It was developed in Australia and is widely implemented throughout the world, including in North America, Australia, New Zealand, and parts of Asia and Europe, including some locations in England, Ireland, and Scotland (Sanders, 2008). It is informed by ecological principles and therefore designed as a tiered, multilevel strategy that targets all families with young children (universal), incorporating five levels of intervention of increasing intensity. The rationale for the levels is based on a recognition of different levels of dysfunction and behavioural problems in children and of parents' differing needs and approaches in receiving assistance (Sanders, 2012).

The first level of intervention is a universal information media campaign (electronic and print media, radio, etc.) directed at all parents and focusing on common parenting problems (Sanders, 2008). Level 2 targets parents interested in parenting education or having specific concerns about their child's behaviour; their need may be addressed through a group seminar or by a brief telephone or face-to-face intervention. At level 3, parents require more information and support. The final two levels provide intensive parent and family programmes for children at risk of more severe behavioural problems (Sanders, 2008, 2012).

Characteristics

The chief characteristic of the programme is its flexible approach to parenting and family support. The central goal is to develop self-regulation in all involved (parents, children, and practitioners). It includes five core principles of positive parenting: providing a safe engaging environment, providing a positive learning environment, setting reasonable expectations, providing assertive discipline, and taking care of oneself as a parent (Prinz *et al.*, 2009). The programme is evidence-based and informed by social learning theories, with an emphasis on prevention and early intervention as well as treatment (Sanders, 2008). The flexibility and the focus on prevention and early intervention mean that, with additional training/education, health visitors can utilise components in their day-to-day work with families.

Evaluation and outcomes

A systematic review and meta-analysis of 101 studies (including 62 trials) concluded that social, emotional, and behavioural childhood outcomes – as well as broad parenting outcomes – can be achieved from the Triple-P parenting intervention (Sanders *et al.*, 2014). Aspects of the Triple-P are in use in several locations across the UK, including Glasgow, Birmingham, and Liverpool. In Birmingham, Triple-P for 4–9 year olds was used alongside other parenting interventions (e.g. Webster Stratton Incredible Years) as part of a Brighter Futures programme; however, with varying degrees of practitioner experience and variable parent attendance, the results were disappointing (Little *et al.*, 2012).

There is some evidence of positive outcomes in programmes carried out by health visitors, including a reduction in maternal anxiety and depression and in negative interactions between mothers and children (Long *et al.*, 2001). It is notable, however, that the most conclusive evidence is found when the health visitor has received additional training and education in a specific parenting intervention or approach (Stewart-Brown *et al.*, 2004; Papadopoulou *et al.*, 2005).

Maternal Early Childhood Sustained Home Visiting (MECSH)

Background

The MECSH programme originated in Australia. It is similar to the FNP programme in that it is targeted and delivers intensive home visiting during the antenatal period through to 2 years. This programme is firmly based on theoretical underpinnings of human ecology and strengths-based approaches to developing family partnerships (Kemp *et al.*, 2008). The key enrolment criterion, though, is high anxiety in the mother during pregnancy, rather than the age of the mother, parity (i.e. not restricted to first pregnancy), or social factors (Kemp *et al.*, 2008). The rationale for targeting this group of mothers is recognition of the importance of stress hormones in influencing brain development in infants (Kemp *et al.*, 2013). In addition to Australia, MECSH is also being worked with in England, Jersey, Australia, South Korea, and Vermont, USA. The England sites include Essex, Plymouth, and Lewisham.

Characteristics

The midwife carries out the initial assessment using well-established assessment tools such as the Edinburgh postnatal anxiety index. Parents eligible for the MECSH programme will be visited by health visitors with additional training in the 'parent advisor' model (Davis *et al.*, 2002). Home visiting starts antenatally and continues until the child reaches 2 years. A child development programme is used to work with parents' strengths to enhance the quality of the home learning environment and parenting capacity (Kemp *et al.*, 2011). In addition, the health visitor will endeavour to put parents in touch with a wider range of social networks and 'mesh' the parent with the local community. As well as helping the parent develop personal support networks, the whole-system approach should also enable greater continuity in care among the services and agencies relevant to each individual family (Whittaker, 2014).

Evaluation and outcomes

An RCT of MESCH with an ethnically diverse population of Australian mothers (aged 15–45 years) demonstrated outcomes of improved child and maternal mental well being, longer breastfeeding, and greater maternal sensitivity to child needs, which supports positive child development (Kemp et al., 2011). Thus far, funding for a UK trial has not been granted; however, when setting up the South of England MECSH sites, the Australian developers established data monitoring systems to collect outcome data and provide evidence of impacts for service commissioners.

Sure Start programmes

Background

While not a home visiting programme, Sure Start is a family support resource which operates in conjunction with home visiting programmes. For this reason, as well as its widespread dissemination in England and Scotland, it is included in this section.

Sure Start local programmes (SSLPs) were developed in 1999, aimed at working with parents and expectant parents to promote the physical and intellectual development of children – initially those under 4 years of age, although this was later extended to under 5 years with the move to Sure Start children's centres programmes as part of the Every Child Matters programme. Social Services funding initially concentrated on the most deprived localities but now provides universal access for all families. In England, the centres have been implemented in three phases, with the aim of having 3400 in place by 2010 – one for every community in England. Since 2010, government austerity measures have meant a cut in the financing of children's centres, although it has been estimated that there were still 3000 in operation in England in 2013 (Rallings, 2014). Scotland Sure Start, however, has now been replaced by the Early Years Framework, delivered through the multiagency Early Years Collaborative, a programme launched in October 2012 to support the transformation of early years (Scottish Government, 2012).

Characteristics

Services include play and early education learning experiences, child care, primary and community health care, support for children with special needs, and parenting and family support through area-based programmes (Audit Commission, 2010; DfE, 2013). There is an emphasis on coordination of services, outreach, and community development to improve services. Family and parenting support is a strong emphasis in SSLPs; this may also include adult learning services and general support. Support is provided either directly by staff or through coordination and referral (Barlow et al., 2007b). Children's centres, by being rooted in specific communities, can also provide innovative services to enable parents to better manage day-to-day life. For example, Barnardo's Benchill children's centre in Wythenshawe, South Manchester works with the local registry office to provide birth registration sessions on site, thus saving parents of newborns a journey to the city centre to register births (Rallings, 2014: 14).

Evaluation and outcomes

The National Evaluation of Sure Start was initially led by Professor Edward Melhuish and colleagues at the Institute for the Study of Children, Families and Social Issues, Birkbeck, University of London. This was an extensive evaluation, addressing the implementation, impact, local context analysis, cost–effectiveness, and support of local programmes. Findings to date suggest some benefits to children and families who participate in Sure Start programmes. The impact of SSLPs on 3-year-olds and their families was assessed through an evaluation of 14 outcomes, including language development, social and emotional development, and physical health. Accidental injury decreased and immunisation rates increased, although improvements were slight (NESS, 2008). In another study of children at age 3, differences in the implementation of SSLPs were examined in relation to effectiveness using a quasi-experimental method (Belsky et al., 2006). The outcomes assessed were mothers' reports of community services, family functioning and parenting skills, child health and development, and children's verbal ability at age 36 months. The results suggested that SSLPs had beneficial effects on non-teenage mothers (i.e. better parenting, better social functioning in children). Evaluation when children were age 7 suggested improvements in 4 of 55 outcomes for children in the SSLP group. Three directly addressed improvement in the quality of the home environment for children (less harsh discipline, more stimulating home learning, and a less chaotic home environment for boys (no differences for girls)). In addition, lone parents and households without a working member reported better life satisfaction (DfE, 2012).

The findings of economic benefit from SSLPs to age 5 are promising with, cost savings estimated at between £279 and £557 per eligible child (Meadows, 2011). More parents in the study area took up paid employment than in comparison areas, and improvements in the quality of the home environment may translate into economic benefit in the future (Meadows, 2011: 1–2). The economic benefit analysis, though, was complicated by the introduction of free early education for 3- and 4-year-olds living in SSLP areas (Meadows, 2011: 2), which meant that the control children received many similar educational and support services to those in the Sure Start programme.

The evaluation of the Sure Start initiative now focuses on the children's centres. A 6-year evaluation project is underway, commissioned by the Department of Education and undertaken by NatCen Social Research, the University of Oxford, and Frontier Economics (Department for Education, 2014). The aim of the Evaluation of Children's Centres in England (ECCE) project is to provide an in-depth understanding of children's centre services, including their effectiveness for children and families and their economic cost in relation to different types of service (Evangelou et al., 2014: 4). The report addressing parenting services (Strand 3) focuses on service users' and providers' perceptions of service usage and user statistics. Services are categorised into four areas of parental need: personal needs of the parent; parent and child; parent and family; and parent and community (Department for Education, 2014: 4).

The findings of the Sure Start initiative are generally positive. Future reports will provide additional understanding of the benefits of children's centres, including outcomes for parents and children.

Summary

The outline of programmes in this section (see Table 4.1) is not intended to be an exhaustive list of all programmes, but rather a few examples of current and/or seminal programmes, indicating what interventions appear to 'work' or not work in supporting young families. Other programmes and approaches have recently been introduced or implemented in some areas in the UK. For example, the Fulfilling Lives: A Better Start initiative has been funded by the National Lottery and introduced within five areas in England to support the use of early preventive approaches during pregnancy and the first 3 years of life. The focus of the initiative is on improving outcomes for children in three key areas of development: social and emotional development; communication and language development; and nutrition. Its fundamental approach to service delivery involves the local health authority, public services, and the voluntary sector working together to put prevention in early life at the heart of service delivery and practice (Big Lottery Fund, 2013). The hope is to see systemic change, with prevention being a central principle governing service design and delivery, as well as thinking by partners. Future evaluations of this and other programmes will contribute to our understanding of what supports are most effective in improving the health and well being of children.

Working with families

The proliferation of programmes does not necessarily mean that they all use different interventions: many programmes appear to be similar in terms of helping interventions but use different terminology. There is recognition of the importance of practitioners developing supportive, trusting relationships with parents and the need to work in partnership with families. For example, providers in children's centres report that the development of relationships with parents is the most popular approach for encouraging and sustaining parents' attendance (reported by 99% of centres) (Evangelou *et al.*, 2014: 5).

These concepts are clearly articulated in many of the programmes outlined in the previous section. They are not particularly 'new' in professional–client relationships, however; nor, many would argue, are they 'new' to health visiting practice. However, the importance of developing supportive relationships when working with young, vulnerable families is now clearly articulated (All Party Parliamentary Group for Conception to Age 2 – The First 1001 Days, 2015).

What is meant by 'supportive relationships' and 'working in partnership'? Research exploring parents' experiences of health visiting by Donetto *et al.* (2013) illustrates that supportive relationships with health visitors include the following features: being known, being given time, being listened to, being offered reassurance and praise (which is consistent with supporting self-efficacy), and knowing that a trustworthy source of help is available if one needs to call on it. Trust is considered the foundation upon which effective practice is built, and it is a necessary part of the health visitor–parent relationship. Working in partnership acknowledges the worth of both parties and sensitivity to issues of power and control. However, the evidence from the Donetto *et al.* (2013) study also affirms concerns that professional

Table 4.1 Child health promotion programmes.

Programme name, location, dates	Key elements	Key findings	Recommendations and comments
First Parent Health Visiting Programme (Child Development Programme) (UK) Developed by Professor Walter Barker of Bristol University in the early 1980s; implemented in the UK	Ante- and postnatal home visits at monthly intervals, by appointment Targeted to disadvantaged children Structured home visiting, with a focus on child development Health visitors work in partnership with families; parents are the 'experts' on their own children	Outcomes assessed at ages 1 and 2 years Few differences between the group receiving first parent services and comparison mothers and children	Evaluation may have been influenced by 'control' health visitors using principles from the programme
Community Mothers' Programme (CMP) (Northern Ireland) Developed in Dublin, 1983	Community mothers (volunteers) monthly visit first-born and (sometimes) second children Emphasis on support, encouragement, and guidance, rather than direct advice	Several positive findings: • For children: primary immunisations, being read to daily, nutrition • For mothers: better diet than controls, less likely to report being tired and miserable, more positive feelings Benefits to children and mothers continued to age 8	With some modifications, the programme is found in a number of areas in the UK, where volunteers provide families with additional support (e.g. the Home Start Programme) Evidence confirms that families perceive personal benefits from volunteer family support Further research is needed to evaluate cost-effectiveness

(Continued)

Table 4.1 (Continued)

Programme name, location, dates	Key elements	Key findings	Recommendations and comments
Family Nurse Partnership (FNP) (England) Based on David Olds' (US) programme; introduced in 2006	Based on ecological, attachment and self-efficacy theories Targeted to vulnerable families from antenatal to age 24 months Structured intensive home visits to build close, supportive relationships and guide parents to adopt healthier lifestyles, improve their parenting skills, and become self-sufficient	Initially piloted at 10 sites; after initial positive feedback, expanded to 20 new sites in 2008 In the third-year evaluation, families were followed until the child was 24 months The findings suggest that the programme goals were being met, parents were satisfied with the programme, and the attrition rate was low during the toddler period A randomised controlled trial (RCT) reported in October 2015 found few differences between FNP and 'usual care' mothers and children	The lead researcher of the RCT considers that the current evidence of outcomes does not justify the continuation of the programme It is not known at this point if differences in child outcomes might be found with longer term follow-up
Flying Start (Wales) Implemented in 2007	Programme targeted to disadvantaged areas and universally available to families with children aged 0 to 4 years Services include enhanced health visiting, parenting support, support for early language development, and free, high-quality, part-time childcare for 2- to 3-year-old children	Evaluations suggest the programme has an impact on parents' uptake of community services, satisfaction with services, and perceptions of support No statistically significant differences were found between Flying Start children and those not in the programme on measures of child cognitive and language skills, social and emotional development, or independence/self-regulation	The researchers raise the issue that the Flying Start Children may have started with lower cognitive and language skills than the comparison children

Programme	Description	Evidence	Additional notes
Triple-P (Positive Parenting Programme) (some locations in the UK) Developed in Australia	Preventive and treatment programme for children from infancy to age 16 years Five levels of intervention, of increasing intensity Core principles of promoting competence and self-regulation and evidence-based interventions	Evaluated in 62 trials: social, emotional, and behavioural childhood outcomes and broad parenting outcomes have been achieved Some research shows positive benefits from health visitors carrying out components of the programme	Aspects of the programme can be delivered by many disciplines
Maternal Early Childhood Sustained Home Visiting (MECSH) Developed in Australia and implemented in parts of England in 2012	Home visiting programme delivered by health visitors or an international equivalent Health visitors use an approach informed by the 'parent advisor' model to work with parents as partners Plan of home visits designed to support positive child development and parental self-efficacy	Trial evidence indicates that following support from a MECSH health visitor in the first 2 years, mothers are more emotionally responsive and sustain breastfeeding for longer than control-group mothers Benefits are also found for mothers who have been identified with psychological distress during the antenatal period	The MECSH programme is designed to provide intensive support in the home and to connect parents with services in the wider community It is suitable for families that need the universal partnership plus level of service offer It differs from FNP in that the mother's age and parity are not used as eligibility criteria for the MECSH service
Sure Start local programmes (SSLPs; now known as Sure Start children's centres) (UK) Developed in 1999	Promote physical and intellectual development of children up to age 5, including play and learning experiences, support for parents, primary and community health care, coordination of services, outreach, and community development Initially, centres were targeted to deprived areas, but now service is universal	Extensive evaluation has addressed implementation, impact, local context analysis, and cost-effectiveness To date, Sure Start and children's centres have resulted in some health improvements; research is ongoing	Specialised supports may also be available to parents, including therapeutic services such as counselling (cognitive behavioural and family therapy) adult learning, and general support

relationships are not always helpful, especially when advice offered during interactions is standardised and nonspecific to the individual needs and circumstances of the client. It highlights how in professional practice, the practitioner still holds considerable power in structuring and directing the interaction (i.e. interview, home visit). It is largely the professional's concept of the client's needs and problems which shapes who is recruited into programmes, how long visits will last, and what will be discussed. When the health visitor carries out an ongoing assessment of the family environment, she or he is also being observed and being judged on her or his attitudes, trustworthiness, friendliness, knowledge, and personal appearance. In addition, the client is aware that the health visitor has information of a personal nature relating to their family and has some power over the fate of the family.

When the health visitor 'delivers' the programme (more or less structured), she or he must also address any needs that the parents consider important. If she or he does not, the parents may withdraw from the interaction and the relationship between the two parties may be impaired – leading to critical life events not being acknowledged and appropriate interventions, including referrals, not being made. It is interesting to reflect on reports of child abuse, spousal abuse, and incest which have come to light months or years after professionals have 'worked with' people but failed to uncover the core problems affecting their well being.

It is also important to acknowledge that, as practitioners, we may impose our reality on the visit. We can see what we want to see, or what we have been taught to expect. As health visitors, our knowledge comes from our own education and experiences, but there is no guarantee that the subjects of our study fully describe the reality of people's lives. Many health visitors have little direct personal experience with the impacts of poverty, relationship breakdown, partner abandonment, beatings, negative cultural views of women in society, low literacy, severe stresses of motherhood (e.g. postpartum depression), lack of family support, and many other stressors.

In recent years, qualitative research approaches have been employed which acknowledge and validate the lived experience of people as they carry out their lives. This knowledge can sensitise health visitors to the types of stressor which families may be facing – without dismissing the fact that there are also strengths. It is helpful – and, we would argue, necessary – to acknowledge these potential impacts as the health visitor begins her or his work with families.

Empirical evidence on relationship development

There is evidence that parents value supportive relationships with their health visitors and other children's services workers (Worth & Hogg, 2000; Russell & Drennan, 2007; Donetto & Maben, 2014; Whittaker et al., 2014). Despite the importance of developing supportive relationships between parents and health visitors, how the process occurs is not explicit (Davis & Tsiantis, 2005). There is little empirical literature which documents just how relationships are developed or what are the outcomes of this process. Some early work on home visiting interactions using observation (videotaping) and follow-up interviews with clients and public health nurses suggests the importance of a friendly, relaxed affect when connecting with community clients and of paying attention to both verbal and nonverbal cues during interactions (Kristjanson & Chalmers, 1990). Trust has been identified as important, enabling the disclosure of sensitive topics (Jack *et al.*, 2002; McIntosh & Shute, 2006; Thompson, 2011).

In an early study of health visiting practice, several issues influenced building and maintenance of the health visitor–mother relationship (Chalmers & Luker, 1991; Chalmers, 1992b). Both health visitors and parents (usually mothers) controlled what they offered to and accepted from each other. The 'offer' had to be something of value to the client, which varied from client to client but might include timely and helpful information, support in the care of the child, and material supports. When the health visitor was seen as 'giving' something helpful, the relationship was able to develop and flourish. When this happened, the health visitor was often able to progress in her or his work with the family and uncover other concerns in need of attention.

More recent work by Bidmead (2013) illustrates how parents attempt to exercise control over their interactions with health visitors, and thus confirms the active role of parents during visits. However, the author suggests that parents' inability to give or ask for information from the health visitor may not be entirely governed by their need to control the conversation but instead be related to a lack of confidence (Bidmead, 2013: 21) Bidmead's work is particularly noteworthy for the method of data collection used: interactions between health visitors and parents were videotaped, and feedback was obtained from both parties. The findings highlight that parents valued continuity of care with a single health visitor and preferred contacts to occur at home, rather than at busy clinics. Health visitors noted that it took time to develop relationships, which was challenging with very busy caseloads in areas of high needs; administrative support was important in this regard, as it freed the health visitors to build client relationships properly. Both groups identified the importance of trust in developing the health visitor–client relationship. You can explore this relationship further in Activity 4.3

Whittaker *et al.* (2014) note the importance of a strengths-based approach when developing relationships, to ensure that client capacities, knowledge, and skills are acknowledged and valued. They also draw on earlier work by Howe (1996), who proposed the concept of 'surface and depth' in work with clients. In the 'surface' approach, practitioners attempt to address the clients' current needs or problems and not the more complex problems underpinning them. There is little focus on the interactions between the practitioner and client in this approach. Examples might include addressing child feeding issues or positive approaches to discipline. In the 'depth' approach, the practitioner uses theoretical knowledge in an attempt to gain a more in-depth understanding of the clients' life experiences. In this approach, the skills the practitioner brings in building relationships and uncovering core life experiences are particularly important. Whittaker *et al.* (2014) used this theoretical perspective in a study of families who repeatedly accessed services providing intensive family support. Interviews with parents and staff emphasised the importance of practical help and of practitioners who engage meaningfully with clients and focus on strengths, and the need for practitioners to try to really understand their clients' life experiences. Whittaker *et al.* (2014) consider that both surface and depth approaches are important when working with families experiencing complex life events and circumstances.

Because of the voluntary nature of the health service, successful recruitment of families (usually mothers) into programmes is crucial if they are to receive their benefits. For example, the FNP is voluntary, and eligible pregnant young women can refuse the service. Whittaker & Cowley (2012) explain that it is not enough merely to have effective programmes in place, as their full benefit will only be realised if parents attend and engage with their content. It is recommended that health visitors appreciate the importance of their role as referral agents, as the initial presentation of a programme or service can influence later attendance and the ongoing relationship between the parent and health visitor. Much more understanding is needed – not only about how to develop supportive relationships and work in partnership with families, but also about the role these relationships play in achieving programme outcomes. Relationships, though, are not the only challenges when attempting to support families; several others may affect the capacity of the health visitor to develop supportive relationships and influence the overall outcomes of the programme. In the next section, these challenges are examined in relationship to planning and delivering services to young families.

Challenges

Working with young families that have high needs can often be challenging, regardless of the programme framework within which the health visitor works. In this section, we examine some of the challenges health visitors face, and some possible underlying reasons for them.

Public health agenda

The public health approach to supporting families is a population health approach focusing on the identification of community-wide needs using various assessment frameworks and statistical data. Targets or goals are then established to 'benchmark' necessary changes and programmes are introduced to improve health indices. These health indices may include breastfeeding rates in the population, smoking rates in pregnant women, school completion for teenage mothers, and so on. The indices and goals are very important in allowing governments and health and social care planners to see the 'big picture'. While the goals and targets are evidence-based, the public health agenda is programme-driven rather than client-driven. The health visitor working within this framework needs to ensure that the stated 'targets' are met. At times, this may conflict with the clients' stated needs and wants from the offered service and influence the capacity of the health visitor to work in partnership with the family. For example, if a programme goal is to reduce prenatal smoking rates, the health visitor who addresses this issue enthusiastically and repeatedly (with accurate but unwanted information on the hazards of smoking) may hinder the development of the relationship with the client, resulting in little engagement around this or other health issues, or even in client withdrawal from the programme. A skilled health visitor has to learn when and how to raise the programme-identified goals in a way that keeps the client engaged.

Level of evidence

To date, the evidence to support positive outcomes from many programmes aimed at young families is mixed. This may be due to a number of factors: poorly designed evaluation studies, overly ambitious 'unreachable' targets in the original programme plan, conceptualisations of service delivery that are difficult to implement fully, and 'importation' of programmes from other jurisdictions which appear promising but do not deliver, to name just a few. Basing programmes on 'what works' in other jurisdictions with vastly different community health care services is problematic even when the programmes are carefully 'adapted' to the local context. The US FNP programme, for example, compared well with usual service in that context (which was very little professional home support). However, 'usual care' in the UK provides considerable midwifery and health visiting support for vulnerable families, which may make it difficult to uncover differences between groups, due to a 'ceiling effect'; that is, home visiting support may improve mothers' health and parenting (in both enhanced and usual care groups), but only up to a certain point (or ceiling). Another issue is that the effect of programmes may take longer to show a benefit than the defined evaluation period. Programmes may be withdrawn by governments before outcomes have been thoroughly evaluated, particularly if earlier findings are mixed. This leaves an 'evidence vacuum' for researchers, policy makers, and practitioners.

The capacity to develop supportive and helpful relationships within the context of particular programmes is a critical skill that health visitors must learn and practise. Programmes may suit some families more than others, and this can affect findings. It is not always clear why some programmes do not deliver the outcomes which were expected (or hoped for). It is important that we continue to learn through qualitative research and process evaluations how to deliver programmes that address the complex and varied needs of parents.

Adhering to the programme criteria

Most programmes in the current health care context are to be delivered according to structured criteria over specific time periods. In the FNP programme, for example, the visit is divided into specific focal areas, with a time allotment for each. Whether this structured approach is the 'best practice' for all families needs further assessment through feedback (research-based) from parents and practitioners. There is some evidence that the implementation of standardised assessments to identify children at risk of abuse has not improved the identification of children at risk; furthermore, this approach may inhibit the development of health visitors' relationships with parents, erode trust, and reduce access to families (Cowley et al., 2013a: 19).

Further, the child health visiting programme literature concludes that many families do not receive the programme according to the stated objectives. For example, families may receive only about half of the intended visits, and 20–67% of families leave programmes prior to the intended termination date (Gomby, 1999). Early evaluations of the FNP programme found that 87% of clients received half or more of the expected visits during pregnancy and early infancy (Barnes et al., 2009). Recent research on the US FNP programme found that more parents were retained over time (compared to controls) when the nurses gave parents more control over the frequency and content of visits (Olds et al., 2015).

Poor attendance affects the strength of the evaluation, yet few studies control for bias caused by dropouts and nonattendance (Whittaker & Cowley, 2012). If families are not receiving the full complement of visits or the visits do not conform to the programme standards, this creates difficulty in evaluating whether outcomes are due to deficiencies in the programme or to the lack of adherence. It is important that programme evaluations build in, when possible, interviews with clients who do not complete the programme (or otherwise do not adhere to the stated objectives) in order to provide helpful information on issues related to retention and programme delivery.

High-needs families

Under the current implementation plan (DH, 2011b), services are directed universally to all children based on families' needs. All young children have access to universal services (newborn visits, developmental assessments, etc.). Those with more needs receive additional visits from the health visitor for targeted and ongoing help and, as required, referral to community services. For services to be beneficial, though, additional diagnostic and supportive services need to be available and the parent needs to access these resources.

The health visitor has an important role in assisting high-needs families to understand and accept additional services and in 'staying connected' to the family while additional supports are being put in place. Many high-needs families might benefit from referrals and additional supports but, for a variety of reasons, not attend the programmes or services. They might have had negative experiences with persons perceived to be 'in authority', be fearful of exposing their parenting to professional criticism, or be overwhelmed with general living concerns. The experience of parent support programmes such as Sure Start and Head Start (in the USA) suggests that the most 'needy' parents are the least likely to participate or the most likely to drop out (Olds et al., 2015); this has been called the 'inverse care law' (see also Chapter 3) (Hall & Hall, 2007). Accurately understanding family need, matching it against available resources, and carefully communicating offers of help are critical steps in helping to put parents, and thereby children, in contact with services (Whittaker & Cowley, 2012). Moreover, making referrals to other community services is a key responsibility of professionals addressing health inequalities (Allen et al., 2013), and, therefore, learning to refer families successfully (i.e. so that the service is used) is an important skill for health visitors to develop.

Practice specialisation

Does a specialised approach (i.e. working in one programme only, such as the FNP) provide the best outcomes for families? This appears to be an assumption underlying the structuring of many programmes. The FNP and other programmes like it are reported to be intensive and demanding on staff and supervisors (Barnes *et al.*, 2009); little is known at present about provider burnout and retention of staff in these programmes.

Other models for health visiting practice, such as the family-centred public health role (Audit Commission, 2010), may entail working across various 'levels'; for example, working with groups and the community (e.g. community development) as well as with families. However, this more 'generic' approach raises questions as to the skill set which health visitors need in order to work effectively at all levels, including the 'community level' (see also Chapter 3). It is likely that many skills, such as in-depth community assessments, community development, and social capital building require advanced knowledge and practice that are gained through specialised education and opportunities to learn in the community. Also, when practitioners work across several areas, the child support programme may take a 'back seat' to other public health priorities, such as mandated communicable diseases control (Woodgate *et al.*, 2007). However, working in only one programme may contribute to service 'silos', in which many practitioners from different agencies provide services to the same family. With the widespread implementation of the CAF (see earlier and Chapter 5), this problem may be lessening.

Concerns about child safety

Despite the importance of building relationships based on partnerships, this is not always easy. Child safety and client denial and blocking of problems have been reported as being particularly stressful for home visitors (Woodgate *et al.*, 2007). Health visitors attempting to work 'in partnership' with clients may encounter instances when they are concerned that a parent is not providing adequate care or is not moving forward in learning appropriate care-giving behaviours. The health visitor needs the skill to communicate expectations concerning level of care clearly to parents in as supportive manner as possible. There is little in the 'partnership' literature on how this process is best learned and managed.

Adequate resources

Programmes supporting the parenting of young children need sufficient resources, including a manageable ratio of families per health visitor. In addition, there must be other community support available, where families can access peer support and other resources, such as Sure Start children's centre programmes. Support from supervisors is also critical (Wallbank & Woods, 2012), and both practitioners and supervisors need adequate in-service training in order to carry out their roles well. This includes training in using new technologies and systems that support mobile working (see Health & Social Care Information Centre, 2016).

It is important that there is sufficient and ongoing in-service education to ensure that health visitors' skills match the needs of vulnerable families. This includes skills in assessment. Evidence based on direct observation of parent–child interactions (interactions were videotaped and subjected to rigorous analysis) suggests considerable variation among health visitors in the identification of problems in the same interactions (Wilson *et al.*, 2010). This study points to the need for adequate resources (both amount and type) to uncover the learning needs of health visitors, regardless of the type of programme in which they work. This is a particular issue for health visitors, given that most of their work takes place in the home, with little opportunity for their assessments to be 'validated' by a supervisor or peers. Also, with the implementation of progressive (now referred to as 'proportionate') universalism in some jurisdictions, it is imperative that practitioners be able to accurately assess the level of need in families in order to allocate ongoing resources (Wilson *et al.*, 2010).

Summary

This chapter examined approaches and programmes aimed at the support of families with young children. Currently, there appears to be political support to invest in programmes which lead to improved outcomes for children and parents. Once available, details of the outcomes of the FNP and other programmes will provide important data for their widespread implementation and adjustment.

Improving the social determinants of health for young families is critical if the long-term impacts on high-needs children and parents are to be ameliorated. However, home visiting and group support programmes are just one component of measures to enhance the well being of vulnerable families. The development of social cohesion at the community level (i.e. social capital) (Rocco & Suhrcke, 2012) is increasingly seen as a key approach to helping mitigate the effects of the social determinants of health and improving health outcomes among the most disadvantaged members of society (Marmot *et al.*, 2010). Health visitors can have a role to play at this broader community level, as well as in the family, and can make a substantial contribution to improving the nation's health.

Note

Some parts of this chapter were adapted from Orr, J. (1992) Assessing individual and family health needs. In: *Health Visiting: Towards Community Health Nursing* (eds K. Luker & J. Orr). Blackwell Science, Oxford. pp. 107–58.

References

Allen, M., Allen, J., Hogarth, S. & Marmot, M. (2013) Working for Health Equity: The Role of health professionals. Report, UCL Institute of Health Equity, London.

All Party Parliamentary Group for Conception to Age 2 – The First 1001 Days (2015) Building Great Britons. Available from: http://www.1001criticaldays.co.uk/buildinggreatbritonsreport.pdf (last accessed 30 March 2016).

Audit Commission (2010) *Giving Children a Healthy Start: Health Report.* Available from: http://www3.lancashire.gov.uk/corporate/enewsviewer/frmDcDnLd.asp?id=9283 (last accessed 30 March 2016).

Ball, M., Barnes, J. & Meadows, P. (2012) Issues Emerging from the First 10 Pilot Sites Implementing the Nurse-Family Partnership Home-Visiting Programme in England. Department of Health, London. Available from: http://www.iscfsi.bbk.ac.uk/projects/files/Issues%20arising%20from%20FNP%20-Evaluation-July-2012.pdf (last accessed 30 March 2016).

Bandura, A. (1977) Self-efficacy: towards a unifying theory of behavioural change. *Psychological Review*, **84**, 191–215.

Barker, W. (1984) Child Development Programme. Early Childhood Development Unit, Senate House, University of Bristol, Bristol.

Barker, W. & Anderson, R. (1988) Child Development Programme: An Evaluation of Process and Outcomes. Early Child Development Unit, University of Bristol.

Barlow J., Davis H., McIntosh E., Jarrett P., Mockford C. & Stewart-Brown S. (2007a) Role of home visiting in improving parenting and health in families at risk of abuse and neglect: results of a multicentre randomised controlled trial and economic evaluation. *Archives of Disease in Childhood* **92**, 229–33.

Barlow, J., Kirkpatrick, S., Wood, D., Ball, M. & Stewart-Brown, S. (2007b) *Sure Start National Evaluation Summary: Family and Parenting Support in Sure Start Local Programmes.* Available from: http://www.education.gov.uk/research/data/uploadfiles/NESS2007SF023.pdf (last accessed 30 March 2016).

Barlow, J., Johnston, I., Kendrick, D., Polnay, L. & Stewart-Brown, S. (2008) Individual and group-based parenting programmes for the treatment of physical child abuse and neglect. *Cochrane Database of Systematic Reviews*, **2008** (4):CD005463.

Barlow, J., Smailagic, N., Ferriter, M., Bennett, C. & Jones, H. (2010) Group-based parent-training programmes for improving emotional and behavioural adjustment in children from birth to three years old. *Cochrane Database of Systematic Reviews*, 2010 (3):CD003680.

Barnes, J., MacPherson, K. & Senior, R. (2006). Factors influencing the acceptance of volunteer home-visiting support offered to families with new babies. *Child & Family Social Work*, **11**, 107–17.

Barnes, L., Ball, M., Meadows, P., McLeish, J., Belsky, J. & the FNP Implementation Research Team (2008) *Nurse-Family Partnership Programme: First Year Pilot Sites, Implementation in England. Pregnancy and the Post Partum Period.* Research Report DCSF-RW051 Department for Children, Schools and Families, London. Available from: http://www.iscfsi.bbk.ac.uk/projects/files/Year-1-report-Barnes-et-al.pdf (last accessed 30 March 2016).

Barnes, L., Ball, M., Meadows, P., McLeish, J., Belsky, J. & the FNP Implementation Team (2009) *Nurse-Family Partnership Programme: Second Year Pilot Sites, Implementation in England. The Infancy Period.* Research Report DCSF-RR166. Department for Children, Schools and Families, London. Available from: http://www.iscfsi.bbk.ac.uk/projects/files/Second_year.pdf (last accessed 30 March 2016).

Barnes, J., Ball, M, Meadows, P., Howden, B., Jackson, A, Henderson, J. & Niven, L. (2011) The Family-Nurse Partnership Programme in England: Wave 1 Implementation in Toddlerhood & a Comparison between Waves 1 and 2a of Implementation in Pregnancy and Infancy. Institute for Study of Children, Families and Social Issues, Birkbeck, University of London. Available from: https://www.gov.uk/government/uploads/system/uploads/attachment_data/file/215837/dh_123366.pdf (last accessed 30 March 2016).

Belsky, J., Melhuish, E., Barnes, J., Leyland, A.H. & Romaniuk, H. (2006) The National Evaluation of Sure Start Research Team Effects of Sure Start local programmes on children and families: early findings from a quasi-experimental, cross sectional study. *British Medical Journal*, **332**, 1476.

Bidmead, C. (2013) Appendix 1: Health visitor/parent relationships: a qualitative analysis. In: Why Health Visiting? A Review of the Literature about Key Health Visitor Interventions, Processes and Outcomes for Children and Families (eds S. Cowley, K. Whittaker, A. Grigulis, M. Malone, S. Donetto, H. Wood, E. Morrow & J. Maben). National Nursing Research Unit, King's College, London. Available from: https://www.kcl.ac.uk/nursing/research/nnru/publications/Reports/Appendices-12-02-13.pdf (last accessed 30 March 2016).

Big Lottery Fund (2013) *A Better Start: Aiming to Deliver a Change to Improve the Life Chances of Children Aged 0–3*. Available from: https://www.biglotteryfund.org.uk/betterstart (last accessed 30 March 2016).

Bowlby, J. (1969) Attachment and Loss, vol. **1**. Attachment. Basic Books, New York.

Bronfenbrenner, U. (1979) The Ecology of Human Development: Experiments by Nature and Design. Harvard University Press, London.

Brown, R.E., Wills, T.A., Aspinall, N., Hunt, C., George, J. & Rudolf, M.C.J. (2013) Preventing child obesity: a long term evaluation of the HENRY approach. *Community Practitioner*, **86**(7), 23–7.

Brown, S. (2014). Clinical update: A small service evaluation of a Solihull approach foster carer training group pilot study. *Practice*, **26**(1), 37–52.

Brugha, T., Morrell, C., Slade, P. & Walters, S. (2011) Universal prevention of depression in women postnatally: cluster randomized trial evidence in primary care. *Psychological Medicine*, **41**(4), 739–48.

Bryans, A., Cornich, E. & McIntosh, J. (2009) The potential of the ecological theory for building an integrated framework to develop the public health contribution of health visiting. *Health and Social Care in the Community*, **17**(6), 564–72.

Bull, J., McCormick, G., Swann, C. & Mulvihill, C. (2004) *Ante-natal and Post-natal Home Visiting Programmes: A Review of Reviews (Report)*. Available from: http://www.healthevidence.org/view-article.aspx?a=20126 (last accessed 30 March 2016).

Cabinet Office XXXX (n.d.) *Progress on Social Exclusion Action Plan: Reaching Out: Progress on Social Exclusion*. Available from: http://www.bristol.ac.uk/poverty/downloads/keyofficialdocuments/Reaching%20out%20progress.pdf (last accessed 30 March 2016).

Calder, M.C., McKinnon, M. & Sneddon, R. (2012). National Risk Framework to Support the Assessment of Children and Young People Scottish Government, Edinburgh. Available from: http://www.gov.scot/Publications/2012/11/7143 (last accessed 30 March 2016).

Carers UK (2014) *Facts about Carers 2014*. Available from: https://www.carersuk.org/for-professionals/policy/policy-library/facts-about-carers-2014 (last accessed 30 March 2016).

Center on the Developing Child at Harvard University (2010) *The Foundations of Lifelong Health Are Built in Early Childhood*. Available from: http://developingchild.harvard.edu/resources/the-foundations-of-lifelong-health-are-built-in-early-childhood/ (last accessed 30 March 2016).

CETHV (1977) An Investigation into the Principles of Health Visiting. Council for the Education and Training of Health Visitors, London.

Chalmers, K.I. (1992a) Working with men: an analysis of health visiting practice in families with young children. *International Journal of Nursing Studies*, **29**(1), 3–16.

Chalmers, K.I. (1992b) Giving and receiving: an empirically derived theory of health visiting practice. *Journal of Advanced Nursing*, **17**(11), 1317–25.

Chalmers, K.I. & Luker, K. (1991) The development of the health visitor-client relationship. *Scandinavian Journal of Caring Sciences*, **5**(1), 33–41.

Christie, J. & Bunting, B. (2011). The effect of health visitors' postpartum home visit frequency on first-time mothers: cluster randomised trial. *International Journal of Nursing Studies*, **48**(6), 689–702.

Collins, F. & McCray, J. (2012). Partnership working in services for children: use of the common assessment framework. *Journal of Interprofessional Care*, **26**(2), 134–40.

Cowley S., Whittaker, K., Malone, M., Donetto, S., Grigulis, A. & Maben, J. (2013a) Why Health Visiting? A Review of the Literature about Key Health Visitor Interventions, Processes and Outcomes for Children and Families. National Nursing Research Unit, King's College, London. Available from: https://www.kcl.ac.uk/nursing/research/nnru/publications/Reports/Why-Health-Visiting-NNRU-report-12-02-2013.pdf (last accessed 30 March 2016).

Cowley S., Whittaker, K., Grigulis, A., Malone, M., Donetto, S., Wood, H., Morrow, E. & Maben, J. (2013b) Why Health Visiting?: Appendices. National Nursing Research Unit, King's College, London. Available from: https://www.kcl.ac.uk/nursing/research/nnru/publications/Reports/Appendices-12-02-13.pdf (last accessed 30 March 2016).

Cowley S., Whittaker, K., Malone, M., Donetto, S., Grigulis, A. & Maben, J. (2014) Why health visiting? Examining the potential public health benefits from health visiting practice within a universal service: a narrative review of the literature. *International Journal of Nursing Studies*, **52**(1), 465–80.

Davis, H. & Tsiantis, J. (2005) Promoting children's mental health: the European Early Promotion Project (EEPP). *International Journal of Mental Health Promotion*, **7**(1), 4–16.

Davis, H., Day, C. & Bidmead, C. (2002) Working in Partnership with Parents: The Parent Advisor Model. London, The Psychological Corporation.

Dawley, K., Loch, J. & Bindrich, I. (2007) The Nurse Family Partnership. *American Journal of Nursing*, **107**(11), 60–7.

DfE (2012) *The Impact of Sure Start Local Programmes on Seven Year Olds and their Families*. Available from: https://www.gov.uk/government/publications/the-impact-of-sure-start-local-programmes-on-7-year-olds-and-their-families (last accessed 30 March 2016).

DfE (2013) *Sure Start Centres Statutory Guidance*. Available from: https://www.gov.uk/government/uploads/system/uploads/attachment_data/file/273768/childrens_centre_stat_guidance_april_2013.pdf (last accessed 30 March 2016).

DH (2004) National Service Framework for Children, Young People and Maternity Services. Department of Health, London. Available from: https://www.gov.uk/government/publications/national-service-framework-children-young-people-and-maternity-services (last accessed 30 March 2016).

DH (2008) Child Health Promotion Programme. Department of Health, London.

DH (2009) Healthy Child Programme: Pregnancy and the First Five Years of Life. Department of Health, London. Available from: https://www.gov.uk/government/publications/healthy-child-programme-pregnancy-and-the-first-5-years-of-life (last accessed 30 March 2016).

DH (2011a) The Family-Nurse Partnership Programme in England: Wave 1 Implementation in Toddlerhood & a Comparison between Waves 1 and 2a of Implementation in Pregnancy and Infancy. Institute for Study of Children, Families and Social Issues, Birbeck, University of London. Available from: https://www.gov.uk/government/uploads/system/uploads/attachment_data/file/215837/dh_123366.pdf (last accessed 30 March 2016).

DH (2011b) Health Visitor Implementation Plan 2011–15: A Call to Action February 2011. London, Department of Health. Available from: https://www.gov.uk/government/uploads/system/uploads/attachment_data/file/213110/Health-visitor-implementation-plan.pdf (last accessed 30 March 2016).

DH (2013) The National Health Visitor Plan: Progress to Date and Implementation Beyond 2013. Department of Health, London. https://www.gov.uk/government/uploads/ system/uploads/attachment_data/file/208960/Implementing_the_Health_Visitor_ Vision.pdf (last accessed 30 March 2016).

DH (2014). *School Nurse Programme. Supporting Implementation of the New Service Offer: Public Health Supporting the Health and Wellbeing of Young Carers.* Available from: https://www.gov.uk/government/publications/school-nursing-public-health-services (last accessed 30 March 2016).

DH & Ellison, J. (2013) *Reducing Obesity and Healthy Eating.* Available from: https:// www.gov.uk/government/policies/reducing-obesity-and-improving-diet (last accessed 30 March 2016).

DH & Public Health England (2015) *Health visitor and 0–5 Commissioning Transfer.* Available from: https://www.gov.uk/government/publications/transfer-of-0-5-childrens-public-health-commissioning-to-local-authorities (last accessed 30 March 2016).

Department of Health, Social Services and Public Safety (Northern Ireland) (2010) Healthy Futures 2010–2015 – The Contribution of Health Visitors and School Nurses in Northern Ireland. Available from: https://www.dhsspsni.gov.uk/publications/ healthy-futures-2010-2015-contribution-health-visitors-and-school-nurses-northern (last accessed 30 March 2016).

Donetto, S. & Maben, J. (2014) These places are like a godsend: a qualitative analysis of parents' experiences of health visiting outside the home and of children's centres services. *Health Expectations*, **18**(6): 2559–69.

Donetto, S, Malone, M., Hughes, J., Morrow, E., Cowley, S. & Maben, J. (2013) Health Visiting: The Voice of Service Users: Learning from Service Users' Experiences to Inform the Development of UK Health Visiting Practice and Services. Department of Health Policy Research Programme, Ref. 016 0058. Available from: https://www.kcl.ac.uk/nursing/research/nnru/publications/Reports/Voice-of-service-user-report-July-2013-FINAL.pdf (last accessed 30 March 2016).

Douglas, H. (2010) Supporting emotional health and wellbeing: the Solihull Approach. *Community Practitioner*, **83**(8): 22–5.

Douglas, H. & Bennan, A. (2004) Containment, reciprocity and behaviour management: preliminary evaluation of a brief early intervention (the Solihull Approach) for families with infants and young children. *International Journal of Infant Observation*, **7**(1), 89–107.

Eckenrode, J., Campa, M., Luckey, D., Henderson, C. Jr, Cole, R., Kitzman, H., Anson, E., Sidora-Arcoleo, K., Powers, J. & Olds, D. (2010) Long-term effects of prenatal and infancy nurse home visitation on the life course of youths 19-year follow-up of a randomized trial. *Archives of Pediatrics & Adolescent Medicine*, **164**(1), 9–15.

Elkan, R., Kendrick, D., Hewitt, M., Robinson, J.J., Tolley, K., Blair, M., Dewey, M., Williams, D. & Brummell, K. (2000) The effectiveness of domiciliary health visiting: a systematic review of international studies and a selective review of British literature. *Health Technology Assessment*, **4**(13), i–v, 1–339.

Emond, A., Pollock, J., Deave, T., Bonnell, S., Peters, T.J. & Harvey, I. (2002) An evaluation of the First Parent Health Visiting Scheme. *Archives of Disease in Childhood*, **86**, 150–7.

Evangelou, M., Goff, J. Hall, J., Sylva, K., Eisenstadt, N., Paget, C., Davis, S., Sammons, P. Smith, T., Tracz, R. & Parkin, T. (2014) Evaluation of Children's Centres in England (ECCE) Strand 3: Parenting Services in Children's Centres. University of Oxford. Available from: https://www.gov.uk/government/uploads/system/uploads/ attachment_data/file/330276/Final_draft_-_ECCE_Strand_3_Parenting_Services_ Study_Report_FINAL.pdf (last accessed 30 March 2016).

FNP National Unit (2015a) *The FNP Information Pack. Section 1 The Case for Family Nurse Partnership. An Information Pack for Local Authorities.* Available from: http://fnp.nhs .uk/sites/default/files/contentuploads/fnp_information_pack_-_an_overview.pdf (last accessed 30 March 2016).

FNP National Unit (2015b) About us. Available from: http://fnp.nhs.uk/about-us (last accessed 30 March 2016).

Feeley, N. & Gottlieb, L.N. (2000) Nursing approaches for working with family strengths and resources. *Journal of Family Nursing,* **6**(1), 9–24.

Garner, A.S. (2013). Home visiting and the biology of toxic stress: opportunities to address early childhood adversity. *Pediatrics,* **132**(Suppl. 2), S65–73.

Gomby, D.S. (1999) Understanding evaluations of home visiting programmes. *Future Child,* **9**, 27–43.

Government of Wales (2013) *National Evaluation of Flying Start: Impact Report.* Social Research no. 74/2013. Available from: http://gov.wales/docs/caecd/research/ 131205-national-evaluation-flying-start-impact-report-en.pdf (last accessed 30 March 2016).

Hall, D.M.B. & Hall, S. (2007) The 'Family–Nurse Partnership': Developing an Instrument for Identification, Assessment and Recruitment of Clients. Department for Children, Schools and Families. Ref: DCSF-RW022. Available from: http://www.education.gov .uk/research/data/uploadfiles/DCSF-RW022.pdf (last accessed 30 March 2016).

Health & Social Care Information Centre (2016) NHS Mobile Working Knowledge Centre. Available from: http://systems.hscic.gov.uk/qipp/mobile (last accessed 30 March 2016).

Hermanns, J.M.A., Asscher, J.J., Zijlstra, B.J.H., Hoffenaar, P.J. & Deković, M. (2013). Long-term changes in parenting and child behavior after the home-start family support program. *Children and Youth Services Review,* **35**(4), 678–84.

HM Government (2003) Every Child Matters. Presented to Parliament by the Chief Secretary to the Treasury by Command of Her Majesty, September 2003 (Cm 5860). The Stationery Office, London. Available from: https://www.education.gov.uk/consultations/ downloadableDocs/EveryChildMatters.pdf (last accessed 30 March 2016).

HM Government (2013) Social Justice: Transforming Lives. One Year On, The Stationery Office Limited, Norwich. Available from: https://www.gov.uk/government/uploads/ system/uploads/attachment_data/file/203041/CM_8606_Social_Justice_tagged-mw.pdf (last accessed 30 March 2016).

HM Government (2014a) *Child Poverty Strategy 2014 to 2017.* Available from: https:// www.gov.uk/government/publications/child-poverty-strategy-2014-to-2017 (last accessed 30 March 2016).

HM Government (2014b) *Carers Strategy: Actions for 2014 to 2016.* Available from: https://www.gov.uk/government/publications/carers-strategy-actions-for-2014-to-2016 (last accessed 30 March 2016).

Holmes, L., McDermis, S., Padley, M. & Soper, J. (2012). Exploration of the costs and impact of the *Common Assessment Framework. Research Report DFE-RR210.* Department for Education, London.

Home Office (1998) Supporting Families: A Consultation Document. The Stationery Office, London. Available from: http://webarchive.nationalarchives.gov.uk/+/http:/ www.nationalarchives.gov.uk/ERORecords/HO/421/2/P2/ACU/SUPPFAM.HTM (last accessed 30 March 2016).

Howe D. (1996) Surface and depth in social work practice. In: Social Theory, Social Change and Social Work (ed. N. Parton). Routledge, London. pp. 77–97.

Jack, S.M., DiCenso, A. & Lohfeld, L. (2002) A theory of maternal engagement with public health nurses and family visitors. *Journal of Advanced Nursing,* **49**(2), 182–90.

Johnson, R. & Wilson, H. (2012) Parents' evaluation of understanding your child's behaviour, a parenting group based on the Solihull Approach. *Community Practitioner*, **85**(5), 29–33.

Johnson, Z., Howell, F. & Molloy, B. (1993) Community mothers' programme: randomised controlled trial of non-professional intervention in parenting. *British Medical Journal*, **29**(306), 1449–52.

Johnson, Z., Molloy, B., Scallan, E., Fitzpatrick, P., Rooney, B., Keegan, T. & Byrne, P. (2000) Community Mothers Programme – seven year follow-up of a randomized controlled trial of non-professional intervention in parenting. *Journal of Public Health Medicine*, **22**(3), 337–42.

Ke, J. & Ford-Jones, E.L. (2015). Food insecurity and hunger: a review of the effects on children's health and behaviour. *Paediatrics and Child Health*, **20**(2), 89–91.

Kemp, L., Harris, E., McMahan, C., Matthey, S., Vimpani, G., Anderson, T. & Schmied, V. (2008). Miller Early Childhood Sustained Home-visiting (MECSH) trial: design, method and sample description. *BMC Public Health*, **8**, 424.

Kemp, L., Harris, E., McMahon, C., Matthey, S., Vimpani, G., Anderson, T., Schmied, V., Aslam, H. & Zapart, S. (2011) Child and family outcomes of a long-term nurse home visitation programme: a randomised controlled trial. *Archives of Disease in Childhood*, **96**(6), 533–40.

Kemp, L., Harris, E., McMahon, C., Matthey, S., Vimpani, G., Anderson, T., Schmied, V. & Aslam, H. (2013) Benefits of psychosocial intervention and continuity of care by child and family health nurses in the pre- and postnatal period: process evaluation. *Journal of Advanced Nursing*, **69**(8), 1850–61.

Kitzman, H., Olds, D.L., Henderson, C.R. Jr., Hanks, C., Cole, R., Tatelbaum, R., McConnochie, K.M., Sidora, K., Luckey, D.W., Shaver, D., Engelhardt, K., James, D. & Barnard, K. (1997) Effect of prenatal and infancy home visitation by nurses on pregnancy outcomes, childhood injuries, and repeated childbearing: a randomized controlled trial. *Journal of the American Association*, **278**(8), 644–52.

Kristjanson, L. & Chalmers, K.I. (1990) Nurse–client interactions in community based practice: creating common meaning. *Public Health Nursing*, **7**(4), 215–23.

Little, M., Berry, V., Morpeth, L., Blower, S., Axford, N., Taylor, R., Bywater, T., Lehtonen, M. & Tobin, K. (2012) The impact of three evidence-based programmes delivered in public systems in Birmingham, UK. *International Journal of Conflict and Violence*, **6**(2), 260–72.

Long, A., McCarney, S., Smyth, G., Magorrian, N. & Dillon, A. (2001) The effectiveness of parenting programmes facilitated by health visitors. *Journal of Advanced Nursing*, **34**(5), 611–20.

Marmot, M., Atkinson, T., Bell, J., Black, C., Broadfoot, P., Cumberlege, J., Diamond, I., Gilmore, I., Ham, C., Meacher, M. & Mulgan, G. (2010) Fair Society, Healthy Lives: The Marmot Review. Marmot Review Team, University College, London. Available from: http://www.instituteofhealthequity.org/projects/fair-society-healthy-lives-the-marmot-review (last accessed 30 March 2016).

McAuley, C., Knapp, M., Beecham, J. & McCurry, N. (2004) Young Families under Stress: Outcomes and Costs of Home-Start Support. Joseph Rowntree Foundation, York. Available from: http://www.jrf.org.uk/sites/default/files/jrf/migrated/files/1859352189.pdf (last accessed 30 March 2016).

McGoldrick, M., Gerson, R. & Petry, S.S. (2008) Genograms: Assessment and Intervention, 3rd edn. W.W. Norton & Co., New York.

McIntosh, J. & Shute, J. (2006) The process of health visiting and its contribution to parental support in the Starting Well demonstration project. *Health and Social Care in the Community*, **15**(1), 77–85.

Meadows, P. (2011) *National Evaluation of Sure Start Local Programmes: An Economic Perspective.* Research Report DFE-RR073. Department for Education. Available from: https://www.gov.uk/government/publications/national-evaluation-of-sure-start-local-programmes-an-economic-perspective (last accessed 30 March 2016).

Molloy, B. (2008) Ireland's community mothers take the pressure off family life. *Prevention Action.* Available from: http://www.preventionaction.org/node/478 (last accessed 30 March 2016).

Munro, E. (2011) Munro Review of Child Protection: Final Report – A Child-Centred System. The Stationery Office, Norwich.

National Assembly for Wales (2014) *Flying Start: Research Note.* Available from: http://dera.ioe.ac.uk/23963/1/rn14-005-English.pdf (last accessed 30 March 2016).

NESS (2008) *The Impact of Sure Start Local Programmes on Three Year Olds and their Families.* Research Report NESS/2008/FR027. Department for Children, Schools and Families, London. Available from: http://www.ness.bbk.ac.uk/impact/documents/41.pdf (last accessed 30 March 2016).

NHS England (2014) *2015–16 National Heath Visiting Core Service Specification.* Available from: http://www.england.nhs.uk/ourwork/qual-clin-lead/hlth-vistg-prog/info/docs-res/ (last accessed 30 March 2016).

NHS Scotland (2011) A New Look at Hall 4. The Early Years Good Health for Every Child. The Scottish Government, Edinburgh. Available from: http://www.gov.scot/Publications/2011/01/11133654/0 (last accessed 30 March 2016).

Olds, D.L., Henderson C.R. Jr, Tatelbaum, R. & Chamberlin, R. (1986) Improving the delivery of prenatal care and outcomes of pregnancy: a randomized trial of nurse home visitation. *Pediatrics,* **77**(1), 16–28.

Olds, D.L., Eckenrode, J., Henderson C.R. Jr., Kitzman, H., Powers, J., Cole, R., Sidora, K., Morris, P., Pettitt, L.M. & Luckey, D. (1997) Long-term effects of home visitation on maternal life course and child abuse and neglect. Fifteen year follow-up of a randomized trial. *Journal of the American Association,* **278**(8), 637–43.

Olds, D.L., Henderson, C.R. Jr, Cole, R., Eckenrode, J., Kitzman, H., Luckey, D., Pettitt, L., Sidora, K., Morris, P. & Powers, J. (1998) Long-term effects of nurse home visitation on children's criminal and antisocial behavior: 15-year follow-up of a randomized controlled trial. *Journal of the American Association,* **280**(14), 1238–44.

Olds, D.L., Kitzman, H., Hanks, C., Cole, R., Anson, E., Sidora-Arcoleo, K., Luckey, D.W., Henderson, C.R. Jr., Holmberg, J., Tutt, R.A., Stevenson, A.J. & Bondy, J. (2007) Effects of nurse home visiting on maternal and child functioning: age-9 follow-up of a randomized trial. *Pediatrics,* **120**(4), e832–45.

Olds, D., Holmberg, J., Donelan-McCall, N., Luckey, D., Knudtson, M. & Robinson, J. (2013) Effects of home visits by paraprofessionals and by nurses on children: follow-up of a randomized trial at ages 6 and 9 years. *JAMA Pediatrics,* **168**(2), 114–21.

Olds, D., Kitzman, H., Knudtson, M., Anson, E., Smith, J. & Cole, R. (2014) Impact of home visiting by nurses on maternal and child mortality: results of a two-decade follow-up of a randomized, clinical trial. *JAMA Pediatrics,* **168**(9), 800–6.

Olds, D.L., Baca, P., McClatchey, M., Ingoldsby, E., Luckey, D, Knudtson M., Loch, J. & Ramsey, M. (2015) Cluster randomized controlled trial of intervention to increase participant retention and completed home visits in the Nurse–Family Partnership. *Prevention Science,* **16**(6), 778–88.

Owen-Jones, E., Bekkers, M-J., Butler, C., Cannings-John, R., Channon, S., Hood, K., Gregory, J.W., Kemp, A., Kenkre, J., Martin, B.C., Montgomery, A., Moody, G., Pickett, K.E., Richardson, G., Roberts, Z., Ronaldson, S., Sanders, J., Stamuli, E., Torgerson, D. & Robling, M. (2013) The effectiveness and cost-effectiveness of the Family Nurse Partnership home visiting programme or first time teenage mothers in England: a protocol for the Building Blocks randomized trial. *BMC Pediatrics,* **13**, 1–24.

Papadopoulou, K., Dimitrakaki, C., Davis, H., Tsiantis, J., Dusoir, A., Paradisiotou, A., Vizacou, S., Roberts, R., Chisholm, B., Puura, K., Mantymaa, M., Tamminen, T., Rudic, N., Radosavljev, J. & Miladinovic, T. (2005) The effects of the European Early Promotion Project training on primary health care professionals. *International Journal of Mental Health Promotion*, **7**, 54–62.

Perry, J., Williams, M., Sefton, T. & Haddad, M. (2014). Emergency Use Only: Understanding and Reducing the Use of Food Banks in the UK. Oxfam. Available from: http://policy-practice.oxfam.org.uk/publications (last accessed 30 March 2016).

Poverty and Social Exclusion UK (2013) *The Impoverishment of the UK. PSE UK First Results: Living Standards*. Available from: http://www.poverty.ac.uk/pse-research/pse-uk-reports (last accessed 30 March 2016).

Prinz, R.J., Sanders, M.R, Shapiro, C.J., Whitaker, D.J. & Lutzker, J.R. (2009) Population-based prevention of child maltreatment: the U.S. Triple P system population trial. *Prevention Science*, **10**, 1–12.

Public Health England (2014) Children and Young People's Benchmarking Tool. Available from: http://fingertips.phe.org.uk/profile/cyphof (last accessed 30 March 2016).

Public Health England (2015) *Rapid Review to Update Evidence for the Healthy Child Programme 0–5*. Available from: https://www.gov.uk/government/uploads/system/uploads/attachment_data/file/429740/150520RapidReviewHealthyChildProg_UPDATE_poisons_final.pdf (last accessed 30 March 2016).

Puura, K. Davis, H., Mäntymaa, M., Tamminen, T., Roberts, R., Dragonas, T., Papadopoulou, K., Dimitrakaki, C., Paradisiotou, A., Vizacou, S., Leontiou, F., Rudic, N., Miladinovic, T. & Radojkovic, A. (2005) The outcome of the European Early Promotion Project: mother–child interaction. *International Journal of Mental Health Promotion*, **7**(1), 82–94.

Rallings, J. (2014). What are children's centres for? Barnardo's. Available from: http://www.barnardos.org.uk/15733_what_are_children_s_centres_for_report_v2_hr.pdf (last accessed 30 March 2016).

Robling, M., Betkers, M.-J., Bell, K., Butler, C.C., Cannings-John, R., Channon, S., Corbacho, B., Gregory, J.W., Hood, K., Kemp, A., Kenkre, J., Montgomery, A.A., Moody, G., Owen-Jones, E., Pickett, K., Richardson, G., Roberts, Z., Ronaldson, S., Sanders, J., Stamuli, E. & Torgerson, D. (2015) Effectiveness of a nurse-led intensive home-visitation programme for first-time teenage mothers (Building Blocks): a pragmatic randomised controlled trial. *The Lancet*, **387**(10014): 146–55.

Rocco, L. & Suhrcke, M. (2012) Is Social Capital Good for Health? A European Perspective. WHO Regional Office for Europe, Copenhagen. Available from: http://www.euro.who.int/__data/assets/pdf_file/0005/170078/Is-Social-Capital-good-for-your-health.pdf (last accessed 30 March 2016).

Russell, S. & Drennan, V. (2007) Mothers' views of the health visiting service in the UK: a web-based survey. *Community Practitioner*, **80**(8), 22–6.

Sanders, M.R. (2008) Triple P-Positive Parenting Programme as a public health approach to strengthening parenting. *Journal of Family Psychology*, **22**(3), 506–17.

Sanders, M.R. (2012) Development, evaluation, and multinational dissemination of the Triple P-Positive Parenting Program. *Annual Review of Clinical Psychology*, **8**, 345–79.

Sanders, M.R., Kirby, J.N., Tellegen, C.L. & Day, J.J. (2014). The triple P-positive parenting program: a systematic review and meta-analysis of a multi-level system of parenting support. *Clinical Psychology Review*, **34**(4), 337–57.

Scottish Government (2012) Early Years Collaborative. Available from: http://www.gov.scot/Topics/People/Young-People/early-years/early-years-collaborative (last accessed 30 March 2016).

Scottish Government (2014) Proposal for the Development of Guidance to Support the GIRFEC Provisions in the Children and Young People (Scotland) Act 2014. The Scottish Government, Edinburgh. Available from: http://www.gov.scot/Topics/People/Young-People/gettingitright/publications (last accessed 30 March 2016).

Stewart-Brown, S., Patterson, J., Mockford, C., Barlow, J., Klimes, I. & Pyper, C. (2004). Impact of a general practice based group parenting programme: quantitative and qualitative results from a controlled trial at 12 months. *Archives of Disease in Childhood*, **89**, 519–25.

Sweet, M.A. & Applebaum, M.I. (2004) Is home visiting an effective strategy? A meta-analytic review of home visiting programs for families with young children. *Child Development*, **75**(5), 1435–56.

The Children's Society (2013) *Hidden from View: The Experiences of Young Carers in England*. Available from: http://www.childrenssociety.org.uk/sites/default/files/tcs/report_hidden-from-view_young-carers_final.pdf (last accessed 30 March 2016).

Thompson, C. (2011) Learning to Trust in Home Visiting: Mothers' Perspective. Iowa State University Graduate Theses and Dissertations. Paper 12108. Available from: http://lib.dr.iastate.edu/cgi/viewcontent.cgi?article=3079&context=etd (last accessed 30 March 2016).

Wallbank, S. & Woods, G. (2012). A healthier health visiting workforce: findings from the Restorative Supervision Programme. *Community Practitioner*, **85**, 20–3.

Whittaker, K. (2014) Supporting parents and parenting practice: the health visitor context. *Journal of Health Visiting*, **2**(5), 2–11.

Whittaker, K. & Browne, K. (2014) Health visiting: standing the test of time and informing a new generation of home visiting in Eastern Europe. *Community Practitioner*, **87**(6), 36–7.

Whittaker, K. & Cowley, S. (2012) An effective programme is not enough: a review of factors associated with poor attendance and engagement with parenting support. *Children & Society*, **26**, 138–49.

Whittaker, K.A., Cox, P., Thomas, N. & Cocker, K. (2014) A qualitative study of parents' experiences using family support services: applying the concept of surface and depth. *Health and Social Care in the Community*, **22**(5), 479–87.

Wilson, P., Thompson, L., Puckering, C., McConnachie, A., Holden, C., Cassidy, C. & Gillberg, C. (2010) Parent–child relationships: are health visitors' judgements reliable? *Community Practitioner*, **83**(5), 22–5.

Woodgate, R.L., Heaman, M.I., Chalmers, K.I. & Brown, J. (2007) Issues related to delivering an early childhood home visiting program. *American Journal of Maternal and Child Health Nursing*, **32**(2), 95–101.

Worth, A. & Hogg, R. (2000). A qualitative evaluation of the effectiveness of health visiting practice. *British Journal of Community Nursing*, **221**(5), 224–8.

Wright, L.M. & Leahy, M. (2013) Nurses and Families: A Guide to Family Assessment and Intervention, 6th edn. FA Davis, Philadelphia.

Activities

Activity 4.1

Using genograms and eco-maps in health visiting

To gain some practice using genograms and eco-maps within health visiting, first draw a genogram relating to your own family or a family you are

(Continued)

Activity 4.1: *(Continued)*

currently visiting, using the symbols shown in Figure 4.3. Place the family at the centre of the page. Draw a dotted line around everyone who currently lives in the same house. Place children from oldest to youngest, left to right. Connecting lines denote whether a relationship is strong (solid, straight line), stressful (wavy line), tenuous/weak (dashed line), or broken (line with a strike through it).

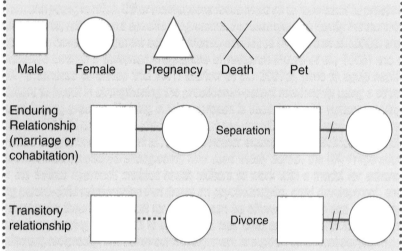

Male   Female   Pregnancy   Death   Pet

Enduring Relationship (marriage or cohabitation)

Separation

Transitory relationship

Divorce

Figure 4.3   Genogram symbols. These are just some of the symbols that can be used when compiling a genogram.

Next, extend the visual to create an eco-map and indicate the range of other relationships the family has within the community. Additional circles/ovals can be included to show wider community facilities (e.g. church, school, clubs, employers) (see Figure 4.2).

Further details on drawing genograms and the use of symbols can be found at the NHS National Genetics and Genomics Education Centre website (www. geneticseducation.nhs.uk).

Activity 4.2

Assessing child health programmes

Think about the child programmes which the health visiting service in your area offers. Answer the questions given in Box 4.1.

Activity 4.3

Health visitor–client interaction

- Reflect on a recent visit with a family.
- Do you feel this was a good interaction? If so, why? If not, why not?
- In either case, is there anything you will do differently during your next contact?

5

Safeguarding Children: Debates and Dilemmas for Health Visitors

Julianne Harlow
University of Derby, Derby, UK

Martin Smith
Liverpool City Council, Liverpool, UK

Introduction

The first 16 years of the new millennium have seen an increase in political and societal demands to tackle various forms of child abuse and so safeguard children. It is widely acknowledged that for all practitioners involved in working with vulnerable children and their families, safeguarding children can be both difficult and challenging, and yet intensely rewarding. A plethora of policies relevant to safeguarding children, underpinned by the United Nations Convention on the Rights of the Child (UNCRC) (UNICEF, 1989), exists at all levels of society. Such policies chart the growing emphasis on safeguarding work and have refocused the roles of numerous professionals and practitioners. For those health visitors who work with children and families, the increased emphasis on safeguarding children has led to both tensions within and a reinforcement of the value of their (public health) role in practice. This chapter will address these tensions in order to contextualise the contemporary role of health visitors as public health practitioners in safeguarding children. It will recognise the importance of leadership in health visiting practice aimed at ensuring the safety and well being of children. Although the chapter will focus on health visiting from the perspective of specialist community public health nursing, it will also be relevant to other key practitioners working in the field of safeguarding children.

Given the emphasis on leadership within specialist community public health nursing (NMC, 2004), it is important that health visitors understand how to work with ambiguity and ethical decision making in complex situations where there may

Health Visiting: Preparation for Practice, Fourth Edition.
Edited by Karen A. Luker, Gretl A. McHugh and Rosamund M. Bryar.
© 2017 John Wiley & Sons, Ltd. Published 2017 by John Wiley & Sons, Ltd.

be competing interests and needs amongst family members. In order to reach these understandings, this chapter will begin with an exploration of some of the key concepts surrounding child abuse and safeguarding children. Initially, consideration of how UK society currently defines a 'child' will be given, as understanding the concept of 'child' has ramifications for health visitors as they seek to practice within a society and a legislative and policy framework that present inconsistencies and tensions. The meaning of 'child abuse' will be explored as a social construct and from a temporal perspective, along with other associated terms. This will highlight how society has come to respond to various forms of child abuse, which constitute a continually evolving phenomenon. In the UK, this response is currently expressed in terms of safeguarding children; the concept of safeguarding and its relationship with child protection will be explored.

Health visiting has had to respond to the changing nature of child abuse, safeguarding, and child protection in contemporary society whilst having been subject to a range of political changes as a profession. Such changes have had an impact upon how the health visiting role has been interpreted at both national and local levels. In terms of the evidence base, there have been a number of descriptive studies undertaken that highlight different aspects of a health visitor's work with child abuse. However, the evidence base for demonstrating the effectiveness of health visiting in this field has been noted to be somewhat limited (Elkan *et al.*, 2000). Furthermore, the short-term nature of political cycles demands evidence of quick change, which presents major challenges for services working with complex and multifactorial needs in families. For example, the evidence relating to the cost-effectiveness of early years services as a whole has been said to be limited (Health Select Committee, 2009). This contrasts with a growing body of evidence of the longer-term benefits that accrue from investment in the health and well being of children. For example, the Center on the Developing Child at Harvard University (2010) refers to the very persuasive economic arguments from studies for an emphasis on prevention to reduce the escalating costs of future adult disease and disability and to support human and economic development.

Nevertheless, there are clear policy drivers that demonstrate an unequivocal recognition that health visitors have an important role in safeguarding children. This role aligns itself with a public health approach which recognises the wider determinants of heath and the impact upon not only children but also the parents and carers of children. Consequently, this challenges perceptions that working with individuals and families in a safeguarding context is separate in some way to a public health role for health visitors.

This chapter places an emphasis on the fact that good leaders are role models for ethical safeguarding practice. Health visitors are required to be accountable for their practice and fit for professional standing. These are statements which underpin the Nursing and Midwifery Council (NMC) standards for safe and effective practice (NMC, 2004). However, accepting them at face value risks minimising the importance of a clear understanding of why accountability and safe practice are essential in safeguarding work. Health visitors therefore need to develop and maintain skills of critical thinking and reflection in order to fulfil their role not only as effective practitioners in a multidisciplinary arena, but also as leaders within the health visiting team and in engaging with other partners. The value of supervision for enabling a reflective, critical approach has been recognised as essential for safe and effective practice (DfE, 2015a). However, as supervision becomes increasingly established in practice, it is equally important to recognise how the quality of supervision impacts upon the quality of both leadership and practice.

Overall, this chapter takes a considered approach to safeguarding children, through an analysis of health visiting practice emphasising the significance of leadership. This is not a reference piece or step-by-step account of how to safeguard, as this information is readily available in existing texts and policy. For example, the process has been explained with a series of very useful descriptors and flow charts, available online (DH, 2013a; DfE, 2015a, 2015b). This chapter is an analytical contribution designed to underpin contemporary health visiting practice and demonstrate:

- how an understanding of policy and legislation is relevant to safeguarding practice;
- the evidence associated with the impact of child abuse;
- the utilisation of supervision to support critical reflection and thinking.

All of these contribute to the development of leadership in practitioners working in the safeguarding arena.

Throughout the chapter, consideration will be given to examples of published inquiries into child deaths and serious case reviews that are particularly relevant for health visiting. The text draws from relevant legislation and policy. Whilst health visitors are not required to be legal experts, they need an understanding of the legislative and policy framework as it relates to their safeguarding role (NMC, 2015: 17.3). This understanding helps to ensure safe, effective, and accountable safeguarding practice and the tailoring of health promotion activities. The continued movement towards integrated services and closer working with other professionals, such as social workers, reinforces this, as legislation forms the basis of joint discussions and decision making regarding vulnerable children and their families. A health visitor's knowledge and confidence in respect of relevant safeguarding and child protection law therefore requires constant updating on policies and practices.

The key concepts

Defining 'child'

Throughout its history, health visiting has been associated with the health and well being of children as the main group and focus for professional practice. This is not without reason, as the promotion of health and the prevention of ill health (CETHV, 1977) are dependent upon the roots for a long and healthy life being established at an early age. It has been argued (e.g. Symonds, 1991) that if health visitors focus on children and families, this detracts from the broader, whole population approach. It is important to recognise, however, that children form a distinct population within the general population. A population of children has its own distinct health and social characteristics, and needs that vary according to age, developmental stage, and a range of genetic, social, and environmental factors. Furthermore, focusing on the health of families with young children means that not only is the health of the current population of children enhanced, but so too is the health of the future adult population (along with the health of the current population of adult family members).

Current legislation, such as the Children Act 1989 and the Children Act 2004, is informed by the UNCRC (UNICEF, 1989) and defines a child as 'anyone who has not yet reached their 18th birthday'. However, within the UK, tensions exist within law and policy on how chronological age and developmental capacity vary as a marker for childhood. Take as an example the unborn child. Policy sets out procedures and timescales for addressing safeguarding concerns regarding unborn children. For example 1010 unborn children in England were the subject of child protection plans in the year ending March 2014 (DfE, 2014); such plans only come into place at birth, as the foetus has no legal rights to protection in respect of even the most extreme of circumstances. *In utero*, however, the foetus may be subjected to a range of harmful exposures and abuses, such as domestic abuse, tobacco smoke, alcohol, and drugs, all of which are known to cause potential harm to foetal health and development.

Just as the beginning of childhood is an ambiguous and contested concept, so too is the point at which childhood ends. In the UK, this may be illustrated by differences in legislation passed as a result of devolution. Although in law a child is a child until they are 18, 16-year-olds can legally have a sexual relationship with a member of the same or opposite sex of the same age or older. In England, Wales, and Northern Ireland, 16 and 17-year-olds may marry or enter a civil partnership with their parents' consent; however, in Scotland, parental consent is not required at 16. Throughout the UK, young people cannot purchase alcohol or cigarettes until 18 or learn to drive a car or motorbike until they are 17. Under current legislation, a person must be 18 or over to vote in the UK, but 16- and 17-year-olds in Scotland were empowered to vote in the referendum on independence in 2014 and proposals to give the Scottish Parliament powers to reduce the voting age were brought in time for its elections in 2016 (White, 2015). In contrast, there are no plans in the legislative proposals for allowing under-18s across the UK to vote in the forthcoming EU referendum. Further tensions exist within specific pieces of legislation and policy. The Sexual Offences Act 2003, for example, deems that sex for children and young people under 16 years of age is illegal. However, young people under the age of 16 may request and be prescribed contraception if they are deemed competent to do so, in line with guidance produced by the National Institute for Health and Care Excellence (NICE, 2014).

Similarly, in respect of decision making for medical treatment, children may give or withhold their consent to that treatment if they are deemed as competent. Increasing importance is given to the child's wishes with increasing age and evolving capacity for understanding. Courts can and do, however, override these wishes when they are deemed not to be in the best interests of the child or young person. Other tensions in respect of service provision and the chronological age of children exist. For example, young people aged 16 or above requiring hospital admission may be considered too old for admission to a paediatric ward and consequently be exposed to adult environments and services which do not cater appropriately for their needs and may potentially be harmful. Whilst analysis of society's use of chronological age in determining when particular behaviours (healthy or not) may be considered legal falls outside the scope of this chapter, the discussion reflects the ambiguities and contentious nature of society's attempts to determine the age at which childhood begins and ends, demonstrating that childhood is frequently used as a political hostage. Activity 5.1 may help you explore the concept of 'child' further and clarify the ambiguities surrounding the definition of 'childhood', which presents challenges for health visitors in their day-to-day practice.

Defining 'childhood'

Difficulties in reaching a consensus in respect of defining 'childhood' are evidenced by contested concepts within the literature. Different forms and sources of literature offer different perspectives on what constitutes a 'child' and are influenced by political, temporal, spatial, and cultural factors. Smith (2010) presents an analysis of the concept of childhood in contemporary society and suggests that perspectives on childhood are subject to disparate positions, with little to support childhood as a 'clear and coherent entity' (Smith, 2010: 194). He suggests that there may be certain universal features of childhood that act as determinants of children's lives, which are:

- physical growth;
- increasing competencies;
- inexperience;
- vulnerability.

He further argues that these features should be considered as principles in relation to the variations of experiences and the child's context, which may be heavily influenced by such factors as history, culture, and genetics. Nevertheless, these features expose the extent to which childhood is commonly viewed in adult terms; that is, as a deficit in preparation for adulthood and, as Smith (2010: 5) suggests, 'a means to an end'. In contrast to these features, Smith considers other perspectives on childhood that recognise the importance of the child's view, the need to understand the child's lived experience, and how the child formulates their own sense of the world in their own terms. Children draw from the source material of the adult world around them; however, their behaviour through play and interaction with others helps them to create their own roles and identities and develop relationships.

These different perspectives on childhood present dilemmas for health visitors, who are often required to draw on their own professional and personal values, as adults, to make judgments based on a biopsychosocial model reflecting the immaturity of children, who are seen as having limited rights and interests. In addition, health visitors need to develop an understanding of the world through a child's eyes and ensure they give a clear priority to the views of children within families and do not rely upon traditional perspectives of childhood, which view children – as Prout (cited in Smith, 2010) sees it – from a standpoint of immaturity and incompleteness (in relation to children and adulthood). For health visitors to be successful in working with children and understanding their needs and experiences, they need to be able to see them and to engage fully, directly, and empathically with them, by utilising their higher-level communications skills and using observation and active listening. This will enable the health visitors to develop robust assessments of children's needs and of the extent to which they feel safe from harm.

A focus of early intervention and practice with those families and children deemed particularly vulnerable has become known as *progressive universalism* (or, as it is referred to by Marmot *et al.* (2010), *proportionate universalism*). This is thought to make a more significant impact on the reduction of health inequalities affecting the lives of children. Progressive universalism has been defined as a 'universal service that is systematically planned and delivered to give a continuum of support according to need at neighbourhood and individual level in order to achieve greater equity of outcomes for all children' (DH, 2007: 8). However, a consultation with Community Practitioners and Health Visitors Association (CPHVA) members found that the concept had not been easily embraced by some health visitors (CPHVA, 2007). It was suggested that the term *'regressive' universalism* could be more appropriate, to reflect the fact that not everyone would get an adequate standard of service. If health visitors were denied the opportunity to build a relationship with all families, they would feel it impossible to provide a service based on progressive universalism. Indeed, other major charitable organisations suggested that the term 'progressive universalism' was just another means to justify the cutting of health visitor numbers at that time (FPI, 2007). Whilst the concept of progressive universalism assists health visitors in focusing services on those with the most recognised need, in the context of safeguarding children, it presents a challenge, as child abuse occurs across all social classes, involves children of all ages, and is likely to be hidden and not easily recognised. Focusing health visiting practice only on those perceived as vulnerable at a neighbourhood or an individual level means that opportunities for identifying and responding to abuse across the population as a whole will be reduced. Indeed, Lord Laming, in his report to the House of Commons (Laming, 2009), highlighted the tensions between health visitors supporting families with complex needs and the health visitor's role in offering a universal service to all. It is through experience and effective supervision that health visitors are able to determine the point at which concerns should be elevated and responsibilities shared. Laming (2009) made the point that the majority of children in the population do not have – or, indeed, need – a child protection plan, and emphasised the universal role of health visitors as crucially important in developing strong relationships with all families and the value of all children being seen in their home environment. This approach underpins the delivery of the universal Healthy Child Programme (HCP) (DH, 2009), which requires a core offer of mandated contacts with the transfer of the commissioning of health visiting to local authorities in October 2015.

Defining 'safeguarding'

Before reading on, it may be useful to consider your own perceptions of the meaning of 'safeguarding' and begin to complete Activity 5.2. Over recent years, the term 'safeguarding children', coined in Section 17 of the Children Act 1989, has increasingly replaced that of 'child protection'. Whilst 'safeguarding', as a term, is now widely represented in the mainstream language of policy and practice, it represents a multifaceted concept that may be open to interpretation by many different groups, agencies, professionals, and individuals. The literature offers various perspectives on 'safeguarding children', but the importance of professionals sharing an agreed definition of what constitutes safeguarding cannot be overstated. Agreed definitions are vital in terms of understanding the aims of safeguarding practice and simultaneously forming a basis for more specific procedural policy that details how safeguarding practice should be carried out. A current definition of safeguarding and promoting the welfare of children is:

> Protecting children from maltreatment; preventing impairment of children's health or development; ensuring that children are growing up in circumstances consistent with the provision of safe and effective care; and taking action to enable all children to have the best life chances.
>
> (DfE, 2015a: 92)

Whilst this definition does not offer any detail on the activities associated with the safeguarding role, or how effective safeguarding practice might be achieved, it does have a number of strengths. One of the most significant is that it reflects the five outcomes identified as being most important to children and young people in the consultation of *Every Child Matters* (DfES, 2004) and subsequently embedded in the Children Act 2004:

- be healthy;
- stay safe;
- enjoy and achieve;
- make a positive contribution;
- achieve economic well being.

The process of consulting with children and young people and allowing them to express their views is compliant with Articles 12 and 13 of the UNCRC. In addition to the process being respectful of children's rights, the content of the five outcomes is also compliant with the rights of children.

In incorporating the five outcomes, this broad definition of safeguarding represents a holistic view that safeguarding children is much more than protecting them from abuse. Defining safeguarding in a holistic way effectively widens the scope of practice, increasing the opportunities for health visitors and school nurses to work proactively in partnership with children and families in order to safeguard and promote all children's welfare. However, as indicated by the placement of the term 'protecting children from maltreatment', child protection is nevertheless a very important part of the work undertaken to safeguard and promote the welfare of children. Equally, protecting children from harm demands much more than just having systems in place to manage child maltreatment. Suggestions highlighted by Puffett (2010) that the term 'safeguarding' be replaced with the term 'child protection' would have been a retrograde step, although, as Parton (2014) acknowledges, in real terms a framing of policy and practice in terms of child protection has re-emerged. Political attempts to manipulate the discourse and subsequent direction of policy detract from the fact that for children, the issue of preventing child maltreatment remains. Therefore, whilst child protection *per se* refers to the activities undertaken to protect those children who are suffering or likely to suffer significant harm (DfE, 2015a), the concept of safeguarding enables a wider, more holistic understanding of the need to protect all children from harm and subsequently aim to reduce the need for child protection activities. A proactive, preventative approach such as this reflects an early intervention approach, which is defined as:

> targeted, preventive activity which supports people who are at risk of experiencing adverse and costly life outcomes, in order to prevent those outcomes from arising. The activity is not early in terms of a particular stage of life, but early in the onset of problems – before the occurrence of such outcomes in order to prevent the costs associated with them.
>
> (EIF, 2015: 19)

Such an approach reinforces the value of prevention, albeit in secondary prevention terms. Whilst primary prevention is at the heart of the health promoting public health role of health visitors, they nevertheless have a major role to play in identifying needs and providing early help and support.

A robust legislative and policy framework underpins the role of the health visitor in safeguarding children and incorporates a range of global, national, professional, and local policies and procedures. This reflects society's recognition of the seriousness of child abuse and neglect as public health issues, and also the value that health visitors bring to a safeguarding role.

According to the World Health Organization (WHO, 2014), the maltreatment of children is a major global issue. Each year, millions of children worldwide are the victims of and witnesses to physical, sexual, and emotional violence. It is estimated that globally 41 000 deaths in children under the age of 15 are attributed to homicide, with those under 4 and those in their adolescent years at greatest risk (WHO, 2014). The WHO goes on to acknowledge that this number underestimates the true extent of the problem, as a considerable proportion of child deaths due to maltreatment are wrongly attributed to falls, burns, drowning, and other causes. For children who survive abuse, there are likely to be lifelong physical and emotional health consequences for their well being and development, not only through childhood but into adulthood too.

Safeguarding children requires a global political response. The development of policy at a national and international level for the protection of children against abuse has, in recent decades, become increasingly child-centred, with a growing recognition of the rights of children. Global safeguarding policy is underpinned by the UNCRC (UNICEF, 1989), which has become the world's most ratified human rights convention, with only one UN member state, the USA, having declined to ratify it (at the time of writing, Somalia remains in the process of finalising ratification). This international treaty consists of 54 articles that detail a range of civil, political, economic, social, and cultural rights which every child is deemed to require in order to live a safe, happy, and fulfilled childhood. The convention was clearly a significant undertaking by the UN, which challenged its member states to recognise the importance of the state in supporting children, meeting their health and development needs, and, if necessary, intervening to protect them from harm. However, without any significant level of accountability, the UK government has ratified the convention but not incorporated it into UK law in the form of a specific Act of Parliament.

Consequently, there may be some difficulty in enforcing children's convention rights. Whilst the UNCRC places emphasis on the rights and needs of children and on the aim of ensuring an optimum state of child well being, UK policy has continued to wrestle with the rights of children and the rights and wishes of parents. Health visitors therefore find themselves working within a policy framework that, on the one hand, espouses the rights and interests of children and, on the other, sees parental choice as key to how children are parented. A health visitor's access to a child is through the parent, who is the gatekeeper to observation and communication with the child.

Although the fact that the UNCRC has not been incorporated into English law by an Act of Parliament may be considered a limitation on the value placed on children's rights in England, there is other evidence concerning the extent to which the seriousness of children's rights are taken. The government for example, is bound to making regular reports to the Committee on the Rights of the Child, a UN monitoring body. In court settings, children's convention rights are referred to and used in legal arguments and decision making, whilst in policy in respect of children, reference is often made to the fact that such policy and guidance reflects the principles of the UNCRC. An example of this in respect of a child-centred approach to safeguarding may be seen in *Working Together to Safeguard Children: A Guide to Inter-Agency Working to Safeguard and Promote the Welfare of Children* (DfE, 2015a: 10).

The UNCRC is clearly a very important document that holds great relevance for health visitors. It can be explored further in Activity 5.3. Of particular significance to the health visitor's safeguarding role is Article 19, which requires that states parties take appropriate measures to protect children from all forms of physical and mental violence, injury, abuse, and neglect. Article 19 therefore acts as a mandate for national safeguarding legislation and policy, which encompass the roles of public sector employees and professionals such as health visitors. Other articles found within the UNCRC may also be considered directly relevant to the health visitor's role in safeguarding children.

Newell (cited in Martell, 1999: 121) stated that health visitors need to see themselves as part of a new 'movement to build a human rights culture for children'. In respect of health visiting practice and children's rights *per se*, this is a laudable goal, and one which health visitors should strive for. However, in the context of the health visitor's role in safeguarding and protecting the most vulnerable children, it becomes an urgent element of essential practice. Parton (2014) argues that combining a children's rights orientation with a broad public health approach to child maltreatment provides the most positive framework for developing future policy and practice. This reinforces the value of the role of specialist community public health nurses and their contribution to safeguarding children. Health visitors therefore need a fundamental awareness and working knowledge of the convention rights that underpin their work with children, families, and the communities in which they live, as well as the ability to act as advocates for children in spite of the challenges they face within every-day practice. Prior to the Health Visitor Implementation Plan 2011–15 (DH, 2011), challenges in health visiting included those brought to light by Unite/CPHVA's (2008) Omnibus survey and subsequently emphasised by Lord Laming (2009), such as large and complex caseloads, staff shortages, and resultant time pressures, which may reduce the effectiveness of child and family interactions and assessment. Despite the recent increase in health visitor numbers as a result of the Health Visitor Implementation Plan, a current major challenge for health visitors is working in a child protection system stretched to its financial limits. The National Society for the Prevention of Cruelty to Children (NSPCC, 2014: 4) recently described the system as 'buckling under pressure', with expenditure for the main areas of public spending relating to child protection and safeguarding in all four nations of the UK relatively unchanged in the financial years from 2006/07 to 2012/13. Furthermore, it should be acknowledged that despite the growth in health visitor numbers, a great proportion of the health visiting workforce is fairly recently qualified and may therefore, even with good quality supervision, still be developing the knowledge, skills, and confidence required to undertake its safeguarding role effectively. This, together with evidence that the demand for child protection services is outgrowing expenditure, means that in respect of their safeguarding and child protection responsibilities, challenges for health visitors remain.

Health visitors face other issues within the context of health visiting practice and the safeguarding of children, too, such as the problem of balancing the needs and rights of children with the competing rights of parents. The European Convention on Human Rights (ECHR) was incorporated into English law through the Human Rights Act 1998. This important piece of legislation confers a range of human rights on all UK citizens and requires all public authorities, including health authorities and therefore health visitors, to perform their duties and enact their roles in accordance with these rights. The Conservative government (Conservatives, 2015) has pledged to replace the Human Rights Act with a British Bill of Rights. Health visitors therefore need to embed their safeguarding practice within their knowledge and understanding of any changes to human rights legislation in the context of their safeguarding and child protection roles. Of particular relevance to – and sometimes causing tension within – child protection activity is Article 8 of the ECHR: the right to respect for private and family life, home, and correspondence. Whilst it is generally unlawful for public authorities to behave in a way that is incompatible with this right, there are a number of exceptions, including activity which is in the interests of public safety, for the prevention of crime, for the protection of health or morals, or for the protection of the rights and freedoms of others. All the exceptions specified are relevant to the role of professionals in protecting children. The challenge for health visitors and other professionals, however, is to ensure that the degree of interference with families' rights under Article 8 is proportionate. It is important to recognise that the rights conferred by the ECHR and Human Rights Act extend not only to adults but to children, too. They therefore add impetus to the UNCRC and to the requirements of health visitors as public servants.

The emphasis on safeguarding children within contemporary society justifies, underpins, and guides the health visitor's role in safeguarding children. Major shifts in national child protection and safeguarding policy generally occur reactively, precipitated by high profile child deaths or scandals involving children and subsequent inquiries. For example, the death of Dennis O'Neill, beaten and starved aged 12 whilst in foster care in Shropshire, precipitated the Monckton Inquiry (Home Office, 1945) and the Children Act 1948. Later, the 1987 crisis in Cleveland, where 121 children were removed from their families following dubious diagnoses of sexual abuse, was detailed in the Cleveland Report (Butler-Sloss, 1988) and gave impetus to the Children Act 1989, which is described as having radically affected all aspects of legal practice concerning children (White *et al.*, 2008); consequently, the practice of all professionals working with children – especially those defined by the Act as being 'in need' of support and/or protection – was also affected. The death of Victoria Climbié in 2000 from severe physical abuse and neglect at the hands of her great-aunt and her partner led to an inquiry (Laming, 2003) and a range of policy and organisational changes, including *Every Child Matters: Change for Children* (DfES, 2004) and its legislative spine, the Children Act 2004. Subsequently, the death of Peter Connelly in 2007 precipitated the commissioning of a report by Lord Laming (2009) on the progress made to implement effective arrangements for safeguarding children and, later, a revision of *Working Together to Safeguard Children* (DCSF, 2010). Such policy changes impact on and present a challenge to the professional practice of health visitors when considered alongside the raft of other policy initiatives being introduced at regular intervals. Activity 5.4 will allow you to explore this further, taking into account local policy initiatives. Keeping an up-to-date working knowledge of policy changes presents a challenge to health visitors, who need to be able to identify new learning needs on a regular basis and access the knowledge and support required to fulfil their safeguarding role.

National policy also informs professional policy. The *Standards of Proficiency for Specialist Community Public Health Nurses* include the safeguarding of children and specify that specialist community public health nurses need 'in depth knowledge of child protection' (NMC, 2004: 15). Driven from a high level by both the NMC as a professional regulator and central government departments, there is no shortage of professional policy and guidance around safeguarding children. Clearly, professional practice and the policy that guides that practice should reflect the principles contained within *The Code: Professional Standards of Practice and Behaviour for Nurses and Midwives* (NMC, 2015). Recently updated, section 17 of *The Code* is explicit in respect of registrants' professional responsibilities to protect all those at risk of harm, neglect, and abuse. Furthermore, it contains a range of other, core professional values that may be applied to health visitors' safeguarding practice. Crucially, this document represents the minimum standard against which professionals are measured in relation to the NMC's function of protecting the public. Thus, it is vital that health visitors have a working knowledge of *The Code* and its application within a safeguarding and child protection context.

Defining 'child abuse'

Although children have been exposed to harmful acts and behaviours from the beginning of time, an understanding of what society considers as child abuse today only began to emerge during the 19th century. At that time, children were seen as the property of adults and not as individuals in their own right. They were often subjected to all manner and types of abuse and neglect. Indeed, a measure of society's value of children was their utility as small individuals who could perform dangerous roles by virtue of their size as factory and mill workers, coalminers, and chimney sweeps. During this time, there was growing political pressure to tackle this and other forms of exploitation of children for economic gain. Legislative change ensued with a series of Factory Acts that increasingly excluded younger children from working and limited the hours that older children could work.

A number of Education Acts gradually introduced compulsory education, whilst legislation such as the Infant Life Protection Act 1872 was designed to tackle the barbaric practice of *baby farming*. This was the term used to describe the taking in of children for a commercial fee, many of whom subsequently lived in over-crowded conditions, were subjected to abuse and neglect, and were frequently murdered. Although baby farming as such no longer exists in contemporary English society, informal, private arrangements between parents and other family members or friends are sometimes still made and may put children at risk. Whilst this practice is not confined to any one ethnic group, in today's multicultural society it is important to acknowledge that in some countries entrusting children to relatives in Europe who can offer educational and other opportunities not available to them at home is not uncommon (Laming, 2003). Where private, unregulated care arrangements are made in an abusive context, children may be used primarily as a mechanism to gain access to financial support, housing, and other benefits, may not have their needs met, and may be at risk of harm. Health visitors need to be alert to these possibilities, and be prepared to share their concerns in a procedurally appropriate manner. Accounts of relevant 19th-century legislation such as those outlined earlier are relevant to society in the 21st century. They show a clear marker for the birth of law and other forms of policy that we would now consider reflect the ethos of safeguarding children in a holistic sense; that is, taking account of the wider socioenvironmental factors that impact upon the lives of children. They also illustrate the fact that despite legislation and policy, abuse and neglect for financial gain still occur.

Despite society's attempts to address the welfare of children, there are also accounts during the 19th century of serious injuries sustained by children as a result of acts of physical abuse and neglect (Kempe & Kempe, 1978). Such accounts were predominantly recognised and interpreted within a medical discourse, through autopsy findings and epidemiological analysis of population data on injuries sustained by children. These data presented a picture of the extent to which children were abused and neglected. The first UK Act of Parliament to recognise the need to address the extent of physical abuse was the Prevention of Cruelty to Children Act 1889, which for the first time allowed the state to intervene between parents and children. This Act was amended in 1894 to acknowledge mental cruelty, create an offence where a sick child was denied medical attention, and allow children to give evidence in court. This can be interpreted as the beginnings of society's recognition of the rights of children to voice their thoughts and opinions, as well as their right to protection from emotional abuse and neglect. It would be many years, however, before the rights and interests of children would be considered more fully, with firmer legislation and stronger penalties for the perpetrators of abuse.

The association of health visiting with child protection arose during the mid–late 19th century, as it became aligned with the maternal and child welfare movement as a result of appalling poverty and insanitary conditions (Robinson, 1982). Indeed, Robinson notes that in 1867, the Ladies Sanitary Reform Association set out the duties of its visitors to include 'teaching' hygiene, child welfare, and mental and moral health and providing social support. These activities clearly align health visiting with an interest in the welfare of children. However, caution needs to be applied in interpreting the drivers for this 'teaching'. Smith (2004) challenges the altruistic and romanticised perception of the origins of health visiting with reference to middle-class fears over the spread of epidemics (Wohl, 1986), concerns over the fitness of the workforce and army recruits (Caraher & McNab, 1997), and a desire for a source of occupation among middle-class women (Cowley, 1996). Whatever the drivers were, health visiting became increasingly aligned with maternal and child welfare, and the basis for what we would now consider a 'safeguarding' role was recognised in legislative terms through the Children Act 1908, where health visitors were appointed as Infant Life Protection Visitors.

According to Robinson (1982), the development of health visiting in the 20th century was influenced both by the development of the National Health Service (NHS) and its relation with other occupational groups. The Children Act 1948 was heavily influenced by the Monckton Inquiry (Home Office, 1945) into the death of Dennis O'Neill, which highlighted how divided administrative responsibilities across departments increased the risk of errors (Robinson, 1982). Robinson presents an analysis of the influence of the Children Act 1948, the development of new children's services, and the NHS Act of 1946 for health visiting, and highlights the degree of ambiguity over its development and the parallel development of the social work profession, both of which were based within local authorities, but with an overlapping set of skills and functions. The point here for health visitors is that, to this day, we continue to see a blurring of the interface between the preventative and reactive roles of both professions. This was highlighted by Lord Laming (2009), who underlined how social workers' caseloads had risen and how, as a result, health visitors were increasingly carrying child protection issues that would previously have been referred on to children's social care services. This demonstrated that the threshold for accepting referrals of children at risk of suffering abuse was not consistent and was dependent in part on resourcing. Whilst Lord Laming acknowledged that this situation was both inappropriate and unmanageable for health visitors, it remains a challenge to be addressed. The situation also serves to illustrate the impact that the under-resourcing of one professional group has on another.

The term that first articulated the concept of child abuse in modern society was 'battered-baby syndrome', which emerged in 1961, having been coined by Kempe (Kempe & Helfer, 1972). The term was emotive and deliberatively provocative, designed to shock paediatricians and society in general out of complacency. Although it succeeded in its aim, it was acknowledged to have several limitations: it was open to interpretation, lacking in clarity, and a cause of confusion. For some, the term represented a narrow interpretation of only the severest forms of physical abuse, whereas for the authors it encompassed the total spectrum of abuse. Whilst the term 'syndrome' was used in the context of referring to a set of symptoms, it also presents connotations of a disease process, which may detract from the often premeditated and deliberate nature of child abuse. Clearly, however, the early recognition of the phenomenon of child abuse was not confined to one particular person, place, or time. Recognising the issue and naming it took a number of intellectuals and professionals from a variety of countries just short of a century.

Different sources of literature offer different terms, definitions, and perspectives on what constitutes child abuse. It is important that health visitors work with definitions of child abuse that are agreed across professional groups, so that a common consensus is reached in working together to prevent, identify, and respond to behaviours, contexts, situations, and settings that may be abusive. The current definition of child abuse aimed at the interagency workforce and offered by recent statutory guidance is:

> A form of maltreatment of a child. Somebody may abuse or neglect a child by inflicting harm, or by failing to act to prevent harm. Children may be abused in a family or in an institutional or community setting, by those known to them or, more rarely, by others (e.g. via the internet). They may be abused by an adult or adults, or another child or children.
>
> (DfE, 2015a: 92)

This is a contemporary definition, and is key for practitioners working with and coming into contact with children. Although neglect is recognised as one of the forms of child maltreatment, it is clearly differentiated in this definition from other forms, which may be further categorised as physical, emotional, and sexual. Highlighting and giving prominence to neglect in this way reflects its significance in terms of its being the most common reason for children being subjected to a child protection plan in England or for being on a child protection register in Northern Ireland, Scotland, and Wales (NSPCC, 2014), as well as increasing recognition of the deleterious impact of neglect on the health and well being of children. Indeed, neglect is often considered as separate from abuse, as it relates to acts of omission rather than commission; that is, it is based on shortfalls in meeting the needs of children, rather than specific acts they are subjected to. This can be seen in the Department for Education (DfE) definition of neglect, which refers to a 'persistent failure to meet a child's basic physical and/or psychological needs likely to result in the serious impairment of the child's health and development' (DfE, 2015a: 93). Highlighting neglect in this way may counteract the problem that it is often not perceived as abuse or maltreatment. That said, it is important to also acknowledge that whilst neglect may be referred to as a passive form of maltreatment by some authors, this does not reflect cases where neglect appears to have been premeditated and actively pursued as a form of child abuse, as for example in the case of Khyra Ishaq (Radford, 2010). Health visitors need to be mindful that differentiating neglect from physical, emotional, and sexual abuse does not diminish its significance, and, indeed, it could be argued that neglect is likely to have the greatest impact on a health visitor's workload.

Defining child abuse and neglect is only the first step for health visitors in applying these concepts to real situations in practice; you can explore this further in Activity 5.5. However, there is a broader context here relating to the formative nature of child abuse and neglect that practitioners need to consider. The concept of child abuse becomes problematic when trying to determine whether an action (or omission) should be considered abusive or not, given that how child abuse is defined and refined is subject to change over time and across different societies in different parts of the world. When we attempt to define child abuse and neglect, we do so at a given point in time and within the broad context of what society considers constitutes satisfactory parenting and what behaviours towards children are considered acceptable.

Different forms of child abuse receive different prominence in different forms of literature (e.g. policy, research, the media) at different times, often as a result of specific child abuse cases or scandals which become highlighted due to various aspects of their shocking nature. The emergence of hundreds of allegations of child sexual abuse perpetrated by Jimmy Savile in 2012 and the subsequent launch of Operation Yewtree, the criminal investigation into Savile and other alleged perpetrators, is one example. The sexual exploitation of at least 1400 children in Rotherham between 1997 and 2013 (Jay, 2014) is another. Child abuse cases and scandals emerge and lie within the broader context of an ever-increasing knowledge and evidence base around child abuse theory, safeguarding, and child protection practice, as well as improvements in investigation techniques. Technological advances, in particular, have had a paradoxical influence on how child abuse is defined. On the one hand, improvements in forensic techniques such as those used by the National Crime Agency's Child Exploitation and Online Protection (CEOP) Centre have underpinned a 'pathologisation' of child abuse by providing a medium for more sophisticated diagnosis and intervention. On the other hand, 21st-century technology, in the form of the Internet, tablets, and mobile phones, has been increasingly used as a vehicle for accessing children: both in grooming and abusing them directly (Jay, 2014) and as a means of sharing information relating to the abuse of children in the form of still or moving images or the written word. Unsurprisingly, it is not only adults who use technology to abuse children. Cyber bullying, recognised as a form of emotional abuse (DfE, 2015a), generated an 87% increase in ChildLine counselling sessions between the years 2011/12 and 2012/13 (NSPCC, 2014). In addition, there is increasing recognition and concern over the growing trend of young people taking and sharing indecent photographs of themselves, their friends, and their partners via mobile phones. Known as *sexting*, the impacts of this behaviour may be 'extremely damaging' and have been associated with suicide (CEOP, n.d.). Whilst such images may not be produced as a result of grooming, CEOP states it is aware of cases where images have found their way on to paedophile chat sites and forums. A further issue for children and young people engaging in sexting is that the behaviours associated with it make them vulnerable not only to sexual abuse and emotional harm, but also to prosecution and criminalisation. Section 45 of the Sexual Offence Act 2003 amended the Protection of Children Act 1978 to make it a criminal offence to take, make, distribute, show, and possess such photographs of any person below the age of 18. Up until recently, such technology did not exist, and this type of activity could not have been imagined as a form of child abuse. Some accepted behaviours and practices, such as allowing children access to social networking sites, may on face value appear harmless, yet they clearly pose known risks in respect of adults accessing and grooming children for the purposes of abuse. These examples illustrate an ever-expanding societal and technological context in which forms and understandings of child abuse continue to evolve. It is important that health visitors remain alert as to what constitutes both existing and newly emerging forms and definitions of child abuse as they seek to interpret behaviours and practices within families and communities. Such behaviours and practices include female genital mutilation (FGM), forced marriage (FM), and so-called 'honour based violence' (scHBV), which have been recognised as abusive and of concern to those seeking to safeguard and protect children from diverse communities in the UK. These issues will be commented on later in this chapter. It is important also to recognise that incidents of abuse, whatever form they take, do not occur in a vacuum within the lives of children, and that survival of abuse has lifelong impacts upon the health and well being of the victim (see Box 5.1).

Box 5.1   The health impacts of child abuse: examples from research

Symptoms of post-traumatic stress disorder (PTSD) are common among adult survivors of childhood abuse, with victims of past traumatic events more vulnerable to current life stressors (Kendall-Tackett, 2000).
PTSD is associated with:

- a significant impact on brain function (Van der Kolk, 1984);
- parental lack of support (Pine & Cohen, 2002);
- witnessing threats to a caregiver (Scheeringa et al., 2006);
- chronic hyper-arousal, associated with abnormal levels of stress hormones and alteration of certain brain structures (Bremner, 1999).

There is an association between neglect and:

- adverse effects on the development of a child's brain (Glaser, 2000);
- maldevelopment of neural systems associated with social and emotional functioning (Perry, 2002);
- reduced brain mass (Perry, 2002).

Adults with four or more adverse childhood experiences (ACE study):

- had higher rates of ischemic heart disease, cancer, stroke, chronic bronchitis, emphysema, diabetes, skeletal fractures, and hepatitis (Felitti et al., 1998);
- were more likely to have had 50 or more sexual partners, and to have had a sexually transmitted disease (STD) (Felitti et al., 2001);
- were more likely to have considered themselves alcoholics, to have used illegal drugs, and to have injected drugs (Felitti et al., 2001).

(Continued)

Box 5.1 *(Continued)*

Survivors of childhood abuse are more likely to:

- smoke (Felitti *et al.*, 2001);
- have higher rates of obesity (Felitti, 1991);
- develop irritable bowel syndrome (IBS) (Talley *et al.*, 1995; Kendall-Tackett, 2000);
- report diabetes or three or more symptoms of diabetes (Kendall-Tackett & Marshall, 1999);
- experience sleeping difficulties, including repetitive nightmares (Teegen, 1999);
- have twice the physical symptoms reported in primary care, require more primary care visits, and undergo twice as much surgery (Hulme, 2000);
- consider themselves alcoholics, have used illegal drugs, have injected drugs, and have attempted suicide (Felitti *et al.*, 2001);
- develop major depression (Briere & Elliot, 1994);
- suffer from conduct disorders, depression, and suicide (Fergusson *et al.*, 1996);
- have children with hyperactivity, conduct problems, and peer or emotional problems (Roberts *et al.*, 2004).

Female survivors of child sexual abuse:

- are 10 times more likely to have a history of drug addiction and twice as likely to have been alcoholics than members of the control group (Briere & Runtz, 1987);
- have a higher risk of sexual activities than non-abused females, with earlier age of first intercourse and higher likelihood of having fifty or more partners, unprotected intercourse, and STIs (Kendall-Tackett, 2002).

Whilst the quality of these studies may vary, there is a clear and consistent pattern that makes the association between child abuse and health issues explicit. This is more so with forms of abuse that are easier to measure/observe (e.g. physical abuse) and less so with sexual abuse, neglect, and emotional maltreatment, which can be more challenging to research. Evidence from various inquiries may be useful in this respect; for example, the Independent Inquiry into Child Sexual Exploitation in Rotherham 1997–2013 (Jay, 2014) found that in just over a third of cases, children affected by sexual exploitation were previously known to services because of child neglect and the need for child protection. There was also a history of domestic violence in 46% of cases, as well as high levels of truancy and school refusal. This points to comorbidity in respect of forms of child sexual exploitation and possible compounding of impacts on children's physical, emotional, and social well being. Despite the variance across the studies, the wealth of evidence to date suggests an association between child abuse and poor health that could be readily applied to Bradford Hill's criteria for causation (Bradford Hill, 1965).

This evidence demonstrates that the health visitor's role in safeguarding is not only to seek to protect a child from harm in the short term, but also to optimise and promote the child's future trajectory for health into adulthood. It is also important to consider when working with parents/adults experiencing the health problems mentioned in this box that they may have been exposed to adverse childhood experiences, or indeed be survivors of child abuse themselves.

Defining 'significant harm'

The concept of 'significant harm' represents a legal definition of child abuse, and was first introduced in Section 31(9) of the Children Act 1989. The concept reflects a threshold that legitimises state intervention into the lives of children and families to safeguard and promote child welfare. Under Section 47 of the Children Act 1989, social workers, as employees of 'local authorities', have a duty to 'make enquiries' or begin investigations, undertaking assessments and gathering information to inform decision making regarding actions that may need to be taken to protect a child who is suffering, or at risk of suffering, significant harm. As part of this process, where the age of the child is relevant to the recent or current work of health visitors, social workers will communicate with health visitors in the investigation process and may draw from health or other assessments. As a result of such activities led by social workers, courts may subsequently make a care order (whereby the child is committed to the care of the local authority) or supervision order (whereby the child is put under the supervision of a social worker or probation officer) where the threshold criterion is reached.

The term 'significant' is not defined in the Children Act 1989, but in deciding what is significant, provision is made for courts to compare the health and development of the child concerned 'with that which could reasonably be expected of a similar child' (Children Act 1989, §31:10). A 'similar child' was defined by the Lord Chancellor at that time as a child with the same physical attributes as the child concerned, and not simply a child of the same background. This notion was contested by Freeman (1992), who argued that whilst the goal of the 'similar child' notion was to be applauded because it emphasised the unique needs of children with disabilities, it overlooked the essential individuality of families and their problems. Health visitors have the opportunity of forming assessments that reflect the individuality of children and families, and courts may use these assessments to decide for themselves what constitutes significant harm. 'Harm' is clearly defined in the Children Act 1989 as 'ill-treatment or the impairment of health or development'. This definition was later extended by Section 120 of the Adoption and Children Act 2002 to include impairment suffered by hearing or seeing the ill treatment of another, in recognition that children exposed to the domestic abuse of others suffer harm. The Children Act 1989 considers 'ill treatment' to mean sexual abuse and abusive actions that are not physical (thus implicating both physical and emotional abuse as abuse). In addition, 'health' is deemed to mean both physical and mental health, and 'development' is taken to include dimensions such as physical, emotional, behavioural, intellectual, and social development. It is essential that health visitors have an understanding of the concept of the risk of significant harm and recognise the value of their contributions to child protection processes. Such contributions include using their knowledge to make appropriate referrals and sharing their well-documented assessments of children's circumstances and experiences, their physical and mental health, and all aspects of their development: physical, emotional, behavioural, intellectual, and social.

The concept of significant harm is, however, ambiguous, subjective, and open to interpretation by individual practitioners and representatives of various authorities. Its effectiveness in protecting the right children at the right moment in time will thus be inconsistent, as individual cases will, by their very nature, vary, as will the knowledge, experience, skills, and confidence of practitioners working with them. Health visitors should be aware that there are no absolute criteria on which professionals can rely when judging what constitutes significant harm. The interpretation of significant harm as a threshold for intervention is not static and depends on a number of factors; you can explore these further in Activity 5.6.

A clear example of the sometimes acutely volatile nature of the threshold for intervention may be seen in response to the case of Peter Connelly, who died in 2007 as a result of extreme physical abuse and neglect. Following Peter's death, there was an unprecedented rise in applications for neglected and abused children to be taken into care (Cafcass, 2010). The demand for care applications has climbed steadily since 2008–09, and applications during 2014–15 were recently described by the Children and Family Court Advisory and Support Service (Cafcass, 2015) as having been at an all time high, with July 2014 producing eleven thousand one hundred and thirty five. Cafcass (2015) suggests that the 2014–15 data may be attributable to a number of factors, including increased awareness of child sexual exploitation leading to a greater number of referrals to local authorities, greater public and professional awareness of child protection issues, and more rigorous reviewing and greater scrutiny of plans within local authorities.

Variations in the threshold for removing the most vulnerable children at risk of – or actually suffering from – significant harm from their families present challenges in practice. When the threshold for intervention is high, it may be difficult for professionals to succeed in getting very vulnerable children into care. Such children may be exposed to continuing risk of abuse and neglect and are more dependent on higher levels of support and supervision within the community. Clearly, this has an impact on health visiting and other family support services.

The concept of significant harm as a threshold for intervention thus presents challenges, both in theory and in practice. Nettleton (1998) and Appleton (1994) both identified the stress on health visitors when working with families in which there are significant concerns about the harms that children may be subjected to, but where a threshold has not been reached to trigger formal intervention by child protection services. The key here is for health visitors to access supervision and to underpin their carefully and clearly written referrals, assessments, and reports with reference to research and the evidence base. Such an approach will help to form the basis of collaborative, critical, evidence-based decision making and so determine whether or not a child is being subjected to significant harm. Despite its ambiguities, Harwin & Madge (2010) acknowledge that the concept of significant harm has largely stood the test of time and that the absence of a clear operational definition is both its strength and its weakness. They consider that it allows for necessary professional discretion, but acknowledge that its vulnerabilities are associated with external pressures that affect its interpretation and suggest that a more confident workforce and greater resources are required.

One advantage of the legal concept of significant harm not being static is of particular interest to health visitors working with families in which there is domestic abuse. As already mentioned, the legal definition of harm includes harm suffered by seeing or hearing the ill treatment of others. This amendment occurred in recognition of society's growing awareness of both the scale of domestic abuse and its negative impact on women, children, and young people. Based on statistics from the 2013/14 Crime Survey for England and Wales, the Office for National Statistics (ONS, 2015) estimates that 1.4 million women aged 16–59 in England and Wales suffered domestic abuse in the years 2013 to 2014. It should be acknowledged that domestic abuse is also perpetrated by women against men – there were an estimated 700 000 male victims in the same time period (ONS, 2015) – and that it also occurs in same-sex relationships. However, it is recognised that the vast majority of acts of gender-based violence are perpetrated by men against women and girls (HM Government, 2011). Furthermore, women are more likely than men to have experienced intimate violence across all headline types of abuse when asked (ONS, 2015). The Department of Health (DH, 2013b) acknowledge that domestic abuse often starts or intensifies during pregnancy, and it has been estimated that at least 750 000 children witness domestic abuse each year (DH, 2002) and that in homes where domestic abuse occurs, children witness approximately three-quarters of incidents (RCPsych, 2014). Hughes (1992) found that in 90% of cases, when domestic abuse occurs, the children are in the same or next room. Thus, even when children do not directly see violent or abusive incidents, they are likely to be exposed to them through hearing both the abuse itself and the reaction of the victim. Furthermore, they will subsequently be exposed to its physical and emotional impact. Being exposed to domestic abuse can cause children harm in a number of ways; for example, seeing and hearing a parent (most likely their mother) being abused can cause children emotional distress; children may sustain physical injuries during violent physical assaults when they attempt to intervene to protect a parent; and children may be forced to take part in various forms of abuse or to witness it (DH, 2009b). Forcing children to take part in or witness abuse reduces them to being used as tools; this behaviour dehumanises children and increases both their own and their mother's suffering. Threats are often made to harm or kill children in an attempt to exert power and control over women. In 30–60% of cases where women are being abused, children are also being physically and/or sexually abused (Edelson, cited in DH, 2009b). This is significant when working with families where domestic abuse occurs; health visitors need to consider that children may be at risk of suffering or may actually be suffering significant harm through both their exposure to the domestic abuse and through other forms of abuse. Likewise, when working with families where there is suspected or known child abuse, the possibility that domestic abuse may be occurring should be considered and explored. Effective identification of domestic abuse remains a challenge, with many women reluctant to disclose their situation (BMA Board of Science, 2014). A literature review conducted by Litherland (2012) reinforced the value of the health visitors' role in the identification of domestic abuse and concluded that the use of routine enquiry using a screening tool increased disclosure rates. Furthermore, Litherland found that recurrent enquiry, giving information to all women following enquiry, knowledgeable and caring practitioners, and supportive environments were all important in eliciting disclosure of abuse. Health visitors therefore need to embrace these approaches so that they may safeguard and promote the well being of women and children alike.

Amendments to the Children Act 1989 in respect of domestic abuse demonstrate the importance of updating legislation to reflect society's growing understanding of concepts of abuse. Updates to policy also chart shifts in understanding. For example, the definition of domestic abuse itself was recently revised to acknowledge findings from various sources that young people aged 16 and 17 may be victims of domestic violence and abuse:

> The cross-government definition of domestic violence and abuse is:
> any incident or pattern of incidents of controlling, coercive, threatening behaviour, violence or abuse between those aged 16 or over who are, or have been, intimate partners or family members regardless of gender or sexuality. The abuse can encompass, but is not limited to:
>
> - psychological
> - physical
> - sexual
> - financial
> - emotional
>
> (Home Office, 2015)

Controlling behaviour

Controlling behaviour is a range of acts designed to make a person subordinate and/or dependent by isolating them from sources of support, exploiting their resources and capacities for personal gain, depriving them of the means needed for independence, resistance and escape and regulating their everyday behaviour.

Coercive behaviour

> Coercive behaviour is an act or pattern of acts of assaults, threats, humiliation and intimidation or other abuse that is used to harm, punish or frighten their victim.
>
> (Home Office, 2015)

A strength of the recent definition is clearly its inclusion of 16- and 17-year-olds, but further it is a cross-government definition, which should assist professionals from various disciplines to share a common understanding of domestic violence, which can then be used as a starting point for effective identification and intervention. However, in respect of safeguarding vulnerable groups, it is not a legal definition, and there is no specific statutory offence of domestic violence. Some of the behaviours associated with domestic violence might amount to a criminal offence, and it may be useful for health visitors to review these behaviours in the *CPS Policy for Prosecuting Cases of Domestic Violence* (CPS, 2009: Appendix A). Sometimes, disclosures made to and recorded by health visitors may be relevant in respect of not only safeguarding children and vulnerable women but also criminal justice proceedings and potential convictions.

Although the definition of domestic violence is not a legal definition, it does include scHBV, FM, and FGM (DH, 2013b). Over recent years, legislation has been introduced that criminalises the behaviours associated with these forms of abuse. FM, scHBV, and FGM are all abuses of human rights and all potentially involve children as victims and therefore raise safeguarding concerns. The question as to whether scHBV should be incorporated into the definition of domestic violence has been contended, with the differences between scHBV and domestic abuse highlighted (Dickson, 2014; Dyer, 2015). As with domestic violence, there is no specific offence of honour based crime. 'scHBV' is regarded as an umbrella term that encompasses various offences covered by existing legislation. It is described by the Crown Prosecution Service (CPS, 2015) as:

> a collection of practices, which are used to control behavior within families or other social groups to protect perceived cultural and religious beliefs and/or honour. Such violence can occur when perpetrators perceive that a relative has shamed the family and/or community by breaking their honour code.

The CPS (2015) goes on to define scHBV as 'a crime or incident that has [been], or may have been, committed to protect or defend the honour of the family and/or the community'. Children and young people have been identified as the age group most at risk of scHBV (Dyer, 2015). Statistics produced by Karma Nirvana (cited in Dyer, 2015), which runs a dedicated line for victims of FM and scHBV, show that in 2013 it responded to 351 cases from victims aged 17 and under. Children and young people may experience scHBV in a number of ways: they can be the direct victim of physical and emotional abuse or FM themselves or, as cases relating to honour based killings (e.g. the murders of Shafilea Ahmed and Rukhsana Naz) demonstrate, they may be forced to watch. Where so-called honour based killings occur, children will also endure the impact of the death of their sibling, parent, or family member, and may remain at risk of becoming a victim or perpetrator themselves. Furthermore, scHBV has been identified as always preceding FM (Sanghera, cited in Dyer, 2015).

The Department for Children, Schools and Families (DCSF, 2009) estimated reported cases of actual or potential FM at between 5000 and 8000 for 2008, although this did not include 'hidden' victims who did not approach agencies for help. Guidance emphasises the importance of distinguishing between an arranged marriage and an FM:

In arranged marriages, the families of both spouses take a leading role in arranging the marriage, but the choice of whether or not to accept the arrangement still remains with the prospective spouses. However, in forced marriage, one or both spouses do not consent to the marriage but are coerced into it. Duress can include physical, psychological, financial, sexual and emotional pressure.

(HM Government, 2014a: 1)

Recent statistics produced by the Forced Marriage Unit (FMU, 2014) show that over a 12 month period, it gave advice or support in 1267 cases, covering all regions of the UK. Where the age of the (potential or actual) victim was known, 22% of these cases involved a child under the age of 18; in 11% of these latter cases, the child was under the age of 16. Statistics relating to 2012 (FMU, 2012) demonstrate the youngest victim that year was aged just 2. FM has recently been criminalised in England and Wales under the Anti-Social Behaviour, Crime and Policing Act 2014, and the first conviction in the UK has just taken place (Family Law Week, 2015). Dyer (2015) reports that victims of FM and scHBV suffer physically and emotionally, experiencing anxiety and depression, and are more at risk of schizophrenia, self–harm, and suicide. Clearly, health visitors and school nurses must increase their knowledge and understanding of scHBV and FM and of the evolving national and local policies that support their practice in working with those at risk.

Unfortunately, the recent successful conviction of a perpetrator of FM has not yet been mirrored in the case of FGM. The Ministry of Justice (MOJ/Home Office, 2015) defines FGM as 'Procedures that include the partial or total removal of the external female genital organs for non-medical reasons' and acknowledges that whilst the age at which girls are subjected to FGM varies, the majority of cases are likely to occur at between 5 and 8. There is international recognition that FGM is a violation of the rights of girls and women, that it has no health benefits, and that it compromises health in a number of ways, causing severe pain and bleeding, problems in urinating, cysts, infections, infertility, childbirth complications, and increased risk of newborn deaths (WHO, 2015). FGM has been a criminal offence in the UK for 30 years, with the Female Genital Mutilation Act 2003 replacing the Prohibition of Female Circumcision Act of 1985. However, despite estimates that over 20 000 girls under the age of 15 are considered at risk of FGM in the UK each year and the possibility of up to 60 000 women living with the consequences of FGM (Dorkenoo et al., 2007), the UK is yet to see a single successful conviction. As a result of this, the Serious Crime Act 2015 has recently amended and strengthened the 2003 Act, with the following provisions:

- Offences of FGM committed abroad by or against those who are habitually resident in the UK irrespective of whether they are subject to immigration restrictions may now be prosecuted.
- Victims of FGM may now be provided with anonymity.
- A new offence for those with parental responsibility of failing to protect a girl under the age of 16 from FGM has been introduced.
- FGM Protection Orders have been introduced.
- Professionals now have a duty to notify police of FGM.

The latter provision is of particular relevance to professionals, including specialist community public health nurses, as it creates a mandatory reporting duty. This means that where, in the course of their professional duties, health visitors and school nurses discover that FGM appears to have been carried out on a girl under the age of 18 at the time of discovery, they must report this to the police. This duty applies both where the professional is informed by the girl that an act of FGM has been carried out on her and where the professional observes physical signs which appear to indicate that an act of FGM has been carried out. In addition, the Secretary of State has issued statutory guidance on FGM. Up-to-date guidance for professionals safeguarding children from FGM (DH, 2015) is available, however, as are more general multiagency practice guidelines concerning FGM (HM Government, 2014b; 2016). Clearly, midwives, health visitors, and school nurses should become conversant with and work in partnership within the realms of such guidance as a matter of urgency. The DH (2015) points out that antenatal and intranatal care afford NHS professionals an opportunity to identify that FGM has been carried out on a mother, indicating potential risk of FGM in a female child, and that safeguarding procedures may have to be in place for many years in order to protect girls at risk.

Although it is clear that strides are being been made in respect of changes to legislation and policy to safeguard and protect vulnerable children, it should be acknowledged that society and legislators may take some time to respond to and accept the changing knowledge base about what constitutes child abuse. Take, as an example, many failed attempts to make child smacking an offence. The repercussions are that the law may not be terribly explicit in safeguarding children from contentious or newly emerging forms of child abuse, leaving some children inadequately provided for. It is vital, therefore, that health visitors place themselves in a position to influence policies affecting health (CETHV, 1977) by lobbying for changes in national legislation to safeguard children, whilst keeping abreast of legislative changes that impact on their everyday practice.

Incidence and prevalence of child abuse

The terms 'incidence' and 'prevalence' hold their own distinct features and can provide useful information on the extent of a given condition in the population. 'Incidence' has been defined as the number of new events occurring within a given population within a specified period of time (Last, 2001). Within the context of child abuse, this refers mainly to those cases that are reported and recorded (Creighton, 2007). 'Prevalence', however, refers to the number of events in a given population at a designated time (Last, 2001). In the context of child abuse, this says more about the extent of abuse in the community, and includes both unreported and reported cases. Data on prevalence rely mainly on survey-based studies to identify 'hidden' unreported cases. This might be done by asking a sample of adults or young people whether they were abused during their childhood, regardless of whether it was reported or not. Consequently, the nature and outcomes of such studies can only provide estimates of the extent of child abuse in the community or population as a whole.

Prevalence studies have been conducted in the USA, UK, and Netherlands over the last 30 years or so, and are mostly confined to child sexual abuse (Creighton, 2007). By virtue of the problems associated with these studies and their inherent biases, prevalence estimates range markedly across them. For example, in relation to child sexual abuse, the percentage of adults and adolescents affected varies from 6.8 to 20.4% in women and girls and from 1.0 to 16.2% in men and boys (Creighton, 2007). Some international studies have shown that, depending on the country, between a quarter and a half of all children report severe and frequent physical abuse, which includes being beaten, kicked, or tied up by parents (WHO & ISPCAN, 2006).

In relation to socioeconomic status, some studies have suggested a relationship between income and harm to children (DH, 1995; Baldwin & Caruthers, 1998; Corby, 2000). However, this predominantly relates to physical harm and neglect: whilst there may be more known cases of physical abuse or neglect amongst families with lower socioeconomic status, studies have been consistent in failing to find differences in the prevalence of sexual abuse (Parton, 1997). Given that most statistics associated with child abuse are based on known and reported cases, this may only reflect that low-income families are more likely to have contact with state agencies and professionals, in a variety of contexts, and as such are susceptible to a greater level of state surveillance than families on higher incomes. Caution needs to be applied when considering data at a population level, as these are not directly attributable to individuals: not every parent on a low income abuses their children and not every abuser will be of low socioeconomic status.

A starting point for determining the threshold at which child abuse is reported to children's services might be the number of Section 47 enquiries that take place. As an example, Table 5.1 shows the number of enquiries that took place in England each year from 2009 to 2014 and the subsequent number of these enquiries that led to initial child protection conferences; as can be seen, these numbers have been steadily increasing during this period (DfE, 2014). The table also shows that whilst Section 47 places a duty on children's services departments to investigate whether there is a need for further action to safeguard a child's welfare, over half of cases do not lead to an initial child protection case conference. This is further evidence of the extent to which health visitors will find themselves working with families with vulnerable children who are exposed to an environment which at the very least lies close to the threshold for recognition as child abuse.

Figure 5.1 demonstrates the rising trend in the recording of child abuse cases, from 26 in 10 000 children under 18 years in 2000 to 34 in 10 000 in 2009. The trend, of course, is not completely linear, and suggests that the recording of abuse is linked to other factors besides the actual number of abused children. For example, the rises in 2002/03 and 2008/09 may be associated with the responses of children's services to the Victoria Climbié and Peter Connolly cases, respectively. Table 5.2 shows similar data for the years 2011 to 2014. These data are taken from the Children in Need census (an annual statutory census for all local authorities), and due to the move from an emphasis on local authorities calculating indicators and returning aggregate-level information to a child-level national return, where indicators

Table 5.1 Section 47 enquiries and initial child protection conferences in England from 1 April 2009 to 31 March 2014.

	2009/10	2010/11	2011/12	2012/13	2013/14
Number of children subject to Section 47 enquiries	89 300	111 700	124 600	127 100	142 500
Number of children who were the subject of an initial child protection conference	43 900	53 000	56 200	60 100	65 200

Source: DFE (2014) Statistical First Release 43/2014.

are calculated by the DfE, it is not possible to make direct comparisons between Figure 5.1 and Table 5.2. Suffice it to say that the most recent statistical reports from the DfE suggest a continued increase in the number and rate of children becoming the subject of a child protection plan (Table 5.2).

Figure 5.2 presents another perspective on the numbers of children recognised as abused and subject to a child protection plan between 2000 and 2009. From 2010, the data were again reported from the Children in Need Census. Health visitors, in particular, will note that the largest group of children is aged under 4 years.

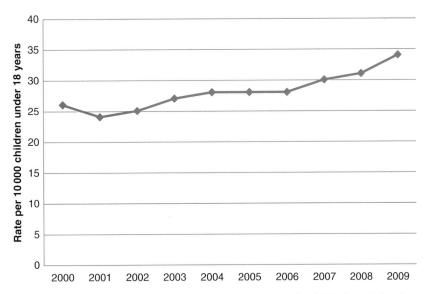

Figure 5.1 Children who became subject to a child protection plan in England during the years 2000–09.
Source: DCSF (2009) Statistical First Release 22/2009. Used under OGL 2.0.

Table 5.2 Number and rate of children who became the subject of a child protection plan during selected years.

	2011/12	2012/13	2013/14
Number	52 100	52 700	59 800
Rate per 10 000 children	46	46.2	52.1

Source: DfE Statistical First Releases 27/2012; 45/2013; 43/2014

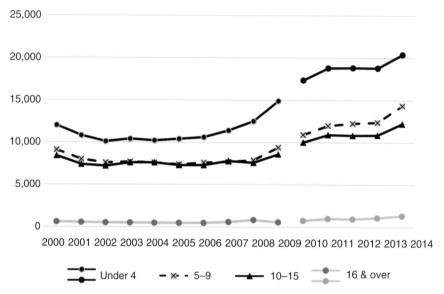

Figure 5.2 Number of children who were the subject of a child protection plan in England by age group at 31 March for selected years.
Source: DfE Statistical First Releases 22/2009; 27/2012; 45/2013; 43/2014. NB: Data since 2010 collected from Children in Need Census.

School-age children in total present an even larger group, which in itself presents challenges for school nursing services. Again, the trend is not linear, with a slight 'U' shape, showing a decrease up to 2002 and a subsequent gradual rise, followed by a steeper rise more recently. The reasons for this are not entirely clear. Changes in trends can be the result of particular events, such as:

- A possible response by services to high-profile cases or scandals, with a resultant tendency to acknowledge behaviour as abusive where it may not previously have been perceived as such.
- Changes in a data source, where data are collated and reported in different ways.
- Changes in policy:
  o The introduction of the Framework for Assessment of Children in Need (DH *et al.*, 2000) meant that some children who would previously have been placed on the child protection register could now be defined as 'in need'.

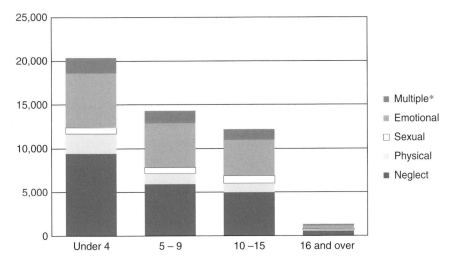

Figure 5.3 Number of children who were the subject of a child protection plan in England by age and category of abuse at 31 March 2014.
Source: DfE (2014) Statistical First Release 43/2014. *'Multiple' refers to instances where there is more than one main category of abuse. These children are not counted under the other abuse headings, so a child can appear only once in this table.

○ The acknowledgement of domestic abuse as a form of child abuse may have contributed to an increase in cases in recent years.

Figure 5.3 goes further and breaks down the age groups into the recognised categories of abuse. It is clear across all the age groups that the predominant form is that of neglect, followed by emotional abuse. The incidence of physical abuse appears to decline with age. Health visitors therefore face difficult challenges in working with families with abused young children, where clearly the emphasis is on fostering good attachment, effective parenting skills, and positive, warm relationships between parents and their children.

Despite the variation across studies, there is a large group of children who are subjected to different forms of abuse that never come to the attention of the authorities. Those that are reported and subsequently recorded as abuse form the 'tip of the iceberg'. The figures in this section have to be placed within the context of the total population of children, where the majority of children are not abused. For health visitors and school nurses, this reinforces the importance of the fundamental and universal nature of their provision, which should remain pivotal to their work with children and families.

Assessment of vulnerable children

In respect of the assessment of vulnerable children, it is important that health visitors are familiar with the legislation and policy that applies to the country they are employed in. Each of the four nations that make up the UK has its own laws, policies, guidance, and systems to help safeguard and protect vulnerable children at risk. The NSPCC (2015) recognises that despite differences in child protection systems in each nation, the principles they are based on are shared. The NSPCC website Child Protection in the UK (NSPCC, 2015) may be a useful starting point to find out more. Clearly these differences may present challenges to health visitors when moving across geographical boundaries. In England and Wales, Section 17 of the Children Act 1989 (see also Section 17 of the Children (Northern Ireland) Order 1995 and Section 22 of the Children (Scotland) Act 1995, as appropriate) is concerned with the duty of local authorities, including health authorities (and therefore health visitors), to safeguard and promote the welfare of children deemed to be 'in need' in their area. Section 17 defines a child in need as follows:

(a) He is unlikely to achieve or maintain, or have the opportunity of achieving or maintaining, a reasonable standard of health or development without appropriate provision for him of services by a local authority under this Part;
(b) His health or development is likely to be significantly impaired, without the provision for him or her of services by a local authority under this Part; or
(c) He is disabled.

(Children Act 1989)

In line with the duty of authorities to safeguard and promote the welfare of children in need, local authorities in each of the four nations of the UK are required to promote the upbringing of children in need by their families by providing a range and level of services appropriate to those children's needs. These provisions reflect an underlying principle of the Children Act 1989, Children (Northern Ireland) Order 1995, and Children (Scotland) Act 1995 that, wherever possible, children should be brought up by their families. It is important to bear in mind, though, that this duty is not absolute. The cost implications of meeting identified needs through resources are huge, and resources need to be allocated effectively. As a result, there is an acknowledgement that resources need to be prioritised according to the assessment of need. Authorities are not required to meet the needs of every single child, but they are required to take reasonable steps to do so and to make provisions as they consider appropriate. The legal provisions for children in need are clearly significant to the work of health visitors across the UK in that they seek to acknowledge the importance of the safety, health, development, and emerging potential of vulnerable children. Health visitors are trained to work with children and families to search for health needs, stimulate awareness of health needs, and facilitate health enhancing activities (CETHV, 1977). However, the effectiveness of this provision in the context of health visiting is weakened by both inadequate resourcing and the retention of health visiting services.

Assessment of children in need and their families

The allocation of resources both to those children in need of support under Section 17 of the Children Act 1989 and to those in need of possible and actual protection is dependent on effective assessment of children's needs. As highlighted in Chapters 2 and 3, a key element of the health visitor's role relates to the assessment of the

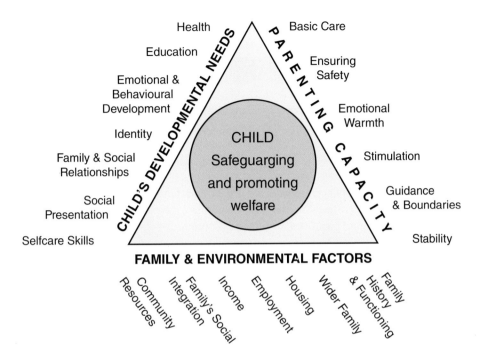

Figure 5.4 Assessment Framework.
Source: DfE (2015a: 22). Used under OGL 2.0.

health needs of children and their families. In offering a universal service, health visitors provide a range of early help, health supporting, and health promoting interventions, which, if effective, may empower families to take control of their children's health and well being, reducing the need for referral on to other services. In respect of supporting all professionals in the process of assessing vulnerable children, the Assessment Framework (DfE, 2015a) ensures a systematic and thorough approach to assessment takes place. It requires consideration of the child's health and development needs, the parents' capacity to parent, and relevant social and environmental factors (see Figure 5.4). These are described as three domains, and the DfE (2015a) defines a good assessment as investigating their interaction.

Health visitors need a working understanding of the Assessment Framework and the ability to demonstrate its critical application by maintaining relevant, contemporaneous records that detail not only areas of concern but also areas of strength and positivity within a child's life, reflecting these critical dimensions. The DfE (2015a) stresses the importance of identifying the impact of what is happening to the child, thus encouraging health visitors to take an empathic, child-centred approach to their assessment work. Behaviours or events that cause concern or constitute significant harm may emerge suddenly or may surface gradually over time. Sudden major concerns relating to significant harm can occur as a result of a single significant event, such as the violent shaking of a neonate or the beating or rape of a child. Conversely, a temporal, gradually unfolding picture of concern may emerge through a combination of seemingly less significant events occurring over a much longer period of time.

The corrosive impact of neglect as a form of child abuse on children's health and well being is a good but not exclusive example of how significant harm occurs in this way. Another example from a parenting perspective relates to those parents who exhibit low warmth towards and high criticism of their children (DH, 1995). In such cases, the realisation that significant harm may be occurring is based on reflection on the significance of both retrospective and current events and knowledge. The Assessment Framework is useful, therefore, in assisting health visitors to articulate their knowledge of unmet need and possible child abuse within a chronological context and supports both their referrals to other agencies and any statutory assessments undertaken by social workers.

The Assessment Framework can provide a useful mechanism to support practice. However, where health visitors have large and/or complex caseloads, practice shifts from the larger population of children who may have some degree of unrecognised, unmet need and who are possibly at risk to a smaller, distinct group of vulnerable children whose needs have already been recognised and prioritised. A silent escalation of risk can occur in the larger population, which eventually crosses the threshold from children in need of support to children in need of protection, resulting in even heavier demands upon services. The utility of the Framework therefore lies in the opportunity for contact with children to provide early help and intervention. Where there is no contact, there is no opportunity to assess and meet unmet need and a greater likelihood of practice becoming crisis-led. Furthermore, even when contact between health visitors and families occurs, barriers to the opportunistic recognition of abuse within practice exist and should be considered. For example, 'routine' top-to-toe examinations of babies during primary visits may no longer occur and babies may be seen and weighed less frequently than they once were. Good leadership and decision making become an essential part of the health visiting role in these circumstances, which calls for innovative practice, political awareness, and the confidence to work in different settings. An example of good leadership might be a health visitor working in partnership with a local faith group to raise awareness of children's needs for safety and protection in a faith setting, with the aim of establishing a safeguarding policy. A strength of such an approach would be that the faith leaders may themselves become partners in identifying vulnerable children at risk of suffering or actually suffering harm.

Common Assessment Framework (CAF)

The *Every Child Matters* strategy (DfES, 2004) introduced the Common Assessment Framework (CAF) following Lord Laming's (2003) report into the death of Victoria Climbié in 2000. The CAF is a useful shared assessment and planning framework for use across children's services and local areas in England (for an example of a CAF form, see www.cwdcouncil.org.uk/caf). At face value, the introduction of 'another' assessment framework may appear confusing. Some clarity on the relationship between the CAF and the Assessment Framework is therefore of value at this point.

The CAF is recognised as a standardised approach to interagency assessment where a child would benefit from the coordinated support of one or more agencies

(DfE, 2015a). This process enables early identification of additional needs and the promotion of a coordinated service response. The CAF is therefore an example of an early help assessment, and in the context of safeguarding aims to identify the assistance that children and families require to prevent their needs from escalating to a point where intervention through a statutory assessment under the Children Act 1989 is needed. In some areas, assessment tools based on the CAF have been developed locally and have now replaced the CAF (see for example the Early Help Assessment Tool (EHAT) (Liverpool City Council, n.d.) or the Early Help Assessment Form (EHAF) (Nottinghamshire County Council, n.d.)).

Early help assessment tools such as the CAF are therefore intended for use by practitioners who are concerned that a child is at risk of not achieving one or more of the five outcomes of *Every Child Matters* and where the support of one or more agencies is required when a practitioner perceives that a child's additional needs cannot be met by the existing service.

The Children's Workforce Development Council (CWDC, 2009) provides a helpful breakdown of the components of CAF:

- a pre-assessment checklist to help practitioners identify children who might benefit from a common assessment;
- a process to enable practitioners to undertake a common assessment and then act on the result;
- a standard form to allow practitioners to record the assessment;
- a delivery plan and review form.

The CAF is *not* for use where practitioners have concerns that a child may be suffering or may be at risk of suffering harm. In these cases, the practitioners' Local Safeguarding Children Board's (LSCB's) safeguarding procedures should be followed immediately, and if necessary advice should be sought from the local safeguarding or child protection team. In these cases, health visitors and other professionals may find it useful to refer to guidance such as *Working Together* (DfE, 2015a) or *What to Do if You're Worried a Child Is Being Abused* (DfE, 2015b). However, where there have been long-standing problems or concerns in families in which child protection concerns emerge, it is likely that other services have been involved and that a CAF is in place. Clearly, assessments undertaken as part of the CAF process should inform work undertaken to protect children who are suffering or are likely to suffer significant harm.

The CAF is a voluntary process and, given the requirements of the Data Protection Act 1998, children and/or their parents/carers must give their consent at the start in order for the assessment to take place. The CAF may be opened before or in support of a referral or subsequent specialist assessment. However, it is not a referral form *per se*. CAFs can be useful in the referral process, ensuring that a referral is relevant and helping reduce the duplication of repeated assessment. Furthermore, a CAF may assist in building up a holistic picture of needs, and as such is likely to carry greater weight in a referral process than a series of partial isolated snapshots. But whilst the CAF can be a tool that supports health visitors' work with children and families, it also presents a challenge for health visitors in respect of the extra work generated in undertaking it (Holmes *et al.*, 2012). In Brandon *et al.*'s (2006) early evaluation of the introduction of the CAF, health and education services were cited as carrying the bulk of common assessments. In addition, Brandon *et al.* identified that some workers highlighted their confidence/skills gap in taking up the role of Lead Professional and chairing meetings. Working with vulnerable children and the CAF process is a good opportunity for health visitors to build their confidence and develop and demonstrate effective leadership skills in a multidisciplinary arena. Although Holmes *et al.* (2012) highlighted that the Lead Professional role was sometimes allocated to health visitors without discussion, this role was highly regarded and valued by parents and carers. Undertaking the lead professional role thus affords health visitors an opportunity to build on their strengths in forming and maintaining effective relationships with children and families. It is important to recognise that whilst assessment tools such as the CAF and the Assessment Framework are the mainstay of effective assessment in practice with children and families, a range of other tools exist. These have been and continue to be developed to respond to specific forms and contexts of abuse and may be used in an integrated way to complement assessments undertaken using the frameworks discussed in this section.

Graded Care Profile (GCP)

One tool that has been adopted by many LSCBs and practitioners for use in practice is the Graded Care Profile (GCP), an assessment tool designed specifically for use in cases of suspected and actual neglect. It is important to recognise that neglect may take various forms (Howe, 2005) and that different perspectives on these forms will influence how they are assessed by practitioners. As highlighted earlier, neglect has a significant impact on health visitors' practice and workload. Ayre (2007) acknowledges that despite knowledge of the deleterious impact of neglect on children, practitioners continue to apply alarmingly high thresholds for intervention. This has been highlighted as a particular concern within health for some time (Srivastava *et al.*, 2003).

The GCP was developed by Dr Prakash Srivastava, a community paediatrician, with the aim of assisting practitioners to quantify in an objective manner the different levels of care offered by any caregiver (for an example of the GCP, see Polnay & Srivastava, n.d.). The tool is based on Maslow's (1943, 1954) Hierarchy of Needs and focuses on four domains of care: physical care, safety, love, and esteem. Assessment outcomes are scored on a summary sheet and are used to form a baseline assessment, set targets for improvements in parenting, and set an agreed threshold for referral to children's services. Srivastava *et al.*'s (2003) account of early evaluation highlights a number of strengths in respect of the GCP, including:

- cost-effectiveness;
- targeted interventions;
- ease and appropriateness of use across professions and agencies;
- popularity with professionals and families as caregivers, children, and young people (may contribute their own evaluations of care given);
- identification of strengths and weaknesses of caregiving;
- decreased subjectivity and increased objectivity associated with the assessment of neglect.

The success of the GCP to date suggests that it has worked well at a local level; more substantive research into its use is eagerly awaited. Evidence-based assessment tools are essential if assessment in practice is to be acceptable to children, families, and the professionals involved in safeguarding children effectively from neglect.

Working together

Evidently, one of the strengths of assessment frameworks is that they provide a mechanism for professionals and agencies to engage with one another to understand the needs of children and assess the degree to which a child might be at risk of harm. Indeed, Section 10 of the Children Act 2004 introduced a requirement that agencies cooperate to achieve the best outcomes for children.

This is clearly very important, as the outcomes of public inquiries and serious case reviews following the deaths of children have consistently highlighted the fact that professionals and agencies from health, children's services, and the police fail to work together effectively. There have been gross errors in communication, which may have contributed to a child suffering harm. Take, for example, the case of Peter Connelly:

> Poor communication and lack of detailed background information about the case also led to delays in making appropriate assessments. For example, at the child protection case conference on 16 March 2007, it was stated in the action points of the case conference that a paediatric assessment was needed. However, the health visitor did not complete a referral for assessment until 10 April 2007. We do not have any information that indicates why the referral took almost a month to be undertaken. It was then delayed further because insufficient information was provided on the referral form. The referral was subsequently rejected by the clinic at St Ann's Hospital until further information was supplied.
>
> (CQC, 2009: 16)

Despite constant messages from inquiry reports that stress the importance of interagency working, this failure suggests that professionals and agencies need to 'learn to learn' from such failures if those children most at risk are to be adequately protected. All too often, assumptions are made between professionals without clarification or evidence of understanding. The case study in Box 5.2 relates to the death of Khyra Ishaq and highlights this point. After reading it, you should carry out Activity 5.7.

> **Box 5.2   Case study: Khyra Ishaq (extracts in *italics* from Serious Case Review (Radford, 2010)**
>
> Khyra was the second youngest child in a family of six children, all born to the same parents. She was 7 years old when she died in May 2008; her mother
>
> *(Continued)*

Box 5.2 *(Continued)*

and mother's partner were later convicted of manslaughter, causing/allowing the death of a child, and five other offences of cruelty in relation to the other children. At post mortem, Khrya was described as severely malnourished, with severe wasting. The evidence indicated that the severe malnutrition was due to inadequate nutrition and that she had suffered starvation over a period of several months.

Para 11.39
26th February 2007 – During Health Visitor 8's contact with mother at the Medical Centre the mother informed the Health Visitor she was very frightened of her ex husband who was very abusive and was inflicting emotional abuse on the children which was having a severe impact on their behaviour. He had asked the children to be uncooperative to their mother and has physically abused them by hitting them if they do not obey him … Health Visitor was clear given the information provided she would need to make a referral to Children's Social Care.

Para 11.40
28th February 2007 – Referral made by Health Visitor 8 to Children's Social Care letter read 'I have referred this family because of concerns raised by the children's mother there is a history of domestic violence in this family the parents are no longer married or have any intimate relations according to mother however, persistent abuse still occurs when he visits children' … The letter continues 'mother feels that her ex spouse's behaviour has had a severe impact on her children's behaviour and in my opinion this family needs an urgent assessment and investigation into father's second family.'

(Paragraphs 11.41–11.84 relate to incidents or concerns arising from other agencies, including the school.)

Para 11.85
30th Jan 2008 Referral and Advice Officer, Children's Social Care contacted the Health Visitor who stated she had had no contact with the family since her referral in 2007 despite her own concerns. Health Visitor was requested to check whether a sibling had received the correct immunisations and discussed issues in relation to mother's mental health.

Para 12.3.9
The health visitor did not maintain any contact or support to the family following the referral, although the health visitor made two unsuccessful attempts to contact mother by telephone following the referral. The health visitor had received a letter from Children's Social Care stating that they had completed an assessment and there were no concerns as the mother was able to protect the children and herself. The father was no longer living with the family at that time.

A consistent finding from every high-profile inquiry into the deaths of children is that children are most effectively protected when those working with them are clear about their own individual professional roles and how they need to work together. France *et al.* (2010: 99) recognise that:

For inter-agency working to be effective professionals need to find ways of overcoming professional boundaries and tensions caused by differences in professional cultures. Involving and engaging a wide range of agencies in safeguarding children is recognized to be challenging but has the potential to support the development of new practices and enhance the decision-making process.

It is therefore vital that health visitors recognise, acknowledge, and discuss professional boundaries and tensions and are able to clearly articulate their role to other professionals and agencies. This forms the necessary basis for effective safeguarding work, and ultimately for the advancement of health visiting practice.

Confidentiality and information sharing

In the context of multiagency working and the safeguarding of children, of those challenges listed earlier, the issues of communication, confidentiality, and information sharing may seem most contentious and anxiety-provoking to professionals in practice. Indeed, Lord Laming's (2009) progress report noted that in some situations, practitioners remained uncertain about when they could share information. There is, however, a range of legislation and policy that helps to guide professional practice. A broad platform for this includes relevant sections of:

- the Human Rights Act 1998;
- the Data Protection Act 1998;
- the Crime and Disorder Act 1998;
- the Children Act 2004;
- the NHS Act 2006;
- the Health and Social Care Act 2012;
- the Common Law Duty of Confidentiality.

Clear and recent guidance on information sharing, such as *A Guide to Confidentiality in Health and Social Care* (HSCIC, 2013), is particularly useful to practitioners. All legislation and policy underpins the professional guidance offered by *The Code* (NMC, 2015), Section 5 of which outlines how registrants may respect people's right to privacy and confidentiality in the context of professional, accountable practice.

The use of higher-level communication skills is an essential part of health visiting practice, and it is in the nature of the health visitor–client relationship that sensitive information may be disclosed by the client during contacts. In many cases, the health visitor will be able to respect and maintain the client's confidentiality; however, health visitors must not give an absolute guarantee of confidentiality as there are times when it cannot be kept, and information should be shared when it is needed for the safe and effective care of an individual (HSCIC, 2013), such as when practitioners have reasonable cause to believe that a child or adult may be suffering or at risk of suffering significant harm. Information sharing should preferably be carried out with the client's consent. Where consent cannot be obtained, it is still possible to share information to protect others. In some cases, court orders are made which require practitioners to share confidential information, unless their employing organisation is prepared to challenge the order. In all cases where information needs to be shared, health visitors must ensure that they follow the most up-to-date guidance and, where necessary, seek support. Even where it is necessary to share information, rules about confidentiality and privacy still apply. This means that only those who have a *need to know* should have access to confidential information, and that that information should be *relevant*. Of particular interest to health visitors working with a wide age range of children in a safeguarding arena are guidelines around obtaining the consent not only of adults but of children and young people too. Where children have the capacity to consent (or not) to information sharing, the process of seeking their views and opinions on matters concerning their welfare may be deemed as children's rights-compliant. Where information sharing is necessary, it is important that only relevant information is shared and that it is appropriately, with only those other professionals and agencies that need to know it.

Supervision

The need for health visitors to work safely and effectively together with vulnerable children and their families in a safeguarding context cannot be overstated. Indeed, safety and effectiveness demand key skills from health visitors, which also depend upon good interagency working and partnerships. In recent years, supervision in the health visitor's safeguarding role has been increasingly recognised as crucial for achieving these aims. It has been described as an elementary requirement of each service (Laming, 2009) and a 'right' of those working with children at all levels of intervention (Brandon *et al.*, 2009). Supervision has been defined as 'an accountable process which supports assures and develops the knowledge, skills and values of an individual, group or team' (Skills for Care & CWDC, 2007: 5). Wallbank & Wonnacott (2015) highlight that the term 'safeguarding supervision' is preferable to 'clinical supervision' or 'child protection supervision' as it reflects the needs of all children beyond universal provision, some of whom need protection. Supervision aims to help health visitors develop the necessary skills, confidence, and judgment to safeguard children effectively, and should be regular and proactive (DCSF, 2010). The extracts in Box 5.3, taken from high-profile inquiry reports into child deaths, demonstrate that whilst the nature of supervision has changed from the 1980s to today, the deaths of these children were underpinned by services that evoked a sense of apathy and lack of prioritisation towards the supervision of staff in protecting children.

Box 5.3 Supervision

Jasmine Beckford Extracts in *italics* from the Panel of Inquiry Report by the London Borough of Brent (1985: 143).

Jasmine was the oldest of three children. She was 4 years old when she died in July 1984, after being subjected to severe physical abuse over a period of time. Her stepfather, Morris Beckford, was found guilty of manslaughter and jailed for 10 years. Her mother, Beverley Lorrington, was jailed for 18 months for neglect.

Miss Tyler, Senior Nurse, told us that the health visitors under her supervision … were expected to recognise their own areas of weakness and of doubt about their responses to individual cases, and to approach her for guidance and assistance. She considered that there was no obligation on her part to monitor the performance of a health visitor. The crux of supervision to her was self-monitoring by the supervised of his or her own performance; once problems were so identified, to seek help from the supervisor.

This Inquiry recommended the need for '*establishing the practice of planning regular discussions between health visitors and their senior nurses, even if she does not consider there to be a problem with which she is able to deal*'.

Peter Connelly Extract in *italics* from a review of the involvement and action taken by health bodies in relation to the case of Baby P (CQC, 2009).

Peter Connelly (known previously as Baby P) died in August 2007, aged 17 months, after suffering months of severe physical abuse, including a fracture/dislocation of the thoraco-lumbar spine. Peter's mother pleaded guilty to causing or allowing his death; her partner (a lodger) was also found guilty of the same charge. Following the Serious Case Review into Peter's death, the Care Quality Commission (CQC) visited four trusts involved in his care and found an absence of child protection supervision.

The Whittington Hospital NHS Trust
Staff reported that there is no formal safeguarding supervision system in place that incorporates reflective practice. However, there are weekly multidisciplinary team meetings for safeguarding and child protection staff. In addition, named professionals have the opportunity to attend monthly peer support meetings but, at present, these meetings have not been given priority due to work commitments.

Paediatric services managed by Great Ormond Street Hospital at North Middlesex University Hospital NHS Trust
While there are weekly multidisciplinary team meetings for safeguarding and child protection staff at the trust, staff reported a lack of safeguarding supervision. In addition, they disclosed a lack of formal one-to-one meetings with their line managers or supervisors. While staff reported having good working

(Continued)

Box 5.3 *(Continued)*

relationships, particularly in the A&E department, some staff reported feeling isolated in their role, and that such supervision would provide an element of support to them.

Paediatric services managed by Great Ormond Street Hospital at Haringey Teaching PCT

A number of staff reported that they were not currently receiving any form of safeguarding supervision. Despite this, staff were aware of the appropriate person to approach if they wanted to discuss a case or raise concerns. In general, staff reported that they felt able to access supervision if they needed it. However, due to time constraints, supervision was not being made a priority. Staff reported feeling isolated at St Ann's Hospital and, due to the low staffing levels, reported that there is little sense of team working. In addition, due to the shortage of staff within St Ann's Hospital, peer supervision does not appear to be a viable option at this time.

The Royal College of Nursing (RCN, 2014) recognise that regular, high-quality safeguarding supervision is an essential element of effective safeguarding practice. Clearly, the ability of practitioners to reflect honestly, critically, and analytically is crucial if they wish to develop their safeguarding knowledge, skills, and expertise and make critical judgments. Such skills can only develop with time and experience, but form the basis for strong and effective leadership in safeguarding practice. However, the quality and thus effectiveness of supervision will be dependent upon a number of factors – not least the knowledge, skills, and expertise of the supervisor, who may be a peer, manager, or named or designated professional. In recent years, the model of restorative supervision (Wallbank & Wonnacott, 2015) has received increasing attention. This model aims to support professionals to think clearly, make decisions, reduce stress and burnout, and increase the pleasure associated with work. Wallbank & Wonnacott (2015) describe a number of key facets of the model:

- Providing a supportive and challenging supervisory environment
- Improving the capacity of the individual to remain resilient in the face of challenging case work through their ability to recognize personal triggers
- Enhancing the ability of professionals to relationship build with other professionals to avoid isolation and reduce difficult collegiate behaviours
- Encouraging the professional to focus on the events and/or situations they can change so they experience less helplessness
- Improve the ability of the professional to communicate issues so they can be escalated effectively

(Wallbank & Wonnacott, 2015: 42)

Recently, this approach has been developed further, and Wallbank & Wonnacott (2015) have proposed a new integrated restorative model which incorporates the $4 \times 4 \times 4$ model (Morrison, 2005). Morrison's model is a framework that combines the functions, stakeholders, and main processes of the supervision cycle. Integrating the two approaches, Wallbank & Wonnacott (2015: 43) assert, 'provides a balanced approach which maintains a focus on the outcomes for the child whilst supporting and challenging the practitioner'. It is important that sufficient resources are invested in the development, updating, and provision of services that provide supervision for health visitors. A significant factor, in addition to the quality of the model and the approach used, is the frequency of and time allocated to supervisory sessions. Too often, health visitors have been reliant upon informal, peer-led supervision in place of formal supervision (Nettleton, 1998). Brandon et al. (2009) cite one health visitor who received 6-monthly safeguarding supervision – clearly, this is inadequate. In the context of the current challenges within the health visiting services, including increased numbers of newly qualified health visitors, large complex caseloads, and health visitors continuing to tackle child protection issues that would once have been referred on to children's social care services, effective resourcing, the use of evidence-based approaches, and the prioritisation of supervision in health visiting practice are vital.

Key findings from interviews held as part of Brandon et al.'s (2009) analysis into serious case reviews include:

- the need for regular and sufficiently frequent supervision;
- the need to monitor and follow up key issues (including missed appointments);
- the need for supervision to consider continuity of approach to the family;
- the provision of extra support for less experienced workers;
- the creation of a structured sharing of uncertainty, in order to reach the best possible response to concerns.

Whilst these points are a necessary aspect of expert-led child protection supervision, there is another aspect that is essential to ensuring that practitioners have the right level of knowledge and skills in 'working together'. A supervisory relationship that encourages the practitioner to be critically reflective is most likely to be productive where the protection of children is concerned.

It is important to consider what is actually meant by 'critical' reflection. It is not just a superficial discussion of practicalities around a case. Critical reflection has been defined as 'A process of reflection which incorporates analysis of individuals' thinking with regard to the influence of socially dominant thinking' (Fook & Askeland, 2006: 41). Therefore, health visitors need to be open to new perspectives on how they work with children who are at risk of being or have been abused and must be ready to challenge their pre-existing, dominant assumptions about abuse and the need for a child-focused response. If utilised effectively within supervision, the health visitor becomes more aware of how broader social factors impact upon the family, develops skills to challenge appropriately, and – equally crucial – understands the boundaries within which she or he can practise safely and effectively.

Therefore, experience alone is not the only prerequisite for a good child protection supervisor. Child protection supervision also requires critical thinking and communication skills that take the supervisory relationship to a new level. In a supportive environment, the supervisee is enabled to confront her or his own values, perceptions, and practice and so form a robust approach to safeguarding. This raises issues and challenges for organisations that need to develop those individuals to take on a supervisory role. Indeed, supervision training should not be a one-off event; rather, there should be opportunities for supervisors to develop their knowledge and skills on an ongoing basis. This leads further to the vital consideration, '*Quis custodiet ipsos custodes*' – Who will guard the guardians? Or, who supervises the supervisors? Child protection supervision requires a structured framework within an organisation with appropriate resourcing in order to safeguard not only the children it aims to protect but also the well being of staff and the integrity of the organisation.

Summary

This chapter has highlighted some of the challenges that may confront health visitors and other practitioners in their safeguarding practice. In recent decades, child abuse and the protection of children under the umbrella term 'safeguarding' have received a higher prominence in society, and as a result the health visitor's role has become underpinned with a plethora of policy and guidance from the international to the local level. The extent and patterning of child abuse across society has enabled an understanding of the burden of child protection work that health visitors face. Health visiting has a long history of association with child welfare and the protection of children from abuse, which has become reinforced with the development of the profession and its duties under the auspices of the NMC.

Key concepts have been considered here as a means of highlighting the tensions that exist when working with vulnerable children. An understanding of those tensions assists health visitors in working their way through the ambiguities of everyday practice. Furthermore, with a working knowledge of legislation and policy, health visitors are able to undertake the safeguarding role in a safer and more effective way. The importance of agreed definitions of what constitutes child abuse has been highlighted, alongside the need for health visitors to keep up to date with emerging forms of child abuse.

Case study material has been utilised to support the discussion and highlight the extent to which poor communication continues to blight the lives of children with gross errors and mis-assumptions between professionals. There is a need for assimilation of messages from serious case reviews and enquiries into child deaths. The role of the health visitor is acknowledged in recent reports as giving added value to safeguarding services. The profession has a duty to respond to that acknowledgement by seeking to develop through research evidence the effectiveness of its function in safeguarding. Furthermore, the importance of supervision that enables health visitors to develop their knowledge, skills, and expertise has been explored, with an emphasis on the quality of supervision and the responsibilities of organisations to support this. At the time of writing, there is significant change occurring within public sector organisations, and it is vital over the coming years that the safeguarding of children remains a key focus of policy and health visiting practice and that the profession makes the most of every opportunity to advocate for the rights of children in an increasingly challenging world.

References

Appleton, J. (1994) The concept of vulnerability in relation to child protection: health visitors' perceptions. *Journal of Advanced Nursing*, **20**, 1132–40.

Ayre, P. (2007) Common ground: child neglect. *Community Care*, 29 March–4 April, 36–7.

Baldwin, N. & Caruthers, L. (1998) Developing Neighbourhood Support and Child Protection Strategies: The Henley Safe Children Project. Ashgate Publishing, Farnham.

BMA Board of Science (2014) Domestic abuse. British Medical Association, London. Available from: http://www.bma.org.uk/-/media/files/pdfs/news%20views%20analysis/po-domesticabusereport-16-12-2014.pdf (last accessed 30 March 2016).

Bradford Hill, A. (1965) The environment and disease: association or causation? *Proceedings of the Royal Society of Medicine*, **58**, 295–300.

Brandon, M., Howe, A., Dagley, V., Salter, C. & Warren, C. (2006) What appears to be helping or hindering practitioners in implementing the Common Assessment Framework and lead professional working? *Child Abuse Review*, **15**, 396–413.

Brandon, M., Bailey, S., Belderson, P., Gardner, R., Sidebotham, P., Dodsworth, J., Warren, C. & Black, J. (2009) Understanding Serious Case Reviews and their Impact: A Biennial Analysis of Serious Case Reviews 2005–07. Department for Children, Schools and Families, University of East Anglia. Available from: http://dera.ioe.ac.uk/11151/1/DCSF-RR129(R).pdf (last accessed 30 March 2016).

Bremner, J.D. (1999) Does stress damage the brain? *Biological Psychiatry*, **45**, 797–805.

Briere, J.N. & Elliot, D.M. (1994) Immediate and long-term impacts of child sexual abuse. *The Future of Children*, **4**, 54–69.

Briere, J.N. & Runtz, M. (1987) Post sexual abuse trauma: data and implications for clinical practice. *Journal of Interpersonal Violence*, **2**, 367–79.

Butler-Sloss, Dame E. (1988) Report of the Inquiry into Child Abuse in Cleveland 1987. Her Majesty's Stationery Office, London.

Cafcass (2010) Cafcass Care Demand – Latest Figures for April–November 2010. Children and Family Court Advisory Service. Available from: https://www.cafcass.gov.uk/media/6296/1011%20care%20demand%20update%20Nov%202010%20Final.pdf (last accessed 30 March 2016).

Cafcass (2015) April Care Demand Statistics and Rates of Application Breakdown by Local Authority. Children and Family Court Advisory Service. Available from: https://www.cafcass.gov.uk/media/241874/april_2015_care_demand_statistics_and_breakdown_by_local_authority.pdf (last accessed 30 March 2016).

Caraher, M. & McNab, M. (1997) Using lessons from health visiting's past to inform the public health role. *Health Visitor*, **70**, 380–4.

Center on the Developing Child at Harvard University (2010). *The Foundations of Lifelong Health Are Built in Early Childhood*. Available from: http://developingchild.harvard.edu/index.php/resources/reports_and_working_papers/foundations-of-lifelong-health/ (last accessed 30 March 2016).

CEOP (n.d.) Association of Chief Police Officers of England Child Protection and Abuse Investigation Lead's position on young people who post self-taken indecent images. Available from: http://ceop.police.uk/Documents/ceopdocs/externaldocs/ACPO_Lead_position_on_Self_Taken_Images.pdf (last accessed 30 March 2016).

CETHV (1977) An Investigation into the Principles of Health Visiting. Council for the Education & Training of Health Visitors, London.

Conservatives (2015) The Conservative Party Manifesto 2015: Strong Leadership A Clear Economic Plan A Brighter, More Secure Future. The Conservative Party, London.

Corby, B. (2000) Child Abuse: Towards a Knowledge Base. Open University Press, Milton Keynes.

Cowley, S. (1996) Reflecting on the past; preparing for the next century. *Health Visitor*, **69**, 313–16.

CPHVA (2007) *Community Practitioners' and Health Visitors' Association Response to 'Facing the Future – A Review of the Role of Health Visitors'*. Available from: http://www .dodsdata.com/Resources/epolitix/Forum%20Microsites/Amicus-Unite/Appendix %203.pdf (last accessed 30 March 2016).

CPS (2009) CPS Policy for Prosecuting Cases of Domestic Violence. CPS Policy Directorate, London.

CPS (2015) *Honour Based Violence and Forced Marriage*. Available from: http://www .cps.gov.uk/legal/h_to_k/honour_based_violence_and_forced_marriage/#a01 (last accessed 30 March 2016).

CQC (2009) Review of the Involvement and Action Taken by Health Bodies in Relation to the Case of Baby P. Care Quality Commission, London.

Creighton, S. (2007) Patterns and outcomes. In: The Child Protection Handbook (eds K. Wilson & A. James), 3rd edn. Bailliere Tindall, London. pp. 31–48.

CWDC (2009) Early Identification, Assessment of Needs and Intervention. The Common Assessment Framework for Children and Young People: A Guide for Practitioners. Children's Workforce Development Council, Leeds.

DCSF (2009) Forced Marriage – Prevalence and Service Response. Department for Children, Schools and Families, London. Available from: http://webarchive .nationalarchives.gov.uk/20101008231326/education.gov.uk/research/data/ uploadfiles/dcsf-rb128.pdf (last accessed 30 March 2016).

DCSF (2010) Working Together to Safeguard Children: A Guide to Inter-agency Working to Safeguard and Promote the Welfare of Children. Department for Children, Schools and Families, London. Available from: https://www.gov.uk/government/publications/ working-together-to-safeguard-children (last accessed 30 March 2016).

DfE (2014) *Characteristics of Children in Need in England, 2013–14*, final. Table A5. Available from: https://www.gov.uk/government/statistics/characteristics-of-children-in-need-2013-to-2014 (last accessed 30 March 2016).

DfE (2015a) Working Together to Safeguard Children: A Guide to Inter-agency Working to Safeguard and Promote the Welfare of Children. Department for Education, London.

DfE (2015b) *What to Do if You're Worried a Child is Being Abused: Advice for Practitioners*. Available from: https://www.gov.uk/government/uploads/system/uploads/ attachment_data/file/419604/What_to_do_if_you_re_worried_a_child_is_being_ abused.pdf (last accessed 30 March 2016).

DfES (2004) Every Child Matters: Change for Children. Department for Education and Skills, London.

DH (1995) Child Protection Messages from Research. HMSO, London.

DH (2002) Women's Mental Health: Into the Mainstream. Department of Health, London.

DH (2007) Facing the Future: A Review of the Role of Health Visitors. Stationery Office, London.

DH (2009a) *Healthy Child Programme: Pregnancy and the First 5 Years of Life*. Available from: https://www.gov.uk/government/uploads/system/uploads/attachment_data/ file/167998/Health_Child_Programme.pdf (last accessed 30 March 2016).

DH (2009b) Improving Safety, Reducing Harm. Children, Young People and Domestic Violence: A Practical Toolkit for Front-line Practitioners. The Stationery Office, London.

DH (2011) *Health Visitor Implementation Plan 2011–15: A Call to Action*. Available from: https://www.gov.uk/government/uploads/system/uploads/attachment_data/ file/213759/dh_124208.pdf (last accessed 30 March 2016).

DH (2013a) *SAFER Communication Guidelines*. Available from: https://www.gov.uk/ government/uploads/system/uploads/attachment_data/file/208132/NHS_Safer_ Leaflet_Final.pdf (last accessed 18 May 2016).

DH (2013b) *Health Visiting and School Nursing Programmes: Supporting Implementation of the New Service Model. No. 5: Domestic Violence and Abuse – Professional*

Guidance. Available from: https://www.gov.uk/government/uploads/system/uploads/attachment_data/file/211018/9576-TSO-Health_Visiting_Domestic_Violence_A3_Posters_WEB.pdf (last accessed 30 March 2016).

DH (2015) *Female Genital Mutilation Risk and Safeguarding: Guidance for Professionals.* Available from: https://www.gov.uk/government/publications/safeguarding-women-and-girls-at-risk-of-fgm (last accessed 30 March 2016).

DH, DfE & Home Office (2000) Framework for the Assessment of Children in Need and their Families. The Stationery Office, Norwich.

Dickson, P. (2014) Understanding victims of honour-based violence. *Community Practitioner*, **87**(7), 30–3.

Dorkenoo, E., Morison, L. & MacFarlane, A. (2007) A Statistical Study to Estimate the Prevalence of Female Genital Mutilation in England and Wales. FORWARD, London.

Dyer, E. (2015) Honour Killings in the UK. The Henry Jackson Society, London.

EIF (2015) Spending on Late Intervention: How We Can Do Better for Less. Early Intervention Foundation, London.

Elkan, R., Kendrick, D., Hewitt, M., Robinson, J.J., Tolley, K., Blair, M., Dewey, M., Williams, D. & Brummell, K. (2000) The effectiveness of domiciliary health visiting: a systematic review of international studies and a selective review of the British literature. *Health Technology Assessment*, **4**(13), 199–230.

Family Law Week (2015) UK's first forced marriage conviction: 16 years' imprisonment for a range of offences. *Family Law Week*. Available from: http://www.familylawweek.co.uk/site.aspx?i=ed145324 (last accessed 30 March 2016).

Felitti, V.J. (1991) Long-term medical consequences of incest, rape, and molestation. *Southern Medical Journal*, **84**, 328–31.

Felitti V.J., Anda, R.F., Nordenberg, D., Williamson, D.F., Spitz, A.M., Edwards, V., Koss, M.P. & Marks, J.S. (1998) Relationship of childhood abuse and household dysfunction to many of the leading causes of death in adults: The Adverse Childhood Experiences (ACE) Study. *American Journal of Preventive Medicine*, **14**(4), 245–58.

Felitti, V.J., Anda, R.F., Nordenberg, D., Williamson, D.F., Spitz, A.M., Edwards, V., Koss, M.P. & Marks, J.S. (2001) Relationship of childhood abuse and household dysfunction to many of the leading causes of death in adults. In: Who Pays? We All Do: The Cost of Child Maltreatment (eds K. Franey, R. Geffner & R. Falconer). Family Violence and Sexual Assault Institute, San Diego, CA. pp. 53–69.

Fergusson, D.M., Horwood, J. & Lynskey, M.T. (1996) Childhood sexual abuse and psychiatric disorder in young adulthood; II: psychiatric outcomes of childhood sexual abuse. *Journal American Academy Child Adolescent Psychiatry*, **34**, 1365–74.

FMU (2012) Statistics January to December 2012. Available from: https://www.gov.uk/government/uploads/system/uploads/attachment_data/file/141823/Stats_2012.pdf (last accessed 30 March 2016).

FMU (2014) Statistics January to December 2014. Available from: https://www.gov.uk/government/uploads/system/uploads/attachment_data/file/412667/FMU_Stats_2014.pdf (last accessed 30 March 2016).

Fook, J. & Askeland, G.A. (2006) The 'critical' in critical reflection. In: Critical Reflection In Health & Social Care (eds S. White, J. Fook, F. Gardner). Open University Press, Berkshire.

FPI (2007) Health Visiting an Endangered Species. Family & Parenting Institute, London.

France, A., Munro, E. & Waring, A. (2010) The Evaluation of Arrangements for Effective Operation of the New Local Safeguarding Children Boards in England. Centre for Research in Social Policy and Centre for Child and Family Research, Loughborough University.

Freeman, M. (1992) Children, their Families and the Law. Macmillan: London.

Glaser, D. (2000) Child abuse and neglect and the brain – a review. *Journal of Child Psychology and Psychiatry and Allied Disciplines*, **41**(1), 97–116.

Harwin, J. & Madge, N. (2010) The concept of significant harm in law and practice. *Journal of Children's Services*, **5**(2), 73–83.

Health Select Committee (2009) Health Inequalities – Third Report. The Stationery Office, London.

HM Government (2011) Call to End Violence against Women and Girls: Action Plan. Cabinet Office, London.

HM Government (2014a) The Right to Choose: Multi-agency Statutory Guidance for Dealing with Forced Marriage. Cabinet Office, London.

HM Government (2014b) *Multi-agency Practice Guidelines: Female Genital Mutilation.* Available from: https://www.gov.uk/government/uploads/system/uploads/attachment_data/file/380125/MultiAgencyPracticeGuidelinesNov14.pdf (last accessed 30 March 2016).

HM Government (2016) *Multi-agency Statutory Guidance on Female Genital Mutilation.* Available from: https://www.gov.uk/government/uploads/system/uploads/attachment_data/file/512906/Multi_Agency_Statutory_Guidance_on_FGM__-_FINAL.pdf (last accessed 18 June 2016).

Holmes, L., McDermid, S., Padley, M. & Soper, J. (2012) Exploration of the Costs and Impact of the Common Assessment Framework. Department for Education, Loughborough.

Home Office (1945) Report by Sir Walter Monckton KCMG KCVO MC KC on the Circumstances which Led to the Boarding Out of Dennis and Terence O'Neill at Bank Farm, Minsterly and the Steps Taken to Supervise Their Welfare. Cmd 6636. Home Office, London.

Home Office (2015) *Domestic Violence and Abuse: New Definition.* Available from: https://www.gov.uk/domestic-violence-and-abuse (last accessed 30 March 2016).

Howe, D. (2005) Child Abuse and Neglect: Attachment, Development and Intervention. Palgrave Macmillan, Basingstoke.

HSCIC (2013) *A Guide to Confidentiality in Health and Social Care: Treating Confidential Information with Respect.* Available from: http://www.hscic.gov.uk/media/12822/Guide-to-confidentiality-in-health-and-social-care/pdf/HSCIC-guide-to-confidentiality.pdf (last accessed 30 March 2016).

Hughes, H. (1992) Impact of spouse abuse on children of battered women. *Violence Update*, August, 9–11.

Hulme, P.A. (2000) Symptomatology and health care utilization of women primary care patients who experienced childhood sexual abuse. *Child Abuse Neglect*, **24**, 1471–84.

Jay, A. (2014) *Independent Inquiry into Child Sexual Exploitation in Rotherham (1997–2013).* Available from: http://www.rotherham.gov.uk/downloads/file/1407/independent_inquiry_cse_in_rotherham (last accessed 30 March 2016).

Kempe, H. & Helfer, R.E (1972) Helping the Battered Child and his Family. Lippincott, Philadelphia.

Kempe, R.S. & Kempe, H. (1978) Child Abuse, the Developing Child. Fontana, London.

Kendall-Tackett, K.A. (2000) Physiological correlates of childhood abuse: chronic hyperarousal in PTSD, depression and irritable bowel syndrome. Invited review. *Child Abuse & Neglect*, **24**, 799–810.

Kendall-Tackett, K.A. (2002) The health effects of childhood abuse: four pathways by which abuse can influence health. *Child Abuse & Neglect*, **6**/7, 715–30.

Kendall-Tackett, K.A. & Marshall, R. (1999) Victimization and diabetes: an exploratory study. *Child Abuse & Neglect*, **23**, 593–6.

Laming, Lord H. (2003) The Victoria Climbié Inquiry: Report of an Inquiry by Lord Laming, CM5730. The Stationery Office, London.

Laming, Lord H. (2009) The Protection of Children in England: A Progress Report. The Stationery Office, London.

Last, J.M. (2001) A Dictionary of Epidemiology. Oxford University Press, Oxford.

Litherland, R (2012) The health visitor's role in the identification of domestic abuse. *Community Practitioner*, **85**(8), 20–3.

Liverpool City Council (n.d.) Early Help Assessment Tool – EHAT (Previously CAF). Available from: http://liverpool.gov.uk/council/strategies-plans-and-policies/children-and-families/early-help-assessment-tool/ (last accessed 30 March 2016).

London Borough of Brent (1985) A Child in Trust. The Report of the Panel of Inquiry Investigating the Circumstances Surrounding the Death of Jasmine Beckford. London Borough of Brent, London.

Marmot, M., Atkinson, T., Bell, J., Black, C., Broadfoot, P., Cumberlege, J., Diamond, I., Gilmore, I., Ham, C., Meacher, M. & Mulgan, G. (2010) Fair Society, Healthy Lives: The Marmot Review. Marmot Review Team, University College, London. Available from: http://www.instituteofhealthequity.org/projects/fair-society-healthy-lives-the-marmot-review (last accessed 30 March 2016).

Martell, R. (1999) 'Getting it right'. *Community Practitioner*, **72**(5), 121–2.

Maslow, A.H. (1943) A theory of human motivation. *Psychological Review*, **50**(4), 370–96.

Maslow, A.H. (1954) Motivation and Personality. Harper, New York.

MOJ/Home Office (2015) Serious Crime Act 2015: Factsheet – Female Genital Mutilation. Available from: https://www.gov.uk/government/uploads/system/uploads/attachment_data/file/416323/Fact_sheet_-_FGM_-_Act.pdf (last accessed 30 March 2016).

Morrison, T (2005) Staff Supervision in Social Care. Pavillion, Brighton.

Nettleton, R. (1998) Child protection: health visiting and supervision. In: Clinical Supervision and Mentorship in Nursing, 2nd edn (eds T. Butterworth, J. Fauguer, P. Burnard). Stanley Thornes, Cheltenham. pp. 132–52.

NICE (2014) *Contraceptive Services with a Focus on Young People up to the Age of 25: NICE Public Health Guidance 51*. Available from: https://www.nice.org.uk/guidance/ph51 (last accessed 30 March 2016).

Nottinghamshire County Council (n.d.) Early Help Assessment Form. Available from: http://www.nottinghamshire.gov.uk/caring/childrenstrust/pathway-to-provision/early-help-assessment/ (last accessed 30 March 2016).

NSPCC (2014) *How Safe are our Children? 2014*. Available from: http://www.nspcc.org.uk/globalassets/documents/research-reports/how-safe-children-2014-report.pdf (last accessed 30 March 2016).

NSPCC (2015) *Child Protection in the UK*. Available from: http://www.nspcc.org.uk/preventing-abuse/child-protection-system/ (last accessed 30 March 2016).

NMC (2004) Standards of Proficiency for Specialist Community Public Health Nurses. Nursing and Midwifery Council, London.

NMC (2015) The Code: Professional Standards of Practice and Behaviour for Nurses and Midwives. Nursing and Midwifery Council, London.

ONS (2015) Chapter 4: Violent crime and sexual offences – intimate personal violence and serious sexual assault. In: Compendium: Focus on Violent Crime and Sexual Offences: 2013/14. Available from: http://www.ons.gov.uk/peoplepopulationandcommunity/crimeandjustice/compendium/focusonviolentcrimeandsexualoffences/2015-02-12/chapter4violentcrimeandsexualoffencesintimatepersonalviolenceandserioussexualassault (last accessed 30 March 2016).

Parton, N. (1997) Child Protection Risk and the Moral Order. Macmillan, Basingstoke.

Parton, N (2014) The Politics of Child Protection. Palgrave Macmillan, Basingstoke.

Perry, B. (2002) Childhood experience and the expression of genetic potential: what childhood neglect tells us about nature and nurture. *Brain and Mind*, **3**, 79–100.

Pine, D.S. & Cohen, J.A. (2002) Trauma in children and adolescents: risk and treatment of psychiatric sequelae. *Biological Psychiatry*, **51**(7), 519–31.

Polnay, L. & Srivastava, O.P. (n.d.) Graded Care Profile (GCP) Scale. Luton Safeguarding Children Board and Luton Borough Council. Available from: http://lutonlscb.org.uk/pdfs/gcp.pdf (last accessed 30 March 2016).

Puffett, N. (2010) Government clarifies ban on *Every Child Matters*. *Children & Young People Now*. Available from: http://www.cypnow.co.uk/cyp/news/1053008/government-clarifies-ban-every-child-matters (last accessed 30 March 2016).

Radford, J. (2010) Serious Case Review under Chapter VIII 'Working Together to Safeguard Children' in Respect of the Death of a Child, Case Number 14. Birmingham Safeguarding Children Board, Birmingham.

RCN (2014) Safeguarding Children and Young People: Every Nurse's Responsibility. Royal College of Nursing, London.

RCPsych (2014) Domestic Violence and Abuse – Its Effects on Children: The Impact on Children and Adolescents: Information for Parents, Carers and Anyone who Works with Young People. Royal College of Psychiatrists, London. Available from: http://www.rcpsych.ac.uk/healthadvice/parentsandyouthinfo/parentscarers/domesticviolence.aspx (last accessed 30 March 2016).

Roberts, R., O'Connor, T., Dunn, J., Golding, J. & ALSPAC Study Team (2004) The effects of child sexual abuse in later family life; mental health, parenting and adjustment of offspring. *Child Abuse and Neglect*, **28**, 525–45.

Robinson, J. (1982) An Evaluation of Health Visiting. CETHV, London.

Scheeringa, M.S., Wright, M.J., Hunt, J.P. & Zeanah, C.H. (2006) Factors affecting the diagnosis and prediction of PTSD symptoms in children and adolescents. *American Journal of Psychiatry*, **163**, 644–51.

Skills for Care & CWDC (2007) Providing Effective Supervision. Skills for Care/Children's Workforce Development Council, Leeds.

Smith, M.A. (2004) Health visiting: the public health role. *Journal of Advanced Nursing*, **45**(1), 17–25.

Smith, R. (2010) A Universal Child? Palgrave Macmillan, Basingstoke.

Srivastava, P., Fountain, R., Ayre, P. & Stewart, J. (2003) The Graded Care Profile: a measure of care. In: Assessment in Child Care: Using & Developing Frameworks for Practice (eds M.C. Calder & S. Hackett). Russell House Publishing, Lyme Regis.

Symonds, A. (1991) Angels and interfering busy bodies: the social construction of two occupations. *Sociology of Health & Illness*, **13**, 249–64.

Talley, N.J., Fett, S.L. & Zinsmeister, A.R. (1995) Self-reported abuse and gastrointestinal disease in outpatients: Association with irritable bowel-type symptoms. *American Journal of Gastroenterology*, **90**, 366–71.

Teegen, F. (1999) Childhood sexual abuse and long-term sequelae. In: Posttraumatic Stress Disorder: A Lifespan Developmental Perspective (eds A. Maercker, M. Schutzwohl & Z. Solomon). Hogrefe & Huber, Seattle. pp. 97–112.

Unite/CPHVA (2008) Omnibus Survey. Unite/Community Practitioners and Health Visitors Association, London.

UNICEF (1989) *The United Nations Convention on the Rights of the Child*. Available from: http://www.unicef.org.uk/Documents/Publication-pdfs/UNCRC_PRESS200910web.pdf (last accessed 30 March 2016).

Van der Kolk, B.A. (1984) Post-Traumatic Stress Disorders: Psychological and Biological Sequelae. American Psychiatric Press, Washington, DC.

Wallbank, S. & Wonnacott, J. (2015) The integrated model of restorative supervision for use within safeguarding. *Community Practitioner*, **88**(5), 41–5.

White, I (2015) Voting Age. Commons Library Standard Note. Available from: http://www.parliament.uk/business/publications/research/briefing-papers/SN01747/voting-age (last accessed 30 March 2016).

White, R., Carr, P. Lowe, N. & MacDonald, A. (2008) The Children Act in Practice, 4th edn. LexisNexis, London.

WHO (2014) Child Maltreatment. Fact Sheet **150**. Available from: http://www.who.int/mediacentre/factsheets/fs150/en/ (last accessed 30 March 2016).

WHO (2015) Female Genital Mutilation. Factsheet No **241**. Available from: http://www.who.int/mediacentre/factsheets/fs241/en/ (last accessed 30 March 2016).

WHO & ISPCAN (2006) Preventing Child Maltreatment: A Guide to Taking Action and Generating Evidence. World Health Organization and International Society for Prevention of Child Abuse and Neglect, Geneva. Available from: http://whqlibdoc.who.int/publications/2006/9241594365_eng.pdf (last accessed 30 March 2016).

Wohl, A.S. (1986) Endangered Lives: Public Health in Victorian England. Dent, London.

Activities

Activity 5.1

Defining 'child'

Reflect on your own past experiences as a child, young person, and professional.

- What additional tensions or ambiguities exist in respect of defining 'child'?
- What implications do these have in respect of the health visitor's role in working with children?

Activity 5.2

Defining 'safeguarding'

- How would you define 'safeguarding'?
- As you network with colleagues from other professional groups or agencies, ask them how they define 'safeguarding'.
- Reflect on the value of this activity. How might gaining different views be helpful?

Activity 5.3

Accessing the UNCRC

Take the opportunity to access the UNCRC online: http://www.unicef.org.uk/Documents/Publication-pdfs/UNCRC_PRESS200910web.pdf (UNICEF, 1989). Consider which of the articles underpin the health visitor's safeguarding role, and why.

Activity 5.4

Accessing local safeguarding children's policies

Locate, list, and read the local safeguarding children's policies that are relevant to your practice.

Activity 5.5

Defining 'child abuse'

Child abuse is broadly categorised as:

- physical abuse;
- emotional abuse;
- sexual abuse;
- neglect.

Review *Working Together to Safeguard Children* (DfE, 2015a) and make sure that you are able to define each of these categories. Identify the abusive behaviours and signs of abuse associated with each. Also, consider any other forms of abuse of particular concern within the context of your local community at the current time.

Activity 5.6

Analysing the threshold criteria for 'significant harm'

In relation to Figure 5.1:

- Consider the meaning of the term 'significant' in relation to harm of children.
- What factors make finding a 'similar child' challenging in contemporary society?
- What factors might influence the threshold for intervention?
- What do you consider constitutes 'reasonable care' in respect of the health of pre-school children?

Activity 5.7

Reflecting on a case study

In relation to Box 5.2, the case study of Khyra Ishaq:

- What positive actions were undertaken by the health visitor?
- What assumptions have been made, and by whom?
- What could have been done better?
- What is the significance of the domestic abuse allegedly perpetrated by Khyra's natural father in the context of her death by manslaughter at the hands of her mother and her mother's partner?

6

Working with Diverse Communities

Sharin Baldwin
King's College London and London North West Healthcare NHS Trust, London, UK

Mark R.D. Johnson
De Montfort University, Leicester, UK

Introduction

Health visitors have a long and honourable history of assisting disadvantaged people to improve the health of their children and families and of combating inequality and the effects of poverty or social exclusion that contribute to poor health and less than optimum outcomes for children (Adams, 2012; Foster, 1988). This role is highlighted in recent National Institute for Health and Care Excellence (NICE, 2014a) guidance on commissioning health visiting services. Health visitors have been instrumental in making use of the principles of health visiting to lobby for and deliver public health improvements (Unite/CPHVA Health Visiting Forum, 2007). In particular, there have been initiatives by health visitors and other professionals over many years to ensure that a better service is experienced by new migrants to Britain, including deliberate outreach and targeted services, research, and both professional and family education (Webb, 1981; Tesfaye & Day, 2015; Abdu et al., 2015). However, there is little recent literature on work by health visitors with minority ethnic or refugee and travelling families, despite their key role in working with such vulnerable families (Cowley et al., 2013). There are many reasons for failure in health improvement, including poverty or lack of resources, and ignorance on the part of both health care users (who do not understand key matters about causes of ill health or how to prevent illness) and professionals (who may not understand the languages or cultures of potential new service users) (While & Godfrey, 1984; Marmot et al., 2010).

This chapter begins with a brief outline of changes in the ethnic makeup of the UK population, looking at religious issues and the implications for health care in general. The concepts of 'cultural competence' and 'institutional discrimination' are introduced, and the meaning of the term 'diverse' is discussed. The chapter then

Health Visiting: Preparation for Practice, Fourth Edition.
Edited by Karen A. Luker, Gretl A. McHugh and Rosamund M. Bryar.
© 2017 John Wiley & Sons, Ltd. Published 2017 by John Wiley & Sons, Ltd.

looks at cultural practices relevant to everyday health visiting practice, such as pregnancy, diet, customs relating to birth and naming, and mental health, with some examples. Finally, it looks at safeguarding in a multicultural setting, paying special attention to genital cutting or female genital mutilation (FGM), and makes a brief reference to matters of communication. Activities are provided to help you apply this information and approaches in your own life and work.

The UK now has one of the most culturally diverse populations in Europe, with 14% of people belonging to an identified ethnic minority (ONS, 2011). It is estimated that black and minority ethnic (BME) communities will represent between 20 and 30% of the UK's population by 2051 (Sunak & Rajeswaran, 2014; Jivraj & Simpson, 2015). Ethnic diversity can lead to culturally rich communities, but also brings challenges to public health and care services. These result from differences in culture, religion, family background, and individual experiences, all of which can impact on an individual's values, beliefs, and behaviours, as well as the way in which they access health services. Health visiting is designed to provide a universal service to all parents with a child under the age of 5, so health visitors need adequate cultural awareness to work effectively with families from diverse communities and to proactively promote health and address health needs. It is essential for health visitors to have some understanding of cultural differences and complexities in order to feel comfortable delivering appropriate individualised client-centred care, as well as carry out community development work (Cowley et al., 2013; see Chapter 3). For many, the lack of such knowledge and comfort leads to anxiety and inappropriate approaches to service delivery (Cuthill, 2014). In order for health care professionals to be 'culturally competent', however, they must have more than just an understanding of different cultures: they also need the right attitudes and systems of practice (Papadopoulos et al., 1998; Papadopoulos & Tilki, 2008).

Culture and migration

The population of the UK has long been enriched by migration. Since the 1950s, it has benefited from many migrants from the territories of the Commonwealth, and more recently from Europe and the Middle East, who have formed thriving and culturally diverse societies across the country. Some groups faced hostility on first arrival. Many originally came to work for the health and social care services. Over 50% of UK's entire minority ethnic population can be found in three major cities – London, Greater Birmingham, and Greater Manchester – but other places also have significant minority populations, and indeed, three cities were identified in the 2011 census as having 'no overall majority' – no single ethnic group formed more than 50% of their population. Leicester, Luton, and Slough are all now described as 'plural cities' (Jivraj & Simpson, 2015). It is estimated that by 2031, there will be 48 such municipalities where there is no single 'majority' population. Local projections and population estimates are generated by local authorities and can be found on the website of the Office for National Statistics (ONS) (ons.gov.uk) or the Centre on Dynamics of Ethnicity (CoDE) (www.ethnicity.ac.uk). To examine the population of your own local authority, complete Activity 6.1.

The main migrant groups identified by the 2011 census are of South Asian background, normally described as 'British South Asian Indian, Pakistani, or Bangladeshi'. There are also significant populations of black African and black Caribbean heritage, and a growing population of dual-heritage (so-called 'mixed-race' groups). Increasingly, many places also have significant populations of European origin, notably Polish-speaking. Within each of these groups there is further diversity, in terms of religion, language, and whether they are first-, second- or third-generation migrants. The Asian-British Indian population contains members of three major religions – Hinduism (45%), Sikhism (22%), and Islam (14%) – whereas the Bangladeshi and Pakistani communities are almost entirely (but not wholly) Muslim. The majority of black Caribbean people are Christian and the majority of black Africans are also Christian, with a significant minority of Muslims (20%) (Sunak & Rajeswaran, 2014). Religious beliefs and practices, as well as historic cultures, have the potential to influence many aspects of life, including childbirth, family life, and parenting. Horwath et al. (2008) highlight the need for health professionals to understand the influence of different religious values in order to be able to advocate for and support members of different faith communities. It is also important for health visitors to understand how religious beliefs and practices influence childbirth and child rearing, in order to assess whether the needs of children are being met appropriately. Table 6.1 provides an outline of the features of the five major religions found in the UK today. A useful short guide to most major religions can be found at www.bbc.co.uk/religion/religions, with guidance on key festivals and practices. See also Cobb et al. (2012) for wider reading.

Cultural sensitivity and competence

There are a number of different definitions of 'cultural competence', which may be succinctly described as 'a set of congruent behaviours, attitudes, and policies that come together in a system, agency or among professionals and enable that system, agency or those professions to work effectively in cross-cultural situations' (Cross et al., 1989: 13). Alternatively, Betancourt et al. (2002: 5) describe it as: 'the ability of systems to provide care to patients with diverse values, beliefs and behaviours, including tailoring delivery to meet patients' social, cultural, and linguistic needs'.

Five elements can thus be seen to contribute to cultural competency, which should be reflected in any individual or organisation's attitudes, structures, policies, and services:

1. valuing diversity;
2. having the capacity for cultural self-assessment;
3. being conscious of the dynamics inherent when cultures interact;
4. having institutionalised culture knowledge;
5. adapting service delivery to reflect cultural diversity.

Cultural competence, however, is not static:

[it] is the synthesis of a lot of knowledge and skills which we acquire during our personal and professional lives and to which we are constantly adding ... of cultural

Table 6.1 Summary of Five Major Religions.

	Islam	Hinduism	Sikhism	Christianity	Judaism
Place of worship	The mosque	The mandir or temple	The gurdwara	The church	The synagogue
Sacred text(s)	The Quran and the Hadith	The Vedas	Guru Granth Sahib	The Bible (New Testament)	The Torah
Main festivals	Id al-Fitr: the end of the fasting month of Ramadan Id al-Adha: the beginning of the Hajj season of pilgrimage to Mecca Mawlid al-Nabi: marks the birth of the prophet Muhammad	Holi (early spring): an ancient fertility ritual celebrated by squirting coloured water and powder Navrati (October/November): similar to a harvest festival celebrated by prayers, sharing of meals, and traditional stick dancing over 10 days Divali (November, usually after Navrati): Hindu New Year	Gurpurbs (throughout the year): significant dates associated with founding gurus of the faith (birth, death/martyrdom) Baisakhi/Vaisakhi (mid-April): anniversary of the foundation of Sikhism Holla Mohalla (mid-March): celebrates the military traditions of Sikhism Bandi Chorrh Divas (at the same time as the Hindu Diwali)	Advent: 4 weeks of preparation for the coming of Christ Christmas (25 December): celebrates the birth of Jesus Good Friday: marks Jesus' death on the cross Easter Sunday: celebrates Jesus' resurrection from the dead	Pesach (Passover) Rosh Hashanah (the New Year) Yom Kippur (the Day of Atonement) Hanukkah (the Festival of Lights)

diversities and similarities in health and illness as well as their underpinning societal and organisational structures.

(Papadopoulos, 2003: 5)

Whilst there are various definitions for cultural competence, they all refer to a set of skills around being understanding of and sensitive to other cultural values, beliefs, and behaviours, whilst being aware of one's own cultural beliefs and practices, and having the ability to deliver care in a nonjudgmental way based on the needs of the individual(s). A number of models of cultural competence have been developed from practice and through research (Betancourt *et al.*, 2002; Quickfall, 2014), but one of the most commonly used is that of Papadopoulos *et al.* (1998), who, in their seminal book, describe the development of cultural competence as a continuous four-stage model and not an end stage. As shown in Figure 6.1, cultural competence results from a combination of cultural awareness, cultural knowledge, and cultural sensitivity, all of which are continuously updated and enhanced (Papadopoulos *et al.*, 1998; Papadopoulos & Tilki, 2008).

The four concepts in Papadopoulos *et al.*'s (1998) model are as follows:

1. *Cultural awareness:* the ability to recognise that there are differences in attitudes, beliefs, and values between different cultures.
2. *Cultural knowledge:* the process of acquiring information and skills (knowledge) about a culture that shapes an individual's or community's behaviours, values, and beliefs.
3. *Cultural sensitivity:* the ability to be aware of cultural differences and to act in a respectful and nonjudgmental way towards other cultures.

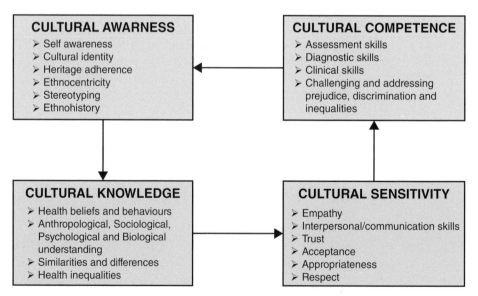

Figure 6.1 The Papadopoulos, Tilki, and Taylor Model for Developing Cultural Competence. Source: Papadopoulos & Tilki (2008).

4. *Cultural competence:* the combination of the skills and knowledge necessary to be culturally aware, knowledgeable, and competent. Being culturally competent does *not* mean having knowledge of every single culture; rather, it is about being open to different approaches and beliefs, and having mutual respect for those with different beliefs. According to O' Hagan (2001: 235), 'Self-awareness is the most important component in the knowledge base of culturally competent practice.'

Some useful tips for developing cultural competence

- Be aware of your own cultural norms, attitudes, values, and beliefs, as well as your own prejudices and biases.
- Understand that cultural differences exist and realise that people's experiences, beliefs, values, and language affect their ways of interacting with others and with the larger community, as well as their health and health-seeking behaviour.
- Treat all people as unique individuals. Be respectful and nonjudgmental of cultural differences (unless there are implications for safeguarding; see Chapter 5).
- Trusting relationships are essential and can only be developed through mutual respect and a desire for understanding.
- Just because some cultural practices may differ, do not allow them to be the basis for criticism and judgments. Do not enforce your own personal beliefs on others.
- Take time to listen: if you do not understand something, ask for an explanation.
- When dealing with specific cultures, having knowledge of some cultural norms and practices can help your sensitivity and understanding, and enables you to provide culturally sensitive information and advice that may be more acceptable to an individual or family. The public health walk in Chapter 3 is a great way to find out more about your local area and community.
- Developing cultural competence is an ongoing process and a lifelong journey – make it part of your continuing professional development (CPD) programme.

Institutional discrimination and organisational cultural competence

One of the key findings from the oft-cited Lawrence Inquiry (Macpherson, 1999) was that the police force was structurally and organisationally discriminating – not necessarily intentionally, but through the operation of its routine policies and practices, which failed to take account of ethnic and cultural specificity. Likewise, the majority of the services in the National Health Service (NHS) were designed around the needs of the population of the time, which was quite different to that today. Migration and cultural change mean that many taken-for-granted assumptions have to be reconsidered and services must be planned to take account of new patterns of living and new social norms. Even if health visitors and other staff have enormous knowledge of cultural diversity and respect for different faiths and traditions, this is rendered meaningless if there is a lack of resources, protocols, and structures to accommodate the distinctive and specific needs of diverse groups in society. A recent example of such a need for cultural change was the introduction of the legal status of 'civil partner' and the legalisation of same-sex marriage. Many agencies have had to redesign their standard registration and recording systems to permit recognition of these new forms of relationship. Similarly, in respect of ethnicity and culture, religious and dietary needs require new menus in hospitals and other places serving food, as well as new diet sheets and advice for parents weaning their children or seeking to follow a healthy diet themselves. There are also certain genuine biological differences between some cultural groups, such as blood-group frequencies and susceptibility to keloid scarring (see PEGASUS, chapter 3, Table 3.4). Certain disease conditions are rare in 'majority' white ethnic groups, whilst others are less common among minority ethnic groups, who might need instead, for example, a blood test for sickle cell anaemia or thalassaemia rather than phenylketonuria (Anionwu & Atkin, 2010). It took many years of campaigning to reach the point where all newborn children are routinely tested for these conditions. A useful exercise is to conduct an audit of your own organisation's preparedness for diversity by examining the 'information' resources available both to service users and to staff.

Understanding different cultural practices

Many treasured cultural practices are associated with significant life events, such as childbirth, marriage, and death (Dobson, 1991). Health visitors supporting families through transition to parenthood and during the early years following birth need to have respect for culturally based values, beliefs, and behaviours. Only then can they effectively assess needs, plan culturally appropriate care, and facilitate health-enhancing activities to achieve positive outcomes for children and families.

In this section, a number of different cultural practices relevant to the field of health visiting are described. However, culture is not static, but is always changing and evolving. Within any culture, families will have their own practices, customs, and views. Health visitors should be mindful of this and not make assumptions based only on ethnic or religious background. Every family should be assessed on an individual basis, asked its views on relevant practices, and treated according to its specific needs. Before reading this section, undertake Activity 6.2.

Pregnancy

Women's experiences of pregnancy, childbirth, and child rearing are influenced by cultural beliefs and practices. Many customs and rituals associated with these significant events shape future mothering behaviour. 'May you bathe in milk and bloom among sons' is a traditional blessing in India, where motherhood – preferably of a son – is highly regarded (Choudhry, 1997; Culley et al., 2007). Traditionally, in India, daughters are seen as a social and economic burden, whilst sons are seen as providers who can not only provide financial security for parents in old age but also perform rites for the souls of deceased family members. Antenatal sex selection, although illegal, is still widely practised on the subcontinent, and some hospitals in the UK have a policy of not telling parents the sex of their baby during routine scans.

Information about local hospital policies can be found on the NHS Choices website (www.nhs.uk; see also 'Can I Find Out the Sex of My Baby?' on that site).

Whilst there are many similarities between the South Asian countries of origin of the British Asian population, religious variations affect the prevalence of some cultural beliefs and practices. Abortion, for example, is regarded as 'haram' (forbidden) by Muslims, and abortion of girls for sex selection is less commonly practised in Bangladesh and Pakistan than in India. The practice of 'Daj' (dowry), however, is widespread across cultures.

Diet in pregnancy is increasingly recognised as important, but there are very many cultural beliefs associated with food. In particular, in many Asian and South Asian cultures, the concept of 'hot' and 'cold' food is prevalent, much as the idea of the 'four humours' (earth, air, fire, and water, representing hot, cold, wet, and dry elements) is prevalent in Shakespeare's plays. Here, 'hot' and 'cold' do not refer to the temperature at which foods are eaten, but to symbolic beliefs associated with them. Generally, hot (garam) foods are seen as being harmful during pregnancy. These include:

- meat, eggs, fish;
- beans, pulses, lentils;
- eggplant (aubergine), onion, garlic, ginger, chillies;
- ghee (clarified butter);
- some fruits, including papaya, banana, and dates;
- jaggery (unrefined cane sugar);
- alcohol, coffee, tea.

Research over many decades has provided evidence of the types of food that are considered hot (Quah, 2015). In a study of 1106 pregnant, lactating, and weaning women in India, Jesudason & Shirur (1980) asked about attitudes to certain foods: 20% of women believed that banana could cause fever and coughing in the mother and was bad for the foetus. Other studies have reported that fish, meat, egg, spices, and salt are often believed to induce abortion (Ferro-Luzzi, 1980; Jeffery et al., 1989; Nag, 1994). Papaya has been reported to have abortive powers, whilst aubergine is considered to be among the most harmful vegetables (Mathews & Benjamin, 1979; Rao, 1985; Pool, 1987; Nag, 1994).

In contrast, cold (thanda) foods are seen as beneficial during pregnancy. These include:

- milk and yoghurt;
- coconut and coconut water;
- wheat and rice;
- green, leafy vegetables.

Cold foods are especially recommended during early pregnancy, to avoid miscarriage (Nag 1994), and milk is considered to have particular benefits (Rao, 1985; Jeffery et al., 1989).

Perceptions surrounding 'hot' and 'cold' foods differ between regions and countries and are common in many cultures. Some mothers use Chinese herbal teas or 'hot–cold' food and drink to recover and balance their 'yin/yang' in the perinatal period.

When working with women from India, it is also important to be aware of the concept of 'eating down': eating less during pregnancy to avoid the risk of a large baby and a difficult delivery (Rao, 1985; Jeffery *et al.*, 1989; Chatterjee, 1991). Many Indian women also fast and ingest herbal medicines during pregnancy in the hope of having a son (Raman, 1988).

These practices can have serious implications for a mother's nutritional intake during pregnancy. In a qualitative study of pregnant British Bangladeshis, Yeasmin & Remi (2013) reiterate the need for an understanding of food practices and beliefs among practitioners and policy makers. D'Souza *et al.* (2015) undertook a review of dietary practices during pregnancy and concluded that migrant women may follow some of these practices but that there is a lack of research on their impact on birth outcomes. The Born in Bradford Cohort Study is one example of the way in which the impact of health in pregnancy in a community with a high migrant population is being assessed (www.borninbradford.nhs.uk). Health visitors need to ensure that all pregnant women are informed and educated about adequate nutritional intake, including adequate intake of iron and vitamin D, since nutritional rickets is a strong risk in dark-skinned population groups (Shenoy *et al.*, 2005). The Asian Feeding Survey (ONS, 1997) found that up to one-third of Indian, Bangladeshi, and Pakistani children had low vitamin D status at age 2. People with darker skin are at increased risk of vitamin D deficiency, as their skin is less efficient at synthesising vitamin D, and therefore NICE Public Health Guidance 56 (NICE, 2014b) recommends that people of African, African Caribbean, and South Asian origins, as well as those who remain covered when outside, should be given vitamin D supplements.

As well as advising women about healthy eating in pregnancy, health visitors have a role in supporting them to access weight-loss programmes following birth if they have a BMI over 30 (NICE, 2015). It is recognised that women from some ethnic groups, including those of South Asian or East Asian origin, may have an increased risk of obesity at a lower BMI, which should also be taken into consideration by health care professionals (NICE, 2015).

Birth customs

There are many different rituals and customs related to childbirth. Whilst there may be variation in practices across people from different countries, they are generally based on religious beliefs; therefore, in this section, the birth customs of four major religions will be discussed. It is not possible for health visitors to know about all the different beliefs and practices that exist, nor is it important to do so – it is more important to be open and ready to have a discussion based on some understanding of the diverse range of beliefs and practices that exist (which are often also mirrored or found in the 'majority' culture). The routine antenatal contact carried out by health visitors as part of the Healthy Child Programme (DH, 2009) is an ideal opportunity to explore and discuss individual customs and practices. Having an understanding of these would enable health visitors to build better relationships with families, which is fundamental to providing effective support during their transition to parenthood and beyond.

Islamic birth customs

There are a number of rituals that a Muslim is expected to perform when a new child is born. Within different cultures, there may be variations, so it is important to remember that not all Muslims will follow all of these in exactly the same way:

- *Adhan:* The 'call to prayer' is whispered into the newborn baby's ear soon after birth. This is usually carried out by the father, or a respected member of the community. The whole ceremony only takes a few minutes. By being aware of this, health professionals can ensure that parents are given adequate privacy to perform this rite.
- *Tahneek:* Soon after birth, a small piece of softened date is rubbed on the baby's upper palate by a respected member of the family. It is believed that some of his/her positive attributes will be transmitted to the baby (Gatrad & Sheikh, 2001). Honey can also be used. Giving honey to a baby before 1 year of age conflicts with health advice given in the UK, due to the risks of botulism (Smith *et al.*, 2010). Health professionals should inform parents about this risk so that they may avoid using honey for this ritual.
- *Taweez:* This is a talisman or charm, most commonly a black piece of string with a small pouch containing Quranic (scriptural) verses, tied around the baby's wrist or neck. The use of *taweez* is believed to protect the baby from any harm and is more common among Muslims from the Indian subcontinent or West Africa.
- *Tasmiyah:* The naming ceremony is traditionally carried out on the 7th day after birth. Muslim names tend to be Arabic in origin, and Muslim children may have nicknames by which they are called at home; it is important to check which name the child is registered under, so that medical records are kept under the official registered name. Commonly used titles include Muhammad, Hussain, Abdul, Ali, Ahmad, and Ullah for boys and Bibi, Begum, and Khatoon for girls. The naming system within some Muslim African communities differs significantly from that of Western communities, including references to the child's grandparents. Therefore, the parents may have different second and third names. In some African communities, the second rather than the last may be regarded as the family name.
- *Aqeeqah or Akeeta:* On the 7th day, the baby's head is ceremonially shaved, the hair is weighed, and an equivalent weight in silver is given to charity. There may be a large family gathering and a lamb or goat may be slaughtered as a sign of gratitude to Allah (God), the meat being shared amongst family, friends, and neighbours and given to the poor.
- *Khitan (circumcision):* Circumcision of male Muslim babies is practised under Islamic law. This can be performed any time before puberty and is seen as a rite of passage into the Muslim community, as well as being carried out for hygiene reasons (Gatrad *et al.*, 2005a). The event is celebrated with friends and family, traditionally by killing and eating a goat or lamb.
- Female circumcision, also known as FGM, is *not* sanctioned by Islamic law. We discuss this later.

Hindu birth customs

Hinduism is the main religion of India and is practised by members of many diverse cultures within the subcontinent. India has so much linguistic and cultural diversity that childbirth customs vary from one region to another, differing between speakers of Punjabi, Gujarati, Bengali, Tamil, and Rajasthani and according to position in the caste hierarchy (brahmin, kshatria, vaishnava, and shudra). We were advised by one informant that:

> In my case (Hindu-Punjabi Kshatria) when my son was born, Father (myself) gave a drop of honey in baby's mouth before starting breastfeeding. Also he was wearing old clothes until his name ceremony which usually happens after 10 days of birth. If I would be in Brahmin caste then both mother and baby was not allowed to be seen by an outsider until 42 days. Mother is also not allowed to enter in kitchen including cooking.
>
> (personal communication, 2015).

Another widespread custom is the whispering of some prayers in the ear of the newborn child, which should be facilitated with discretion (see *Adhan* in the preceding section). This may be accompanied by writing the sacred 'Om' symbol in charcoal behind the ear (see also Gatrad *et al.*, 2004).

It is clear that the most sensible approach is to ask sensitively about the family's own expectations and preferences, and to be prepared to learn – and to recognise that many families will pick and mix between cultural practices to suit their own lifestyles.

Sikh birth customs

There are no formal requirements to be observed in the Sikh community, beyond an expectation that the child will be presented at the gurdwara (temple) soon after birth. Parents may also wish to read sacred verses and administer sweetened water (Nesbitt, 2012). Naming traditionally follows a set procedure using the sacred book, Guru Granth Sahib, and Sikh names are given equally to males and females. Gender is signified by the titles *Singh* ('lion') and *Kaur* ('princess'), to avoid use of 'caste-specific' names. At a later stage, Sikhs may decide to follow a stricter religious regime ('Khalsa' or 'Amrit-Dhari' – 'Baptised' Sikh). The observance of the 'five Ks' – (*kanga* (comb), *kesh* (uncut hair), *khacca* (undergarment), *kara* (iron bangle), and *kirpan* (sword)) is common; shaving or cutting hair may present particular problems in childcare (Gatrad *et al.*, 2005b).

Christian birth customs

Christianity does not require any special practices at birth, but many parents, including those who are not otherwise religious, may plan for a baptism or 'christening' (naming ceremony). Increasingly, some churches hold a thanksgiving or dedication service instead, and delay baptism until adulthood. In an emergency such as the imminent death of a newborn child, any believer can perform a short baptismal dedication, which may give comfort to certain Christian parents.

Confinement following birth

Belief systems surrounding the necessity of confinement for a specific period of time after giving birth inform many cultures, and were prevalent in the UK until the 1950s. In the modern world, it is increasingly unusual that these traditions are observed fully. Sikh women traditionally observed a period of 40 days of seclusion after birth, when the mother is considered ritually unclean. During this time, women have a rich diet (a mixture of nuts, ghee, and sugar) and are not expected to cook or leave their home. On the 40th day, following a ritual bath, both mother and baby attend the Sikh temple and are reintegrated back into the community (Dobson, 1991; Rait, 2005). Similarly, Hindu women would be expected to stay at home following birth, usually in their mother's house, in order to rest and refrain from any housework. Whilst there is no Islamic law that women should stay at home for 40 days following birth, many women will follow this tradition in order to rest and concentrate on the care of the newborn. Similar traditions of 'sitting the month' are also followed by some Chinese mothers, who may avoid exercise and hair washing (Tighe *et al.*, 2014).

Mothers observing a period of confinement after birth may be unlikely to attend child health clinics. It is important to check with every family whether they have any cultural or religious beliefs or rituals that might prevent them from attending any necessary appointments. Health visitors could either see the mother and child at home for routine checks or arrange an appointment outside the confinement period.

Breastfeeding

Breastfeeding is a priority for improving children's health and reducing health inequalities, and exclusive breastfeeding for the first 6 months of a baby's life is advised (DH, 2009, 2013). The 2010 national infant feeding survey showed that the proportion of babies breastfed at birth had risen by 5% in the previous 5 years, from 76 to 81% (HSCIC, 2012), but many cultural practices can impact on breastfeeding.

In Muslim cultures where *tahneek* is practised (and other South Asian cultures), the baby's first taste is likely to be softened date or a sweet substance, not breast milk. In many cultures, colostrum is not considered milk and is withheld from the baby; it is thought to be inferior, 'dirty', and not good for babies because it has been in the breast during pregnancy. A survey of 120 cultures showed that in 50, delay in implementing breastfeeding due to beliefs around colostrum was more than 2 days (Morse *et al.*, 1990). There is evidence from different countries that these types of attitudes persist, but they are changing; for example, in Vietnam, Lundberg & Thu (2012) found some women continued to discard colostrum but others understood its health benefits. McFadden *et al.* (2013) suggest from their study of Bangladeshi women and health practitioners in West Yorkshire and the North East of England that health practitioners may apply outdated stereotypes (e.g. regarding migrant women's attitudes to colostrum), which can mean that they fail to provide the support needed to initiate breastfeeding. Liampattong (2010) explores these issues further, taking a cross-cultural/public health approach to gaining understanding of the wide range of infant feeding practices throughout the world. Interestingly, whilst in the last national infant feeding survey (HSCIC, 2012), exclusive breastfeeding rates at birth were higher for all ethnic minority groups compared with white mothers, this difference was no longer evident at 1 week, where the rates for ethnic minority and white mothers were similar (46% white, 48% Asian, 49% black and Chinese or other ethnic groups). Mothers from ethnic minority groups were also less aware of the health benefits of exclusive breastfeeding compared to white mothers – 78% of white mothers were able to name a health benefit, compared to 64% of Chinese and other ethnic groups, 63% of black, and 59% of Asian mothers (HSCIC, 2012). This survey only categorised the ethnicity of mothers in five groups, however – white, mixed, black, Asian, and Chinese or other – which means that there are likely to be wide-ranging cultural practices within each of these categories. For example, Somalian women have strong beliefs in breastfeeding, but mixed feeding tends to be more common than exclusive breastfeeding (Graham et al., 2007). Many Somali families living in the UK have experienced refugee camps, malnutrition, or life-threatening diseases, such as tuberculosis. A fat baby is considered a healthy one – demonstrably free of malnutrition and disease – and as a result, children tend to be both breastfed and supplemented with formula.

It is important to be aware that a woman's decision to breastfeed will be influenced by her own experiences, beliefs, and cultural norms and may be affected by a lack of information or education. Health visitors should educate all mothers about the value of colostrum and the benefits of exclusive breastfeeding in a sensitive and respectful manner, enabling them to make informed choices. Research on the benefits of breastfeeding can be found from the UNICEF Baby Friendly Initiative (UNICEF, n.d.).

Family members' opinions, especially those of older female members, can have a great influence on breastfeeding initiation and continuation (MacDonald, 1991). Negative attitudes among partners and family members are significant influencing factors for women not starting or giving up breastfeeding (Arora et al., 2000). As well as working to inform and educate the mother, health visitors need to consider fathers and other family members. Where fathers are well informed and supportive of breastfeeding, overall breastfeeding rates are higher (Pisacane et al., 2005). Cultural sensitivity needs to be exercised, however, to ensure that the father is comfortable discussing breastfeeding with a health visitor.

Muslim mothers – indeed, many Asian mothers – may be embarrassed to breastfeed in public places due to the need to protect their modesty. Mothers may be reluctant to attend a breastfeeding group or seek assistance with breastfeeding if it involves having to breastfeed in front of a stranger. Health visitors should be mindful of this and consider having a breastfeeding room or a private screened-off area where mothers can breastfeed when attending group sessions or busy clinics in the community setting.

Diet, weaning, and feeding practices

Feeding practices and dietary intake are influenced by culture and religion. For Hindus, beef is forbidden, and many Hindus refrain from eating meat altogether and are vegetarian. When giving nutritional advice around parents' or a child's diet, it is important to know what types of food to suggest to ensure that the family is receiving a balanced diet. It is particularly important to ensure that vegetarian children are receiving iron-sufficient food. Whilst the Sikh family diet is varied, observant baptised Sikhs tend to be vegetarian and do not eat any fish, meat, or eggs, or any other meat products. Other Sikhs will eat meat, but most avoid eating beef. Milk is used, but 'Indian' cheese (*paneer*) is very different from the traditional European Cheddar or soft cheeses.

Muslims follow *halal* (permitted) dietary rules: they are forbidden to eat pork or drink alcohol, and meat must be slaughtered in a prescribed way. Jews also do not eat pork or any type of shellfish, and require their meat to be *kosher*; that is, slaughtered by a licensed Jewish slaughterer (*shochet*). Jews are also forbidden to eat milk and meat products together, and food is prepared with utensils and cooked in an oven that has only been used for kosher food. Both Muslim and Jewish parents may refuse medication containing gelatin, as it is derived from non-halal or non-kosher animal products. Some Muslims may also refuse medicines containing alcohol, even if the percentage is very low.

When advising on healthy eating and suitable foods for weaning, health visitors should always enquire whether the family has any special dietary requirements so that they can provide culturally sensitive information and food options, and avoid causing any offence. Being familiar with the types of food eaten in the family will also enable them to provide culture-specific weaning advice and recipes incorporating the family foods. Hogg *et al.* (2014) found that routine health visiting advice and information was often difficult to understand and use in traditional Pakistani or Chinese households. One mother stated, 'They don't have Chinese style recipes. So it's difficult because we are not familiar with British ingredients, like custard? That's why I just bought the readymade baby food' (Hogg *et al.*, 2014: 6). In such cases, providing families with recipes containing ingredients they are familiar with is likely to be more effective (see Box 6.1). It is, however, important not to make assumptions, as families from similar ethnic backgrounds may have very different food preferences and practices. Equally, it is important not to give the wrong advice just to be culturally sensitive. One health visitor commented on how she gave inappropriate advice to a Chinese family: 'They don't like to give children cold foods, I'd been stressing things like yoghurt that is completely inappropriate' (Hogg *et al.*, 2014: 6).

Each family situation should be assessed in its own right, as families are likely to adopt aspects of Western cultures to varying degrees. Having awareness of an individual family's needs, preferences, and cooking methods, whilst checking the suitability of advice given, is a more effective way of providing culturally sensitive care than trying to learn every aspect of every culture.

Box 6.1 Resources for healthy and culturally diverse recipes

- First Steps Nutrition Trust: http://www.firststepsnutrition.org/pdfs/Eating%20Well%20Recipe%20Book_July%202014.pdf
- The *NHS Recipe Book 2001* has a useful chart on page 27 listing main foods and their acceptability for different faiths, and also some

(Continued)

Box 6.1 *(Continued)*

> multicultural recipes designed to serve 100 people, which could be adapted: http://www.hospitalcaterers.org/better-hospital-food/downloads/recipe_book.pdf
> - The NHS in Scotland also maintains a selection of useful resources: http://nhsforthvalley.com/health-services/health-promotion/nutrition/multi-cultural-nutrition/
> - Change4Life: http://www.nhs.uk/Change4Life/Pages/meal-planner-recipe-finder.aspx

Eating practices may also vary. Some Asian families use their right hand to eat food (the left hand is traditionally regarded as 'dirty' and is used for toilet purposes). This is the practice in many Muslim, Hindu, and Sikh households. Chinese families may prefer using chopsticks. Children from such households may not know how to use a knife and fork, which might be problematic when they start school. In these instances, the health visitor can work with the family and inform them about the importance of *also* (not *instead*) teaching their child to use cutlery in order to avoid difficulties at school age.

Kumanyika (2008) reviewed the ethnic and cultural influences on childhood obesity and concluded that several influences increase the risk of obesity for children from minority ethnic groups, including greater maternal type 2 diabetes in pregnancy, parental feeding practices, consumption of high-calorie food and drink, and lower levels of physical activity. As we have already noted, in many cultures a fat baby is considered a healthy baby. As a result, children tend to be breastfed and topped up with formula, and become overfed, making obesity and diabetes more likely. It is important to challenge such behaviours and inform parents about the dangers of overfeeding. Culture also plays an important part when introducing children to solid foods. The recommended time for weaning a child is from 6 months (26 weeks) (DH, 2009), and early weaning (before 4 months) has been associated with an increased risk of respiratory illness and eczema. Early weaning is practised across many cultural groups, based on previous experiences, peer pressure, or myths around 'baby being ready for solids if they are waking throughout the night'. Regardless of culture, if any practice is likely to cause harm or is not in the best interest of the child's or parents' health, the health visitor must raise this with the family and discuss it openly, without fear of causing offence. Health visitors must also be competent in challenging behaviours that are not in line with medical evidence or recommended practice, and to do this they must keep themselves up to date with national evidence-based recommendations. NICE produces evidence-based recommendations on a wide range of topics, from preventing and managing specific conditions to improving health and managing medicines in different settings, as well as providing social care to adults and children and planning broader services and interventions to improve the health of communities. These recommendations, in particular Clinical Guideline 110, 'Pregnancy and Complex Social Factors' (NICE, 2010), can be accessed at www.nice.org.uk/Guidance.

Maternal mental health

Transition to parenthood and maternal perinatal mental health have been identified as two of the six high-impact areas where health visitors can have a major effect in improving outcomes for children and families (DH, 2014a,2014b). Whilst health visitors are ideally placed to support parents during this transition, for them to effectively detect and manage perinatal mental health problems, they must have an understanding of cultural influences.

Depression is found in mothers from all cultural backgrounds – it affects 11.8% of women antenatally at around 18 weeks of pregnancy (Evans et al., 2001) and 10–15% in the postnatal period (NICE, 2010). A meta-analysis of 59 international studies concluded that the international prevalence rate of postnatal depression was 13% (O'Hara & Swain, 1996). This prevalence rate was almost the same in another study carried out across countries and cultures in 2004, which reported the rate of depression in the postnatal period to be 12.3% (Gorman et al., 2004). Whilst the prevalence of depression in the perinatal period may be comparable across different cultures, detection can be difficult, due to a variety of cultural beliefs and practices. For example, it is common practice for many Asian women in the UK to live with their husband's family within an extended family setting, which is often seen by health visitors as a source of additional support (Baldwin & Griffiths, 2009). But while living within an extended family may appear supportive, it can create a number of difficulties, including increased levels of conflict with family members and high demands to fulfil a 'tripartite role' of mother, wife, and daughter-in-law (Sonuga-Barke & Mistry, 2000; Oates et al., 2004). Research exploring the relationship between family structure and the mental health of South Asians in the UK highlights increased levels of anxiety and depression among mothers living within extended families, compared with nuclear families (Shah & Sonuga-Barke, 1995; Sonuga-Barke & Mistry, 2000; Oates et al., 2004; Cooper et al., 2006). The mother-in-law being overintrusive, controlling, and overbearing has been strongly related to maternal depression and anxiety (Unger & Cooley, 1992; Chase-Lansdale et al., 1994; Sonuga-Barke et al., 1998; Oates et al., 2004).

Another cultural factor that may be important for understanding and managing depression is the issue of language. In some languages, such as Urdu, Thai, and those spoken in Cambodia and Nigeria, there is no direct translation for the word 'depression'. A study in Uganda concluded that the term 'depression' was not culturally acceptable (Gordon, 2013), whilst one in Nigeria found people responded to those with a mental illness with fear, avoidance, and anger (Arboleda-Florez, 2002). A common South Asian cultural metaphor used to describe the condition is 'sinking heart' (Krause, 1989; Aradhana & Cochrane, 2005) – sometimes experienced as a result of excessive heat, exhaustion, worry, or feelings of social failure. In Nigeria, Kabir et al. (2004) found major causes of depression were thought to be drug misuse (34.3%), divine wrath and the will of God (18.8%), and witchcraft or spiritual possession (11.7%). Depression may be managed in culture-specific ways – such as by relying on religious beliefs or seeking help from religious counsel and traditional healers (Amankwaa, 2003).

Mental illness in the perinatal period may be kept hidden due to the stigma attached to it. Stigma relating to mental illness is common in most cultures, including Western culture. Women in the perinatal period may be reluctant to seek help due to fear of being labelled a 'bad mother' or fear of the involvement of social services. Chew-Graham *et al.* (2002) describe the concept of *izzat* in their study, a term commonly mentioned in South Asian cultures that refers to 'family honour'. Mental health and other issues may not be discussed with strangers or anyone outside the family (including health professionals) in order to preserve and maintain the family *izzat* (Chew-Graham *et al.*, 2002). There may also be reluctance amongst general practitioners (GPs) from the same community to diagnose postnatal depression because of stigma (Chew-Graham *et al.*, 2009).

Whilst cultural beliefs and practices relate to mental health, health visitors should not shy away from addressing mental health issues in women from any minority group. A comprehensive review found that mental health programmes which fail to take cultural factors into account risk poor engagement and the drop-out of BME parents (Barlow, 1999). On the other hand, where services have attempted to understand and meet the needs of minority groups and provide culturally sensitive care, there have been noticeable improvements in service uptake and compliance with treatment (Rack, 1982; Webb-Johnson & Nadirshaw, 1993; Hussain & Cochrane, 2004). Box 6.2 provides information on ways in which health visitors can identify and support mothers with mental health problems.

Box 6.2   How health visitors can promote and support mothers' mental health and well being

- Routinely ask women about their experience of becoming a mother. Explore feelings and expectations, both antenatally (if possible) and at the new-birth visit.
- Educate both parents about postnatal depression, so that they are able to access help if they notice any signs and symptoms in themselves or their partner.
- Routinely assess for risk and signs of mental health problems by asking the depression and anxiety identification questions recommended by current NICE guidance (NICE, 2014c). Questioning must be supported by other skills, such as observation, listening, and clinical judgment, to determine whether the mother is at risk. An assessment tool may be used to support findings, such as the Edinburgh Postnatal Depression Scale (EPDS), a self-report questionnaire available in 58 different languages (available in Cox *et al.*, 2014).
- Use properly qualified interpreters, rather than family members, especially when discussing mental health matters.
- Raise awareness of mental health issues by engaging with the community to encourage people to accept treatment.

Further information on mental well being is available from the following sites:

- iHV Good Practice Points for Health Visitors: http://ihv.org.uk/for-health-visitors/resources/good-practice-points/;
- iHV Top Tips for Parents: http://ihv.org.uk/families/top-tips/;
- Postnatal Depression (PND) Development Wheel: A Guide to Postnatal Depression (PND) in Mothers and Fathers: http://www.kmpublications.com/KMPublications/DevWheel14.htm.

Safeguarding, domestic violence, and abuse

The health visitor has a critical role in safeguarding, since both children and women in or recently after pregnancy are by definition vulnerable. No amount of cultural deference can justify ignoring clear signs of abuse – the Victoria Climbié case demonstrated clearly how professional anxiety about engaging with what is thought to be 'normal' cultural behaviour can lead to a child's death (Laming, 2003). There is no major religion which sanctions such abuse, and rights to life and well being are generally accepted as being sanctioned by major religions above traditional ritual practices: reliance on stereotypes and fear of interference when harm is a genuine possibility are not evidence of 'cultural sensitivity'. If in doubt, seek advice – but do not 'silence' concerns: the professional requirement of the Nursing and Midwifery Council Code is clear (NMC, 2015) (see also Chapter 2, Box 2.2 concerning the UN Convention on the Rights of the Child).

Of increasing concern is FGM, believed to be a cultural practice that predates Islam. Illegal in the UK since 1985 and across the EU, it is considered internationally to be both physical and sexual abuse. Despite this, FGM continues to be practised in some cultures in the name of Islam – being documented in 28 countries in Africa, the Middle East, and Asia, including Egypt, Iraq, Pakistan, and Malaysia (UNICEF, 2013). In the UK, health care professionals and others working with children have safeguarding responsibilities to all children, but in relation to girls under 18 there is now a mandatory reporting duty, applied from 31 October 2015 onwards, which 'requires regulated health and social care professionals and teachers in England and Wales to report "known" cases of FGM in under 18s which they identify in the course of their professional work to the police' (Home Office, 2015: 2). There is additional guidance published by the Department of Health and the Health & Social Care Information Centre (DH & HSCIC, 2015) as part of the FGM Prevention Programme to support the implementation of this mandatory reporting duty. This guidance and other useful resources are provided in Box 6.3. Health visitors play a key role in identifying and supporting girls and young women who may be at risk of, or have been subjected to, FGM. A particular risk is that young girls may be taken abroad for a 'holiday', during which they will be 'cut'. It is important to work collaboratively with GPs, school nurses, teachers, other health professionals, and multiagency and multiprofessional organisations to ensure consistency in care provision for these girls and young women.

Box 6.3   Resources relating to female genital mutilation (FGM)

- FGM Guidance for Professionals: http://www.nhs.uk/NHSEngland/ AboutNHSservices/sexual-health-services/Pages/fgm-for-professionals .aspx (includes video about the mandatory reporting of FGM)
- FGM: Mandatory Reporting in Healthcare: https://www.gov.uk/ government/publications/fgm-mandatory-reporting-in-healthcare (includes a poster for health organisations to display regarding their duty, a training presentation that organisations can use to provide updates to staff, and information leaflets for patients)
- E-learning to Improve Awareness and Understanding of FGM: http://www .e-lfh.org.uk/programmes/female-genital-mutilation
- Combating Female Genital Mutilation (FGM): http://ihv.org.uk/for-health-visitors/resources-for-members/resource/minority-groups/combating-female-genital-mutilation-fgm/

Researchers at Coventry University have created Petals, a new (free) mobile phone or iPad app, endorsed by the National Society for the Prevention of Cruelty to Children (NSPCC), to educate young people about FGM, with support from other charities. It is only available in English but is designed to be accessible and young person-friendly: a quick-link button will delete the app from the browser history if someone is concerned about being discovered researching the issue. It also provides details of where to go to get help and advice and enables users to access the NSPCC National FGM Helpline at the touch of a button. The Petals app is available at petals.coventry.ac.uk.

There are a number of other local projects and national campaigns which exist to combat the scourge of FGM. It is good practice to work with (and within the parameters of) communities, which are experts in the issues of concern to their members. For example, the Foundation for Women's Health Research and Development (FORWARD: www.forwarduk.org.uk) campaigns for and supports gender equality issues for African women and girls. The Institute of Health Visiting (iHV) has developed a useful mnemonic to help health visitors combat FGM (see Box 6.4).

Box 6.4   Health visitor mnemonic for combating female genital mutilation (FGM)

H Health of persons: Health promotion is core to the HV's [health visitor's] role. They can promote healthy knowledge of anatomy and prevent untoward behaviour against girls and women's genitalia. HVs should act to eradicate this practice, safeguard normal female anatomy and foster respect for womanhood.

E Exploring the motivations behind FGM: HVs need to endeavour to understand the different belief and value systems that perpetuate FGM practice within communities living in the UK in order to provide adequate preventative measures to combat the practice.

A Avoid judgement: HVs should adopt a non-judgemental line of enquiry to avoid alienating affected and at-risk communities (Dike & Umoren, 2014). Inclusion of men as fathers, family heads, husbands, partners and relatives is important to effect behavioural change.

L Legislation: Legislation should be implemented through information sharing and collaborative reporting by communities and professionals to strengthen the campaign against FGM (Moeed & Grover, 2012).

T Turn the trend: HVs, working in partnership with other organisations are crucial to reducing the prevalence rate of 23 000 British-born children under age 15 being at risk of FGM.

H Health education, promotion and support groups are vital to effect behavioural change in FGM and FGC [female genital cutting]. Sure Start, Early Intervention, Healthy Child Programme and Outreach Programmes are accessible avenues for HVs to reach at-risk populations (DfE, 2014).

V Vision: Entails foresight in knowing and committing to care of children and families.

I Interested and informed on health promotion, illness and injury prevention.

S Serving to safeguard communities and individuals.

I Involved within statutory duties to enhance health and well being.

T Teaching to ensure robust holistic functionality.

O Organised outreach to communities.

R Role model of responsible caring.

S Sensitivity to the needs of marginalised communities.

Source: Dike (2014). Reproduced with permission of the Institute of Health Visiting.

More guidance on safeguarding is provided in Chapter 5.

Communication

The health visitor–client relationship is one of the core components of health visiting (Cowley *et al.*, 2013), and communication is key to building effective relationships. This can be challenging in different cultural contexts, however. Gestures are used in many different ways amongst different cultures. For example, in some cultures, people use gestures to express their emotions, whereas in others they may not show any emotion at all. In India (and Turkey), shaking the head from side to side communicates being in agreement and means 'yes', whereas in other cultures shaking the head from side to side means 'no'. This can cause a great deal of confusion when nonverbal signs are interpreted incorrectly. It is always worth checking that you have understood a response and concern accurately. For example, one of the authors remembers an aunt, practising as a health visitor in East London in the 1950s, describing a newly arrived family who had been traumatised by 'creatures' in their kitchen – which turned out to be snails, unknown in their own homeland!

In Western culture, one of the signs of good communication is good eye contact. In some other cultures, making direct eye contact is regarded as being disrespectful. Physical contact may also be prohibited or seen as inappropriate in some cultures, especially between people of different genders. Therefore, a greeting involving physical contact, such as a handshake, may not always be acceptable. It is always best to exercise caution and greet by saying, 'Hello' (or, if possible, using an equivalent in the preferred language of the client), especially during the first contact. After this, you will have a better idea about the preferences and customs of the individual family, based on which you will be able to adjust the way you communicate with them in the future.

When visiting families at home, it is important to be respectful of their customs. Many families do not wear shoes indoors, to ensure that the home is kept clean. For this reason, some families may ask you to remove your shoes at the door during home visits. As a rule, it is always best to check the family's preference before entering the home to avoid causing any offence.

Being aware that there are communication differences between cultures will enable you to be more effective in building trusting relationships with parents and families, which in turn will enable better detection of their health needs and the delivery of more effective care (see Activities 6.3, 6.4, and 6.5). Some advice on the most recent guidance on communication can be found in Baughan & Smith (2013), and Seal (2013) discusses the development of communication skills as part of the process of addressing inequalities. A free online resource produced for the NHS, Toolkit: Improving Access to Healthcare for Migrants, provides resources for health care staff (http://ts4se.org.uk/migrants-healthcare.html). It includes wider information about migration and good practice in using interpreters.

Other communities

This chapter has focused on some of the main religious and ethnic minority groups in the UK, but these are not the only groups that health visitors need to be aware of. Throughout the country, there are various minority ethnic communities whose needs may be different from or even greater than those of the general population. There are large groups of Orthodox Jewish communities in the UK, whose childbirth and child rearing practices are very specific, and whose needs therefore differ from those of the general population. Similarly, there are important health needs that are often not addressed within Traveller and Gypsy communities, attributed to poor accommodation, poor access to health services and education, discrimination, and lack of understanding by health professionals (Francis, 2010). In her work, Francis (2010) identifies the need for health staff to have improved understanding of the Gypsy Traveller culture through cultural competency training, as well as opportunities for staff to have open and honest professional forums in which they can explore their biases and prejudices relating to this community. In addition, there are increasingly large communities of Eastern/Central European origin that have distinctive languages, cultures, and experiences (see Jayaweera (2014) for more epidemiological information on these groups and Tesfaye & Day (2015) on health visitor experiences in working with European migrants in one part of England).

It is important to remember that cultural diversity also includes diversity in terms of gender and sexuality and that families in the UK may include same-sex parents or transgender family members. Whilst this chapter has not explored these families, it is crucial that health visitors embrace diversity and work within a model of cultural competence, such as the one outlined earlier.

Case studies

The chapter concludes with two case studies, one of health visitors working with a Somali community and one with an Orthodox Jewish community. These aim to show you how health visitors can work with, learn from, and support families in different communities. Once you have read these case studies, undertake Activity 6.6 on the evidence in your own organisation concerning engagement with minority groups.

Case study 6.1: Breastfeeding support project for Somali mothers in Harrow

This project was set up by a lead health visitor for breastfeeding in Harrow, recognising that exclusive breastfeeding rates were low in the local Somali population, due to strong beliefs that breast milk was not adequate for their babies. Colostrum is not considered milk and is thought not to be good for babies, because it has been in the breast during pregnancy, so bottles of formula milk were given for the first 3 days after birth. An intervention was designed to promote the value of colostrum and the benefits of exclusive breastfeeding.

Initially, in 2006, six Somali peer supporters were trained as breastfeeding peer supporters in Harrow, supported by a Local Area Agreement with the Harrow Somali Voluntary Organisation (HASVO) and run by the Harrow Breastfeeding Project. Training explored the cultural influences on women's decision making on infant feeding. Initially, it was difficult to engage the women in the programme, as there was no payment available for their work. Successful community events included a meeting, attended by 50 women and children, where Somali food was provided and children did drawings about breastfeeding. An imam from a local mosque emphasised that the Holy Quran also promoted the importance of breastfeeding for 2 years.

(Continued)

Case study 6.1: *(Continued)*

In 2011, one Somali peer supporter was trained and began meeting mothers in the antenatal clinic and giving them the key messages of breastfeeding from birth and the value of colostrum, and of the benefits to mother and child of exclusive breastfeeding and child spacing.

In 2013, two Somali peer supporters started work on the Antenatal Intervention Project, where they see six to eight women every week in the African women's antenatal clinic and keep in touch with them until after their babies are born. This work is supported by the Public Health Breastfeeding Service Specification. All Somali women referred to the project are linked with a peer supporter and offered one-to-one support.

HASVO volunteers work with breastfeeding peer supporters to promote breastfeeding in the Somali community groups. Through this project, all generations of women who might be influential in breastfeeding decision making can now be accessed. As many Somalis do not have good spoken English and do not read Somali, using oral methods (word of mouth) is very important in explaining the key messages.

Dr Alison Spiro, Specialist Health Visitor for Breastfeeding

A fuller PowerPoint presentation by Dr Spiro can be located at https://www.regonline.com/builder/site/Default.aspx?EventID=1363872.

Note: frequent postings and updates on the Facebook page Birth & Babies in Brent & Harrow (https://www.facebook.com/BirthBabiesBrentHarrow) have also pointed mothers to this service (and others).

Case study 6.2: New ways of delivering health visiting services for Orthodox Jewish community in Hackney

The Orthodox Jewish community in North East London is the largest such community in Europe. According to the 2011 census, 6.3% of Hackney residents are Jewish, which is higher than the London average (1.8%) and the national average (0.5%). The Orthodox Jewish community has a very large young population (18.5% are aged under 5 years), and the Mayhew Study (Mayhew *et al.*, 2011) estimated the size of the Orthodox Jewish population in Hackney had grown by 14% since the study in 2007, which reflects the continuing high fertility and high birth rates in this community.

Whilst Orthodox Jewish mothers typically have large families, their engagement with and uptake of health visiting services is fairly poor. A study in 2004 reported that both the Orthodox community and the health visiting service in Hackney viewed Orthodox Jewish mothers as being self-sufficient; the role of the health visitor was thus unclear and undervalued, and the relationship between health visitors and Orthodox mothers was often distant (Abbott,

2004). The lack of engagement with health visiting services meant that uptake of the Healthy Child and Immunisations programmes was relatively low. For example, immunisation rates within the Orthodox community were low in spite of relatively high rates for other ethnic groups in the area. Overall rates of children aged 1 being immunised with the 5-in-1 vaccine were 87%, compared to 70% in the Orthodox Jewish population. The number of infants who die due to vaccine-preventable disease is very small, but the number of children who suffer illness and long-term disabilities due to vaccine-preventable illness makes a considerable impact on families, the NHS, and other local services. Findings from a local survey of the views of Orthodox Jewish service users and the views and experience of providers concerning the health visiting service in 2007 (repeated in 2011), indicated that there was a need for better communication between the providers and service users, for provision of services in culturally appropriate settings, and for cultural awareness sessions for health visitors, to help them better understand and meet the needs of the community (City and Hackney Primary Care Trust, 2007).

This led to a health visiting service redesign, working in partnership with the Orthodox Jewish Health Inclusion Nurse and Norwood (a leading Anglo-Jewry children and family services charity) and its Norwood Children and Family Centre (which has a strong track record in providing services for the Orthodox and wider Jewish community in Hackney). A pioneering range of expert health care and advisory services were developed to meet the needs of the Orthodox Jewish community in Hackney: 'Wellbeing at Bearsted'. Health visiting services were taken out of the traditional health centres and children's centres and delivered from a dedicated clinic at Norwood, including child health clinics, immunisation sessions, and development health reviews for children. Other health services were delivered also from Norwood, including speech and language therapy, hearing screening, and family health and exercise classes. This has had positive outcomes for children, parents, and health visitors, as there has been improved uptake of the immunisation and healthy child programmes by the Orthodox Jewish community.

> We feel that we our being listened to and our needs are now being met
>
> Orthodox Jewish mother
>
> Relaxed, pleasant environment which is culturally appropriate and I feel comfortable coming to
>
> Orthodox Jewish mother

Additional cultural awareness training was provided to members of the health visiting staff, to help them better understand and meet the needs of the community:

> Providing services from here has given me an insight into the needs of the local Orthodox Jewish Community and it has made it much easier to build up the services
>
> Health visitor

> **Case study 6.2:** *(Continued)*
>
> *Marcia Smikle, Head of Safeguarding Children, Homerton University Hospital NHS Foundation Trust*
> Further information can be found at http://www.norwood.org.uk/Page/Wellbeing-at-Bearstead.

Summary

The population of the UK (and, indeed, of Europe) has changed considerably over the past 20 years – and continues to change – in its ethnic and cultural makeup. Uniformity and stability cannot be guaranteed, and this will have implications for all health sector workers, who must meet new challenges and not seek to enforce a single model of 'good practice'. Everyone has some cultural patterns that are important to them but appear strange to others. Some practices are very important for the maintenance of identity and tradition at the time of childbirth, including naming practices and diet, which may have implications for mental health. Questions around safeguarding and practices almost universally regarded as abusive or illegal persist, and these may be the exception to the general rule that one should be culturally sensitive and respectful of the traditions of other people. Communication is always important, not only with respect to 'other' languages and the use of an interpreter, but also in regard to the terms we use, what we see as 'normal', and how we relate to other people.

References

Abbott, S. (2004) Lay and professional views on health visiting in an orthodox Jewish community. *British Journal of Community Nursing,* **9**(2), 80–5.

Abdu, L., Stenner, K. & Vydelingum, V. (2015) Exploring the health visiting service from the view of South Asian clients in England: a grounded theory study. *Health and Social Care in the Community,* doi 10.1111/hsc.12233.

Adams, C. (2012) The history of health visiting. *Nursing in Practice.* Available from: http://www.nursinginpractice.com/article/history-health-visiting (last accessed 30 March 2016).

Amankwaa, L.C. (2003) Postpartum depression among African-American women. *Issues in Mental Health Nursing,* **24**(3), 297–316.

Anionwu, E. & Atkin, K. (2010) The Social Consequences of Sickle Cell and Thalassaemia: Improving the Quality of Support. Better Health Briefing 17. Race Equality Foundation, London.

Aradhana, S.A. & Cochrane, R. (2005) The Mental Health Status of South Asian Women in Britain: A Review of the Literature. Sage, New Delhi.

Arboleda-Florez, J. (2002) What causes stigma? *World Psychiatry,* **1**(1), 25–6.

Arora, S., McJunkin, C., Wehrer, J. & Kuhn, P. (2000) Major factors influencing breastfeeding rates: mother's perception of father's attitude and milk supply. *Pediatrics,* **106**(5), e67.

Baldwin, S. & Griffiths, P. (2009) Do specialist community public health nurses assess risk factors for depression, suicide, and self-harm among South Asian mothers living in London? *Public Health Nursing*, **26**(3), 277–89.

Barlow, J. (1999) Systematic Review of the Effectiveness of Parent-Training Programmes in Improving Behaviour Problems in Children Aged 3-10 years. Health Services Research Unit, Oxford.

Baughan, J. & Smith, A. (2013) Compassion, Caring and Communication: Skills for Nursing Practice, 2nd edn. Routledge, Abingdon.

Betancourt, J.R., Green, A.R. & Carrillo, J.E. (2002) Cultural Competence in Health Care: Emerging Framework and Practical Approaches. The Commonwealth Fund, Massachusetts.

Chase-Lansdale, P.L., Brooks-Gunn, J. & Zamsky, E.S. (1994). Young African-American multigenerational families in poverty: quality of mothering and grandmothering. *Child Development*, **65**, 373–93.

Chatterjee, M. (1991) Towards Better Health for Indian Women: The Dimensions, Determinants and Consequences of Female Illness and Death. A paper prepared for the Economic Development Institute Work on Women and Health. World Bank, Washington, DC.

Chew-Graham, C., Bashir, C., Chantler, K., Burman, E. & Batsleer, J. (2002) South Asian women, psychological distress and self-harm: lessons for primary care trusts. *Health and Social Care in the Community*, **10**(5), 339–47.

Chew-Graham, C.A., Sharp, D., Chamberlain, E., Folkes, L. & Turner, K.M. (2009) Disclosure of symptoms of postnatal depression, the perspectives of health professionals and women: a qualitative study. *BMC Family Practice*, **10**, 7.

Choudhry, U.K. (1997) Traditional practices of women from India: pregnancy, childbirth, and newborn care, *Journal of Obstetric, Gynecologic, and Neonatal Nursing*, **26**(5), 533–9.

City and Hackney Primary Care Trust (2007) A survey of Orthodox Jewish service users' and providers' views and experiences of the health visiting service. Unpublished.

Cobb, M., Puchalski, C. & Rumbold, B. (2012) The Textbook of Spirituality in Healthcare. Oxford University Press, Oxford.

Cooper, J., Husain, N., Webb, R., Waheed, W., Kapur, N., Guthrie, E. & Appleby, L. (2006) Self-harm in the UK: differences between South Asians and Whites in rates, characteristics, provision of services and repetition. *Social Psychiatry and Psychiatric Epidemiology*, **41**(10), 782–8.

Cowley, S., Whittaker, K., Grigulis, A., Malone, M., Donetto, S., Wood, H., Morrow, E. & Maben, J. (2013) Why Health Visiting? A Review of the Literature about Key Health Visitor Interventions, Processes and Outcomes for Children and Families. National Nursing Research Unit, King's College, London.

Cox, J., Holden, J. & Henshaw, C. (2014) Perinatal Mental Health: The Edinburgh Postnatal Depression Scale (EPDS) Manual, 2nd edn. Royal College of Psychiatrists, London.

Cross, T., Bazron, B., Dennis, K. & Isaacs, M. (1989) Towards a Culturally Competent System of Care. National Technical Assistance Centre for Children's Mental Health, University Child Development Centre, Georgetown, Washington, DC.

Culley, L., Hudson, N., Johnson, M.R.D., Rapport, F. & Katbamna, S. (2007) 'I know about one treatment where they keep the egg somewhere': British South Asian community understandings of infertility and its treatment'. *Diversity in Health and Social Care*, **4**(2), 113–21.

Cuthill, F. (2014) Understanding the ways in which health visitors manage anxiety in cross-cultural work: a qualitative study. *Primary Health Care Research and Development*, **15**(4), 375–85.

DfE (2014) Sure Start Children's Centres: Guidance for Local Authorities. Department for Education, London. Available from: https://www.gov.uk/guidance/sure-start-childrens-centres-local-authorities-duties (last accessed 30 March 2016).

DH (2009) Healthy Child Programme: Pregnancy and the First Five Years of Life. Department of Health, London.

DH (2013) Improving Outcomes and Supporting Transparency Part 1A: A Public Health Outcomes Framework for England, 2013–2016. Available from: https://www.gov.uk/government/uploads/system/uploads/attachment_data/file/263658/2901502_PHOF_Improving_Outcomes_PT1A_v1_1.pdf (last accessed 30 March 2016).

DH (2014a) Early Years High Impact Area 1 – Transition to Parenthood and the Early Weeks, Maternal Mental Health. Available from: https://www.gov.uk/government/uploads/system/uploads/attachment_data/file/413128/2903110_Early_Years_Impact_1_V0_2W.pdf (last accessed 30 March 2016).

DH (2014b) Early Years High Impact Area 2 – Maternal (Perinatal) Mental Health. Available from: https://www.gov.uk/government/uploads/system/uploads/attachment_data/file/413129/2902452_Early_Years_Impact_2_V0_1W.pdf (last accessed 30 March 2016).

DH & HSCIC (2015) Understanding the FGM Enhanced Dataset-Update Guidance to Support Implementation. Department of Health, London.

Dike, P. (2014) Combating Female Genital Mutilation (FGM): Good Practice Points for Health Visitors. Institute of Health Visiting, London.

Dike, P. & Umoren, I. (2014) Combating female genital cutting in the UK: the role of the health visitor. *Journal of Health Visiting*, **2**(5), 260–5.

Dobson, S.M. (1991) Transcultural Nursing. Scutari Press, London.

D'Souza, L., Jayaweera, H. & Pickett, K.E. (2015) Pregnancy diets, migraton, and birth outcomes. *Health Care for Women International*, doi: 10.1080/07399332.2015.1102268.

Evans, J., Heron, J., Francomb, H., Oke, S. & Golding, J.; the Avon Longitudinal Study of Parents and Children Study Team (2001) Cohort study of depressed mood during pregnancy and after childbirth. *British Medical Journal*, **323**(7307), 257–60.

Ferro-Luzzi, G.E. (1980) Food avoidances of pregnant women in Tamilnad. In: Food Ecology and Culture: Readings in the Anthropology of Dietary Practices (ed. J.R.K. Robson). Gordon and Breach Science Publishers, New York. pp. 101–8.

Foster, M. (1988) Health visitors perspectives on working in a multi-ethnic society. *Health Visitor*, **61**, 275–8.

Francis, G. (2010) Developing the Cultural Competence of Health Professionals Working with Gypsy Travellers. Available from: http://www.qni.org.uk/docs/Gill%20Francis%20Cultural%20Competence%20Gypsy%20Traveller%20MS%20Project%20Report%202010.pdf (last accessed 30 March 2016).

Gatrad, R. & Sheikh, A. (2001) Muslim birth customs. *Archives of Diseases in Childhood Fetal Neonatal Edition*, **84**, F6–8.

Gatrad, R., Ray, M. & Sheikh, A. (2004) Hindu birth customs. *Archives of Disease in Childhood*, **89**(12), 1094–7.

Gatrad, R., Khan, A., Shafi, S. & Sheikh, A. (2005a) Promoting safer male circumcisions for British Muslims. *Diversity in Health and Social Care*, **2**(1), 37–40.

Gatrad, R., Jutti-Johal, J., Gill, P.S. & Sheikh, A. (2005b) Sikh birth customs. *Archives of Disease in Childhood*, **90**(6), 560–3.

Gordon, A. (2013) Mental Health Remains an Invisible Problem in Africa. Think Africa Press.

Gorman, L.L., O'Hara, M.W., Figueiredo, B., Hayes, S., Jacquemain, F., Kammerer, M.H., Klier, C.M., Rosi, S., Seneviratne, G. & Sutter-Dallay, A. (2004) Adaptation of the structured clinical interview for DSM–IV disorders for assessing depression in women during pregnancy and post-partum across countries and cultures. *British Journal of Psychiatry*, **184**(46), s17–23.

Graham, E.A., Haq, A., Musa, S. & Abdullahi, A. (2007) Breast Feeding Support for Somali Mothers. Available from: http://ethnomed.org/clinical/pediatrics/breast_feeding_soma_mothers.pdf/view?searchterm=somali%20breastfeeding (last accessed 30 March 2016).

Hogg, R., Kok, B., Netto, G., Hanley, J. & Haycock-Stuart, E. (2014) Supporting Pakistani and Chinese families with young children: perspectives of mothers and health visitors. *Child Care, Health and Development*, **41**(3), 416–23.

Home Office (2015) Mandatory Reporting of Female Genital Mutilation – Procedural Information. Home Office, London.

Horwath, J., Lees, J., Sidebotham, P., Higgins, J. & Imtiaz, A. (2008) Religion, Beliefs and Parenting Practices: A Descriptive Study. Joseph Rowntree Foundation, York.

HSCIC (2012) Infant Feeding Survey 2010: Summary. The Information Centre, Dundee. Available from: https://www.nct.org.uk/sites/default/files/related_documents/Infant%20Feeding%20Survey_uk_2010_summary.pdf (last accessed 30 March 2016).

Hussain, F. & Cochrane, R. (2004) Depression in South Asian women living in the UK: a review of the literature with implications for service provision. *Transcultural Psychiatry*, **41**(2), 253–70.

Jayaweera, H. (2014) Briefing – Health of Migrants in the UK: What Do We Know. Migration Observatory, Centre on Migration, Policy and Society (COMPAS), Oxford. Available from: http://www.migrationobservatory.ox.ac.uk/briefings/health-migrants-uk-what-do-we-know (last accessed 30 March 2016).

Jeffery, P., Jefferur, R. & Lyon, A. (1989) Labour Pains and Labour Power and Childbearing in India. Zed Books, New Delhi.

Jesudason, V. & Shirur, R. (1980) Selected socio-cultural aspects of food during pregnancy in the Telengana region of Andhra Pradesh. *Journal of Family Welfare*, **27**(2), 3–15.

Jivraj, S. & Simpson, L. (eds) (2015) Ethnic Identity and Inequalities in Britain – The Dynamics of Diversity. Policy Press, Bristol.

Kabir, M., Iliiyasu, Z., Abubaker, I.S. & Aliyu, M.H. (2004) Perception and beliefs about mental illness among adults in Karfi village, northern Nigeria. *BMC International Health and Human Rights*, **4**(3), 1–5.

Krause, I.B. (1989) Sinking heart: a Punjabi communication of distress. *Social Science and Medicine* **29**(4), 563–75.

Kumanyika, S.K. (2008) Environmental influences on childhood obesity: ethnic and cultural influences in context. *Physiology and Behaviour*, **94**, 61–70.

Laming, Lord H. (2003) *The Victoria Climbié Inquiry: Report of an Inquiry by Lord Laming*, CM5730. The Stationery Office, London.

Liampattong, P. (ed.) (2010) Infant Feeding Practices: A Cross-Cultural Perspective. Springer, New York.

Lundberg, P.C. & Thu, T.T.N. (2012) Breast-feeding attitudes and practices among Vietnamese mothers in Ho Chi Minh City. *Midwifery*, **28**(2), 252–7.

MacDonald, M. (1991) Spreading the health message among elderly Asian people. *Health Visitor*, **64**(6), 196.

Macpherson, W. (1999) The Stephen Lawrence Inquiry: Report of an Inquiry. Home Office, London.

Marmot, M., Atkinson, T., Bell, J., Black, C., Broadfoot, P., Cumberlege, J., Diamond, I., Gilmore, I., Ham, C., Meacher, M. & Mulgan, G. (2010) Fair Society, Healthy Lives: The Marmot Review. Marmot Review Team, University College, London. Available from: http://www.instituteofhealthequity.org/projects/fair-society-healthy-lives-the-marmot-review (last accessed 30 March 2016).

Mathews, C. & Benjamin, V. (1979) Health education evaluation of beliefs and practices in rural Tamil Nadu: family planning and antenatal care. *Social Action*, **29**, 377–92.

Mayhew, L., Harper, S. & Waples, S. (2011) Counting Hackney's Population Using Administrative Data – An Analysis of Change between 2007 and 2011. Neighbourhood Knowledge Management, Hackney.

McFadden, A., Renfrew, M. & Atkin, K. (2013) Does cultural context make a difference to women's experiences of maternity care? A qualitative study comparing the perspectives of breast-feeding women of Bangladeshi origin and health practitioners. *Health Expectations*, **16**(4), 124–35.

Moeed, S.M. & Grover, S.R. (2012) Female genital mutilation/cutting (FGM/C): survey of RANZcOG fellows, diplomates & trainees and FGM/C prevention and education program workers in Australia and New Zealand. *Australian and New Zealand Journal of Obstetrics and Gynaecology*, **52**(6), 523–7.

Morse, J.M., Jehle, C. & Gamble, D. (1990) Initiating breastfeeding: a world survey of the timing of postpartum breastfeeding. *International Journal of Nursing Studies*, **27**(3), 303–13.

Nag, M. (1994) Beliefs and practices about food during pregnancy: implication for maternal nutrition. *Economic and Political Weekly*, **29**(37), 2427–8.

Nesbitt, E. (2012) Sikhism. In: Oxford Textbook of Spirituality in Healthcare (eds M. Cobb, C. Puchalski & B. Rumbold). Oxford University Press, Oxford. pp. 89–96.

NICE (2010) Pregnancy and Complex Social Factors. Clinical Guideline 110. National Institute for Health and Care Excellence, London. Available from: http://www.nice.org.uk/Search?q=Pregnancy+and+complex+social+factors (last accessed 30 March 2016).

NICE (2014a) Health Visiting. NICE advice [LGB22]. National Institute for Health and Care Excellence, London. Available from: http://www.nice.org.uk/advice/lgb22/chapter/Introduction (last accessed 30 March 2016).

NICE (2014b) Vitamin D: Increasing Supplement Use among At-Risk Groups. NICE Guidance PH56. Available from: https://www.nice.org.uk/guidance/ph56 (last accessed 30 March 2016).

NICE (2014c) Antenatal and Postnatal Mental Health: Clinical Management and Service Guidance. National Collaborating Centre for Mental Health, London.

NICE (2015) Nutrition: Improving Maternal and Child Nutrition. *NICE Quality Standard* **98**. Available from: http://www.nice.org.uk/guidance/qs98 (last accessed 30 March 2016).

NMC (2015) The Code: Professional Standards of Practice and Behaviour for Nurses and Midwives. Nursing and Midwifery Council, London. Available from: https://www.nmc.org.uk/globalassets/sitedocuments/nmc-publications/nmc-code.pdf (last accessed 30 March 2016).

O' Hagan, K. (2001) Cultural Competence in the Caring Professions. Jessica Kingsley, London.

O'Hara, M. & Swain, A. (1996). Rates and risk of postpartum depression – a meta-analysis. *International Review of Psychiatry*, **8**, 37–54.

Oates, M.R., Cox, J.L., Neema, S., Asten, P., Glangeaud-Freudenthal, N., Figueiredo, B., et al. (2004) Postnatal depression across countries and cultures: a qualitative study. *British Journal of Psychiatry*, **184**(46), s10–16.

ONS (1997) Infant Feeding Practices in Asian Families: Early Feeding Practices and Growth (Social Survey Report). Office for National Statistics, London.

ONS (2011) Census 2011. Office for National Statistics, London.

Papadopoulos, I. (2003) The Papadopoulos, Tilki and Taylor model for the development of cultural competence in nursing. *Journal of Health, Social and Environmental Issues*, **4**(1), 5–7.

Papadopoulos, I. & Tilki, M. (2008) The Papadopoulos, Tilki and Taylor Model for Developing Cultural Competence. Leonardo da Vinci Partnership Project (IENE) Intercultural Education of Nurses and Medical Staff in Europe. Available from: http://www.ieneproject.eu/download/Outputs/intercultural%20model.pdf (last accessed 30 March 2016).

Papadopoulos, I., Tilki, M. & Taylor, G. (1998) Transcultural Care: A Guide for Health Care Professionals. Mark Allen Publishing, Wiltshire.

Pisacane, A., Continisio, G.I., Aldinucci, M., D'Amora, S. & Continisio, P. (2005) A controlled trial of the father's role in breastfeeding promotion. Pediatrics, 116(4), e494–8.

Pool, R. (1987) Hot and cold as an explanatory model: the example of Bharuch district in Gujarat, India. Social Science and Medicine, 25(4), 389–9.

Quah, S.R. (ed.) (2015) Routledge Handbook of Families in Asia. Routledge, London.

Quickfall, J. (2014) Cultural competence in practice: the example of the community nursing care of asylum applicants in Scotland. Diversity and Equality in Healthcare, 11, 247–53. Available from: http://diversityhealthcare.imedpub.com/cultural-competence-in-practice-the-example-of-the-community-nursing-care-of-asylum-applicants-in-scotland.pdf (last accessed 30 March 2016).

Rack, P. (1982) Race, Culture and Mental Disorders. Tavistock, London.

Rait, S.K. (2005) Sikh Women in England: Their Religious and Cultural Beliefs and Practices. Trentham Books, UCL Institute of Education Press, London.

Raman, A.V. (1988) Traditional practices and nutritional taboos. Nursing Journal of India, 79(6), 143–66.

Rao, M. (1985) Food beliefs of rural women during the reproductive years in Dharwar, India. Ecology of Food and Nutrition, 16, 93–103.

Seal, J. (2013) Exploring perceptions of listening, empathy and summarising in the health visitor-parent relationship. Journal of Health Visiting, 1(4), 226–32.

Shah, Q. & Sonuga-Barke, E.J. (1995) Family structure and the mental health of Pakistani Muslim mothers and their children living in Britain. British Journal of Clinical Psychology, 34(11), 79–81.

Shenoy, S.D., Swift, P., Cody, D. & Iqbal, J. (2005) Maternal vitamin D deficiency, refractory neonatal hypocalcaemia and nutritional rickets. Archives of Disease in Childhood, 90(4), 437–8.

Smith, J.K., Burns, S., Cunningham, S., Freeman, J., McLellan, A. & McWilliam, K. (2010) The hazards of honey: infantile botulism. BMJ Case Reports, doi: 10.1136/bcr.05.2010.3038.

Sonuga-Barke, E.J. & Mistry, M. (2000) The effect of extended family living on the mental health of three generations within two Asian communities. British Journal of Clinical Psychology, 39(2), 129–41.

Sonuga-Barke, E., Mistry, M. & Qureshi, S. (1998). The mental health of Muslim mothers in extended families living in Britain: the impact of intergenerational disagreement on anxiety and depression. British Journal of Clinical Psychology, 37(4), 399–408.

Sunak, R. & Rajeswaran, S. (2014) A Portrait of Modern Britain. Policy Exchange, London.

Tesfaye, H.T. & Day, J. (2015) Health visitors' perceptions of barriers to health and wellbeing in European migrant families. Community Practitioner, 88(1), 22–5.

Tighe, M., Chan, E., Tran, L. & Lam, S. (2014) Working with Chinese Families in the UK: Good Practice Points for Health Visitors: Working with Minority Groups. Institute of Health Visiting, London.

Unger, D.G. & Cooley, M. (1992) Partner and grandmother contact in black and white teen parent families. Journal of Adolescent Health, 13, 546–52.

Unite/CPHVA Health Visiting Forum (2007) The Distinctive Contribution of Health Visiting to Public Health and Wellbeing. Addressing Public Health Priorities using the Principles of Health Visiting. Unite, London.

UNICEF (2013) Female genital mutilation/cutting: a statistical overview and exploration of the dynamics of change. Available from: http://www.childinfo.org/files/FGCM_Lo_res.pdf (last accessed 30 March 2016).

UNICEF (n.d.) Breastfeeding research – an overview. Available from: http://www.unicef.org.uk/BabyFriendly/News-and-Research/Research/Breastfeeding-research---An-overview/ (last accessed 30 March 2016).

Webb, P. (1981) Health problems of London's Asian and Afro-Caribbeans. *Health Visitor*, **54**, 141–7.

Webb-Johnson, A. & Nadirshaw, Z. (1993) Good practice in transcultural counselling: an Asian perspective. *British Journal of Guidance and Counselling*, **21**(1), 20–9.

While, A. & Godfrey, M. (1984) Health visitor knowledge of Asian cultures. *Health Visitor*, **57**, 297–8.

Yeasmin, S.F. & Regmi, K. (2013) A qualitative study on the food habits and related beliefs of pregnant British Bangladeshis. *Health Care for Women International*, **34**(5), 395–415.

Activities

Activity 6.1

Examine the statistics for your local authority, using either your local authority's own website or the CoDE 'profiler' at www.ethnicity.ac.uk. What changes in the composition of the population have occurred over the past 10 years?

Activity 6.2

Think about your own family traditions at childbirth, or in another 'life event'. What are the roots of your family traditions?

Explore and reflect:

- What are your own values, beliefs, customs, behaviours, biases, and prejudices?
- Do you know about others' values, beliefs, customs, behaviours, biases, and prejudices?

Activity 6.3

Explore and reflect:

- Do your own values, beliefs, customs, behaviours, biases, and prejudices differ from those of others? What are the similarities and what are the differences?

- How do others' cultural health beliefs and behaviours differ?
- Do you need any additional cultural awareness, understanding, skills, or knowledge?

Activity 6.4

Explore and reflect:

- Are you open to cultural differences?
- How comfortable do you feel communicating with those from other cultures?
- Are you able to act in a nonjudgmental manner around those from different cultures? If not, what are the challenges? How can you overcome these?

Activity 6.5

Explore and reflect:

- Are you understanding of and sensitive to other cultural values, beliefs, and behaviours? How do you demonstrate this in practice?
- Can you adapt in order to work effectively in different cultural contexts, being respectful and nonjudgmental?

Activity 6.6

Explore and reflect:

- Does your place of work/clinic have information in languages other than English? Is a check made on their use?
- Do illustrations in posters and leaflets show a diversity of ethnic backgrounds (e.g. Sikh clothing, African hairstyles, Chinese faces)?
- Are staff and those organising events aware of the dates of key religious or cultural festivals and local community events, such as a carnival or mela, and do they make use of local culturally specific media and community venues (e.g. 'Asian radio', displays in public areas of a gurdwara or mosque)?

7
Evaluating Practice

Karen A. Luker
The University of Manchester, Manchester, UK

Gretl A. McHugh
The University of Leeds, Leeds, UK

Introduction

Evaluation is an important but often neglected component of health care planning and is examined here in the general context of health visiting and public health. Taking into account the developments in evidence-based practice and the interest in evaluation as part of quality improvement (Health Foundation, 2015), health care can be described as the application of best current knowledge in the context of the condition and values of an individual patient or client, family or population – sometimes referred to as evidence-based practice or policy making (Muir Gray, 2004). Health care and health maintenance can be seen to be the concern of the individual, especially in a society where self-care is advocated for the management of a number of long-term conditions (DH, 2005a, 2009a, 2010a; DHSSPS 2015). One of the main challenges facing the health care system is in caring for people with two or more long-term conditions, referred to as 'multimorbidity' (DH, 2014a). Some long-term conditions, such as obesity and type 2 diabetes, are preventable, and a number of professional groups, including health visitors, have a responsibility to provide health advice and health care services to individuals, families, and communities to support prevention of these conditions.

Skill mix is a permanent feature of health visiting teams. Teams vary, but comprise both experienced and recently qualified health visitors, as well as health visitors with specialist interests (e.g. in child protection). In addition, other practitioners – including community staff nurses, nursery nurses, and health care assistants – may undertake aspects of the work that was once considered the traditional role of health visitors, such as running baby clinics or home visiting. Whilst acknowledging this heterogeneity within health visiting teams, for simplicity we have tended to use the term 'health visitor' in this chapter to refer to all these team different members.

Health Visiting: Preparation for Practice, Fourth Edition.
Edited by Karen A. Luker, Gretl A. McHugh and Rosamund M. Bryar.
© 2017 John Wiley & Sons, Ltd. Published 2017 by John Wiley & Sons, Ltd.

The greater emphasis now placed on the evaluation of health care services stems from the escalating public demand for quality services and lower costs, brought about by increased expectations, technological advances, and service complexity, plus the pressure on public finances (DH, 2005b, 2010a, 2012a; NHS England, 2013). The increased complexity of the service has, in part, been a response to the political pressure to improve the efficiency and quality of the National Health Service (NHS). There has been an increasing trend towards specialisation, initiated by medicine and mirrored in nursing, which has resulted in greater competition for limited resources. The uncertainty generated by the fact that demand exceeds supply, in terms of finance, has meant that doctors and nurses alike are forced to look for verifiable facts to assist them in establishing a convincing case worthy of continued or additional financial support. Historically, most policy decisions in the health care field have simply followed a logical appraisal of the options of the people involved in the decision making and may not have involved an analysis of available data. In order to justify society's continued support and commitment to health care, it is necessary to demonstrate effectiveness. Over the past several years, there has been an increase in funding for effectiveness research and for research that seeks to identify whether data on effectiveness exist (Cowley *et al.*, 2013).

In this chapter, we present the key sources of evidence available to health visitors in evaluating their practice, including the different types of evaluation and suggested ways to approach evaluation, such as the 'care planning process' and target setting using the 'SMART' approach. In addition, we provide examples of evaluation of practice and optional activities.

Sources of evidence for practice

The National Institute for Health and Care Excellence (NICE) is the expert organisation which evaluates new and existing medicines, treatments, and procedures in the UK and recommends or does not recommend their adoption by the NHS in England (via the devolved administrations) in Wales, Scotland, and Northern Ireland. It also provides evidence-based guidance on the treatment and care of people with specific diseases and conditions (see www.nice.org.uk). Clinical guidelines of relevance to health visiting practice concerning the postnatal care of women and their babies were developed by the National Collaborating Centre for Primary Care (NCCPC) on behalf of NICE (NCCPC, 2006), with an addendum regarding sudden infant death syndrome in 2014 (NICE, 2014a). There has also been a considerable amount of guidance from NICE around public health, with several of its published guidelines of relevance to health visitors, such as *Community Engagement* (NICE, 2008a), *Maternal and Child Nutrition* (NICE, 2008b), *Reducing the Differences in the Uptake of Immunisations* (NICE, 2009a) and *Maintaining a Healthy Weight and Preventing Excess Weight Gain among Adults and Children* (NICE, 2015). Joint publications from NICE and the Social Care Institute for Excellence (SCIE; see www.scie.org.uk), such as *Looked-After Children and Young People* (NICE & SCIE, 2010a) and *Strategies to Prevent Unintentional Injuries among Children and Young People Aged Under 15* (NICE & SCIE, 2010b) also provide relevant guidance to health visitors in their practice. Another guideline, which extends into the domain of health visiting, relates to helping people to change their behaviour at the population, community, and individual levels (NICE, 2014b). NICE also offers health professionals guidance on how to implement changes in practice, which is often difficult. In addition, some of the guidelines have 'audit guidance' on achieving improved standards; for example, improving immunisation targets (NICE, 2009b). New topics in the area of public health and social care are emerging on a regular basis. NICE has also produced guidance specifically about health visiting as a local government briefing for local authorities and other agencies (NICE, 2014c). It is clearly important for health and social care practitioners to regularly check the NICE and SCIE websites in order to keep up to date with evidence-based practice guidance. It might be useful to locate some of the existing guidance of relevance to health visitors; this can be explored by completing Activity 7.1.

Since 2009, NHS Evidence (see www.evidence.nhs.uk) has provided individuals working in health and social care with access to information, guidelines, and NHS policy with the aim of improving the quality of care for patients and service users. The NHS Improving Quality initiative, established in 2013 (www.nhsiq.nhs.uk), is driving the agenda on quality. In Scotland, the NHS quality-improvement hub (www .qihub.scot.nhs.uk) includes a knowledge network (www.knowledge.scot.nhs.uk) which provides evidence and community tools to staff working in health and social care, along with a portal that enables practitioners to search for the evidence for use in practice (www.evidenceintopractice.scot.nhs.uk). This is all part of Scotland's quality-improvement strategy for health care.

Another good source of evidence is *Effectiveness Matters*, produced by the Centre for Reviews and Dissemination (CRD), which provides information on the development and promotion of evidence-based care, including health promotion interventions, in terms of what was and was not effective in the past (see http://www.york .ac.uk/crd/publications/effectiveness-matters/). There are also evidence briefings produced for commissioners of services, such as guidance on supporting women with postnatal depression through psychological therapies (http://www.york.ac.uk/ crd/publications/evidence-briefings/). CRD used also to publish the *Effective Health Care Bulletin*, which included summaries of systematic reviews and syntheses of the research evidence on health care interventions. This ceased publication in 2004, but the archives are still available online (http://www.york.ac.uk/crd/publications/ archive/). The CRD continues to publish high-quality systematic reviews that evaluate the effects of health and social care interventions (see http://www.york.ac.uk/crd/), including from the Health Technology Assessment programme (HTA), which provides completed and ongoing health technology assessments (see http://www.crd .york.ac.uk/crdweb/). HTA reports are also available from the National Institute for Health Research (NIHR) Journals Library (http://www.journalslibrary.nihr.ac.uk/hta). The Database of Abstracts of Reviews of Effects (DARE), which included abstracts of systematic reviews, quality assessment of reviews, and details of Cochrane reviews and protocols, and the NHS Economic Evaluation Database (EED) were previously part of the CRD; these ceased in 2015 but can still be accessed online. An NHS

Dissemination Centre is now established, which focuses on the dissemination of evidence in health and social care (www.dc.nihr.ac.uk). These are all important sources of evidence for health visitors, and they can be explored further using Activity 7.2.

There is very little evidence concerning the effectiveness of health visiting interventions (discussed later and in Chapter 3) when compared to interventions provided by other health professionals. For example, for some activities (e.g. health promotion interventions), a national scoping exercise of the contribution of nurses, midwives, and health visitors to child health and child health services found very little outcome data demonstrating that these interventions had sustained effects on negative health behaviours or other health outcomes (While *et al.*, 2005). A more recent narrative review examined the literature on key health visitor interventions for children and families (Cowley *et al.*, 2013) and found some evidence of beneficial outcomes from health visiting practice (in particular, structured home visiting and early interventions), but the changes were small. In addition, there have been a number of systematic reviews around health visiting practice which have found conflicting evidence concerning the interventions delivered by health visitors, public health nurses, and other community health workers (Elkan *et al.*, 2000; Ciliska *et al.*, 2001; Shaw *et al.*, 2006).

The only systematic review conducted of the effectiveness of health visiting was over 15 years ago (Elkan *et al.*, 2000). At that time, there was a limited amount of evidence supporting some of the interventions which health visitors undertook. However, there was positive evidence for home visiting to support parents in improving breastfeeding and immunisation rates. Other, later systematic reviews focused more on home visiting programmes, with one reporting that within the scope of public health nurses in Canada, visiting pre- and postnatal clients in their own homes could produce significant benefits, especially with interventions of high intensity and clients considered at 'risk' (Ciliska *et al.*, 2001). An analysis of nine systematic reviews on home visiting programmes found some evidence to support home visiting in the antenatal and postnatal periods, namely in reducing rates of childhood injury and in the identification and management of postnatal depression (Bull *et al.*, 2004). In a more recent meta-ethnographic systematic review of four studies examining programmes for parents of children with behavioural difficulties, two of the studies involved health visitors delivering the programme (Kane *et al.*, 2007). The recently published early evaluation of the effectiveness of the Family Nurse Partnership (FNP) programme (discussed in Chapter 4) is an example of a pragmatic randomised controlled trial (RCT), with women assigned to receiving FNP compared to usual care, which enabled an evaluation of whether the provision of this programme should be continued (Robling *et al.*, 2015).

There is variability by employing authority even within England, despite the NHS Core Service Specification (NHS England, 2014a) delineating what health visitors do, who they visit, and the content of interactions. However, home visiting is only one aspect of their work, and there is a need to examine further the role and function of health visitors in the UK.

For over 25 years – first highlighted in the 1990 National Health Service and Social Care Act, now superseded by the Health and Social Care Act 2012, which came into operation on 1 April 2013 – evaluation has been firmly on every professional's agenda, but unfortunately it has been a very neglected area of study, especially in community nursing services and health visiting. According to the Queen's Nursing Institute (QNI, 2008), there are a number of reasons why community nurses and health visitors need to be skilled in evaluating their services or changes to their services, namely:

> As registered professionals, they have a duty to provide the best possible care, and to do this they need to know the impact of their work on those it's intended to benefit. The increase in competition to provide services means that professionals need to be able to show how and why their service, or new way of working is effective.
>
> (QNI, 2008: 1)

The Nursing and Midwifery Council (NMC) has standards of proficiency for specialist community public health nurses (SCPHNs), several of which focus on the need for health visitors to be involved in evaluation (NMC, 2004); these standards have not been superseded. They are based on 10 key public health principles (Skills for Health, 2008) and the four domains of health visiting (CETHV, 1977; Twinn & Cowley, 1992). There are three public health principles, which focus on evaluation within health visiting practice, covering two domains in health visiting (see Table 7.1). In Wales, the nursing and midwifery strategy has a focus on research and development, with one specific aim of reviewing practice through audit and service evaluation (Public Health Wales NHS Trust, 2014). NICE's (2014c) guidance to those commissioning health visiting services focuses on what health visitors can achieve:

Table 7.1 NMC standards of proficiency for entry on to register.

Principle	Domain: Influence on policies affecting health
Developing health programmes and services and reducing inequalities	Work with others to plan, implement, and evaluate programmes and projects to improve health and well being
	Identify and evaluate service provision and support networks for individuals, families, and groups in the local area or setting
Research and development to improve health and well being	Develop, implement, evaluate, and improve practice on the basis of research, evidence, and evaluation
Principle	**Domain: Facilitation of health-enhancing activities**
Strategic leadership for health and well being	Apply leadership skills and manage projects to improve health and well being
	Plan, deliver, and evaluate programmes to improve the health and well being of individuals and groups

Source: NMC (2004: 11–12)

(i) building resilience and reducing costs in later life; (ii) identifying families with additional needs and providing support; (iii) improving wider factors that affect health and well being; (iv) reducing numbers of children dying prematurely and living with preventable harm and ill health; and (v) supporting people to live healthy lifestyles and make healthy choices.

The mere recognition of evaluation as a neglected area of practice will not be sufficient to promote the activity, however. A better understanding of what evaluation might entail is discussed in the next section; this may encourage health visitors to focus on this element of their work.

Evaluation – the problem of definition

The word 'evaluation' is widely used, and for the most part its meaning is taken for granted. Few attempts have been made to formulate a conceptually rigorous definition of 'evaluation' or to analyse the meanings behind its use. The lack of a clear definition has meant that the word 'evaluation' is used interchangeably with other terms, such as 'assessment', 'appraisal', and sometimes 'audit'. We talk of 'assessment' or 'evaluation' in the context of client or community needs, and indeed assessment is said to be the first stage in care planning and evaluation the last. We hear nurse managers talk of staff appraisal, performance and development reviews, and evaluation, and this relates to how well individual practitioners are functioning in their particular role. It is evident, then, that confusion may arise if we use the word 'evaluation' in a casual way. In addition, there may be confusion about the difference between 'evaluation', 'research', and 'audit' (QNI, 2008). Educational toolkits are available to assist practitioners in understanding the differences between research, audit, and service evaluations (Brain et al., 2011).

Taking into account the common usage of the term 'evaluation', there is a distinction to be made between evaluation of everyday practice by a practitioner and evaluation research, such as the evaluation of pilot schemes:

- a pilot evaluation of the text4baby mobile health program (Evans et al., 2012);
- evaluation of a public health nurse visiting programme for pregnant and parenting teens (Schaffer et al., 2012);
- a mixed-methods study evaluating health visitor assessment of mother–infant interactions (Appleton et al., 2013);
- an RCT of a guided Internet behavioural activation treatment: Netmums Helping with Depression (O'Mahen et al., 2013, 2014).

'Evaluation', when used in a general way, tends to refer to the everyday occurrence of making judgments of worth. Although this interpretation implies some form of logical or rational thought, it does not presuppose any systematic procedures for presenting objective evidence to support the judgment. When used in this way, 'evaluation' refers only to the process of assessment or appraisal of worth. The Health Foundation (2015) discusses evaluation as the capturing of insight which might be lost, with the generation of new knowledge so that lessons can be learned.

Evaluation has been defined by St Leger *et al.* as:

> The critical assessment, on as objective a basis as possible, of the degree to which entire services or their component parts (e.g. diagnostic tests, treatments, caring procedures) fulfil stated goals.
>
> (St Leger *et al.*, 1992: 1)

Two important elements of this definition are highlighted by the authors: first, the reference to goals, which explicitly requires a comparison with some standard, and, second, the importance of objectivity, which ensures the findings of the evaluative process are independent of judgments or prejudices on the part of those undertaking and commissioning the evaluation.

Evaluative research, on the other hand, implies the utilisation of scientific methods and techniques for the purpose of making an evaluation. Inherent in the term 'evaluative research' is an emphasis on the measurement of change and the generation of new knowledge. The distinction made between 'evaluation' and 'evaluative research' may seem irrelevant or daunting to some practitioners who consider that they will never become involved in research as a primary activity, but, nevertheless, practitioners may be involved in generating research questions or become engaged in data collection for others. Many research questions are developed from an observation in practice. However, in their everyday work, health visitors are constantly involved in making judgments of worth. For example, if we simply say that we believe that visits to families with a disabled child are a good idea, this is an unsubstantiated judgment. If, on the other hand, we say that visits to families with a disabled child are good because they reduce the incidence of loneliness and depression in the mother, this may be a substantiated judgment (i.e. based on evidence of the impact of visits on loneliness and depression). If we have some insight into the criteria used as the basis of the statement, this does not make it research, but it does imply that we have some evidence to support our position, and may suggest possible outcome measures to be used in measuring the impact of home visits and in research.

In the past 10 years, a great deal has been written about the importance of being able to measure the outcomes of care. This has largely been driven by the evidence-based practice movement and the international financial situation. There is a desire to measure the effectiveness or adequacy of care (DH, 2008a). The Darzi Report (DH, 2008a) emphasised the need to improve effectiveness of care throughout the patient journey, with personal care, quality, and safety high on the agenda. The Commissioning for Quality and Innovation (CQUINS) is in place to improve services for people, and nurses are a part of ensuring services and targets are being met (NHS England, 2014b; RCN, 2012). In addition, there have been developments in the NHS in the use of patient-related outcome measures (PROMS) to measure the effectiveness of care (DH, 2008b). Policy has highlighted the need to focus on improving health care outcomes, with a more widespread use of PROMS where available, and on learning from patient/client experience surveys and real-time feedback (DH, 2010a). There has been more focus on experiential elements within the NHS patient experience framework, which includes such essential components of the patient experience as integration and coordination of care (DH 2012b). The important insights provided by patient/client experiences of health care and information collected on what is good and what could be improved with regard to services ultimately assists in forming judgments about performance and accountability. Before reading on, take some time to consider your own practice and begin to complete Activity 7.3.

Conceptualising evaluation

There are different types of evaluation. The Health Foundation (2015) provides an overview of four main ones:

- *Summative*: usually carried out at the end of the intervention when data is available to determine whether the goals or objectives have been met and any improvements and how the benefits compared to the costs.
- *Formative*: enables us to shape an intervention and used as the intervention is evolving, so it is useful to take into account any changes that need to be made before implementation.
- *Rapid Cycle*: an example of a formative evaluation which helps with determining if an intervention is effective, but goals are often fixed and enable improvements in the intervention to be made. Often used for large-scale changes for example a new service.
- *Development*: an example of a formative evaluation but goals can often be changed and enables real-time feedback to the intervention team, often involving close working with those doing the evaluation.

(Health Foundation, 2015)

In conceptualising the various approaches to evaluation, the goal-attainment model stands out as being particularly appealing to those involved in the evaluation of health care. The notion of goal attainment is embodied in the target-setting approach adopted by many Trusts; two good examples are the immunisation and cervical screening targets set as goals for general practices and the targets set in the health visitor service specification. Target setting is also used in identifying service priorities. Targets should be specific, measurable, achievable, realistic, and time-bound, summarised in the mnemonic 'SMART'. This framework was developed by Doran (1981) as a management tool and has been used widely in health care and in health care education (Bovend'Eerdt *et al.*, 2009; Sidhu *et al.*, 2015).

The starting point for any evaluation is to be clear about the aims of the service; that is, the benefits expected to be accrued by the service's recipients. There is general agreement amongst those concerned with evaluation that the most important – and yet most difficult – phase is the clarification of goals and objectives. The emphasis on goals and objectives stems from a conceptualisation of evaluation as a measurement of the success or failure of an activity insofar as it reaches its predetermined objectives. One way to avoid this conundrum is to evaluate the service from the perspective of the service user or client. This is a more open-ended approach to evaluation, which seeks to capture the experience of the service user in terms of the perceived benefits and disbenefits of the service. An example of this approach is Russell & Drennan's (2007) Web-based study of 4665 mothers' views of the health visiting service in the UK. Using Netmums (www.netmums.com), an online parenting organisation that currently has 1.7 million users (mostly mothers), Russell & Drennan conducted a survey over concern that the health visiting service was increasingly difficult to access. They found that mothers valued the health visiting service, particularly health visitors' knowledge and expertise concerning child development and parenting, but felt that some recent changes to the service, such as a focus on those families most in need, were making health visitors less accessible to them (Russell & Drennan, 2007). Another example is a questionnaire examining parents' perceptions and experiences of the health visiting service (McHugh & Luker, 2002). Although the service was valued by those who received it, and health visitors provided much needed support and advice, the study highlighted high client expectations, and the need for information based on research and evidence, to allow the service to deliver higher-quality interventions in the community. Such a use of evidence to inform practice and safe health visiting interventions resulted in Tower Hamlets developing an evidence-based toolkit, the priorities of which were developed using a modified Delphi approach: infant stimulation and early speech and language, obesity prevention, and a focus on stressed and unsupported families (Bryar et al., 2013; Barts Health NHS Trust, 2014). The provision of support and guidance in these areas enabled health visitors to focus their practice on these particular health needs of the local population.

A narrative review of service users' views on health visiting found that a trusting relationship between client and health visitor was key to providing valued support; qualitative data highlighted the positive experiences of health visiting services, but showed that those with negative experiences tended to disengage from the service (Donetto et al., 2013). Organisational features of the health visiting service which caused disruption to the care experience were also seen to be an issue (Donetto et al., 2013). The Department of Health's (DH, 2011) service vision for health visiting has been to increase the number of health visitors, in order to provide increased support and evidence-based service to all families, rather than just to those considered at-risk. There is a focus on investing in services for children and families around the following areas, which provide for the development of standards that can be used to evaluate health visitors' impact:

- Improving access to services
- Improving the experience of children & families
- Improving health and well being outcomes for under fives
- Reducing health inequalities.

(NHS England, 2014a)

The process of evaluating can be complex and may be open to subjective influences. Different people want to know different things. Evaluation involves a combination of basic assumptions underlying the activity to be evaluated and the personal values of those engaged in the activities being evaluated. Hence, the process of evaluation always starts with recognition of values, which may be either explicit or implicit, before moving on to goal/objective setting and goal measuring, putting goal activity into operation (programme operation), and finally assessing the effect of the goal operation (programme evaluation) (first described by Suchman, 1967).

Example: tackling childhood obesity

With reference to a goal/objective attainment evaluation process, we will explore possible ways of evaluating a health programme. Let us suppose that we are health visitors who wish to tackle the growing problem of obesity in the under 5s. We have observed that there appear to be a number of overweight children attending the child health clinic for their 2-year check. Our observations will reflect our values. We believe that to be overweight in childhood is not good; we may hold different views on why this is undesirable. Some of us may believe that overweight children experience more upper respiratory tract infections, may be more prone to obesity later in life, and are at an increased risk of developing type 2 diabetes. Others may be of the opinion that children with obesity do not look as attractive as those of average or light build, and that this may lead to an internalisation of a negative self-image or bullying by other children. In part, these value judgments reflect the beliefs and values of the society in which we live and work. However, our views may also be based on literature on childhood obesity we have read or on our use of weight-monitoring charts. In any case, in response to this perceived need, we decide to set up a healthy eating club for parents of under 5s. The underlying rationale for this action is that we believe that it would be beneficial for families to learn about healthy eating, and furthermore we believe it would benefit society if the next generation were fit and healthy.

The objectives of the club will probably be wider than just getting parents to understand about healthy eating in childhood, although this will, of course, be the major focus. First, we may have to convince the parents of the importance of healthy eating to a child's healthy weight and that having an overweight child is undesirable and a potential threat to future health and well being. Second, as health visitors, we see ourselves as health promoters and facilitators, and it is likely that we will use the healthy eating club to teach the parents of children under 5 about the nutritional value of food and the value of a balanced diet. We may even go so far as to teach family members how to cook nutritious food. There are plenty of resources on this, such as those produced by First Steps Nutrition Trust (www.firststepsnutrition.org), which can help provide the informational basis of sessions on eating well, fussy eating, portion sizes, or healthy cooking, depending on the needs of the group. There is also scope for individual practitioners to think of additional objectives, which may be more or less important than those already stated.

After identifying our objectives or goals, the next stage of the evaluation process is to clarify how we will determine when a goal has been achieved. Looking back at our objectives, we can identify a number of possible criteria on which we can base our judgment concerning the success or failure of the programme. First, the number of parents who attend the programme, and the frequency of their attendance. This may give us some indication as to whether the programme was seen as useful by the parents. However, we have to be careful in how we interpret these data, because whether parents attend the programme or not depends to some extent on structural factors – we will return to this topic when thinking about programme planning. Second, any increase in the activity levels of children in the programme, or whether children reduced weight gain. In addition, once the club has ended, whether there is sustained healthy eating or whether the child's target weight is achieved. Unlike most areas of health visiting, we are fortunate in having truly objective criteria in this context. Third, the difference between what parents knew before they attended the healthy eating club and what they know following exposure to our learning materials and teaching sessions on the nutritional value of food. This information may best be obtained by giving the parents a questionnaire to fill in on the first visit and then a follow-up questionnaire after the sessions on nutrition have concluded. This will give us some indication of their knowledge level and some feedback as to whether or not our teaching sessions have been successful.

In order to achieve our goals, the evaluation process suggests that we devise a strategy for setting up our healthy eating club. It is important to work with parents in the planning and implementation of this initiative and to learn from the successes of other, similar initiatives. First, it would be helpful to know how many parents would be interested in coming to the club. We can find out this information by putting a poster in clinics or by informing other health visitors that this initiative is being developed, so that they can inform parents during home visits. The next step is to decide how the programme will be run. Will there, for example, be a formal session every week? Will other health professionals be asked to take part, such as a dietician or a cookery expert? Will there be a session on increasing activity in young children? It is also important to look at the evidence around the effectiveness of weight management interventions and those studies which take into account the child's perspective around obesity and weight management, such as the systematic reviews by Whitlock *et al.* (2008, 2010), Rees *et al.* (2009), Waters *et al.* (2011), and Bleich *et al.* (2013). There is also guidance and a framework to enhance a practitioner's effectiveness in tackling obesity specifically through the Healthy Child Programme (HCP) (Hunt & Rudolf, 2008; Rudolf, 2010), and NICE has developed guidelines for healthy weight management in children and adults (NICE, 2015). Training for health professionals is also available via the charity HENRY (Health, Exercise & Nutrition for the Really Young; www.henry.org.uk), which equips practitioners to support families to develop healthier lifestyles. HENRY's evidence-based intervention focuses on three elements: information about food and activity, parenting skills, and behaviour change.

Once the programme has been devised, we then have to meet the challenge of putting it into action. We may find that in the early stages that we need to make modifications. For example, we may find that it is better to put the formal talk first and the demonstrations afterwards. Perhaps it will be necessary to enlist the support of some colleagues and do more group work. There are always teething problems when launching any new programme, and time is well spent in the early stages making adjustments and modifications. Evaluation of the programme is best thought about at the development stage, in order to show its benefits and that it has achieved its specific goals/objectives. It is important to remember that it is usual to evaluate a programme in terms of its goals, and the goal-measuring criteria are the key to the evaluation. In addition, we may wish to collect supplementary information which might help us with future planning. We could, for example, ask those attending the sessions to suggest ways in which we could improve the healthy eating club. Our evaluation – that is, our judgment about whether or not the programme was a success or failure – may feed back into future programmes. Activity 7.4 provides you with an opportunity to start thinking about designing a new programme to be implemented within health visiting practice.

Evaluation and evaluative research

Although the evaluation component of the care planning process is able to substantiate its claims, there are two reasons why it cannot be said to constitute evaluative research. First, in evaluative research, the main thrust of the activity is directed towards measuring how far intervention has achieved or not achieved its goals, whereas in the care planning process the measurement of the effectiveness of care is subsidiary to the primary goal of giving care. Owing to the secondary purpose of evaluation in the care planning process, goal statements may not be recorded; however, health visitors and other practitioners are involved in making judgments of worth about the care which they give, whether they record it or not. Many of these value judgments will be made on the basis of systematically collected data and experience, and the evaluation criteria may vary between individuals. Second, in evaluative research, data are collected on a predetermined target population, and therefore findings may be related to more than one individual, whereas in the evaluative component of the care planning process the health visitor evaluates the care she gives to each individual and is not in a position to determine her clients in the same way as a researcher determines the sample.

All in all, evaluation may best be viewed as a continuum. The evaluation component of the care planning process can be placed almost anywhere along this continuum, depending upon the way in which the data are collected (systematically or otherwise) and recorded (see Figure 7.1). Data which have been systematically collected and recorded during the execution of care planning may be used retrospectively by health practitioners for research purposes. The retrospective use of the material may be referred to as 'evaluative research', because evaluation and not care giving has become the main thrust of the activity and the researcher is able to determine the population to be studied.

Evaluation of health care

Concern for the measurement of the quality of health care provided to patients/clients and attempts at evaluating care are not new. It may be possible to get agreement on the importance of evaluation. There is less agreement, however, about what will be evaluated and how the evaluation will take place. The US Agency for Healthcare Research & Quality (AHRQ) provides guidance on improving quality to those involved in designing or evaluating new interventions, aimed at improving care coordination. It discusses five key elements: (i) assessment of needs for coordination; (ii) identification of options for improving coordination; (iii) selection and implementation of one of the alternatives; (iv) evaluation to determine effects on care coordination and outcomes of care; and (v) amendments, if required (McDonald et al., 2007).

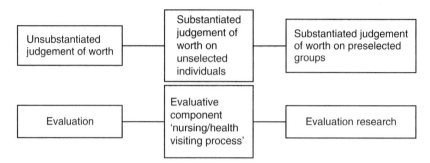

Figure 7.1 Continuum of evaluation.

The North American literature on evaluation dates back to Derryberry (1939), who, in a report concerning the accomplishments of nursing, stated:

> In the past, evaluation of nursing services have been based upon volume and intensity of service ... Evidence of the more elusive quality of service as expressed by the changing state of the patient has been sought in the present analysis.
>
> (Derryberry (1939: 2035)

It is interesting that more than 75 years have passed since Derryberry made this plea to move away from evaluations based on volume and intensity of service in favour of focusing on patient/client outcome. Within the context of health visiting, we have unfortunately failed to move very far forward. It is only with policy recommendations on improving and measuring the effectiveness of care and the drive towards quality in health care that there has been a push towards using defined outcomes measures or PROMS. This has been taken up by the NHS Health & Social Care Information Centre (HSCIC) in measuring quality from the patient's perspective, largely focusing on clinical procedures, and using PROMS to measure health gain after surgical treatment. This will be expanded to more areas of health care in the future (see www.hscic.gov.uk/proms).

Data of relevance to health visiting work are limited. There is often little feedback to health visitors on the activity data they record for client contact. The data most commonly used to provide insight into the work of health visitors at both a national and a local level are the statistical data which relate to frequency of health visitor visits as part of the service specification. With the increase in the number of health visitors between 2010 and 2015, NHS England developed indicators for monitoring service delivery. These are referred to as 'health visitor service delivery metrics'; the most recent data available are provided in Table 7.2. These indicators record data from providers based on health visitors' activity on specific metrics such as percentage of antenatal contacts and percentage of new birth visits. It is possible for these statistics to be used to demonstrate the contacts made by health visitors, which may be useful to managers, policy makers, and commissioners. This information is collected quarterly, and local data can be compared with national data. However, caution must be taken, since collection of these data is not complete and, despite validation checks, they may have some inaccuracies. The data presented in

Table 7.2 Health visitor service delivery metrics. Source: NHS England (2015): Health Visitors Service Metrics Q2 2013/14 to Q2 2014/15 (© Crown Copyright. Reproduced by kind permission).

Indicators	2013/14 Q2 (%)	2013/14 Q3 (%)	2013/14 Q4 (%)	2014/15 Q1 (%)	2014/15 Q2 (%)
1st antenatal visit 28 wks or above	74	88	94	93	95
New birth visit within 14 days	77	91	96	93	94
New birth visit after 14 days	74	90	96	91	93
12 mth developmental reviews	73	87	95	94	97
12 mth developmental reviews complete by 15 mths	54	74	84	84	88
2–2.5 yr reviews completed	74	83	88	89	96
Sure Start Advisory Boards with HV presence	57	78	77	86	81

Table 7.2 demonstrates that there has been an increase in health visiting contacts for these indicators over the course of a year.

Other sources of data that might be of assistance to health visitors and others include routinely collected statistics from the Office for National Statistics (ONS) and the Public Health Observatories (now part of Public Health England), which provide statistical data pertaining to the health of the population and an overview of the health problems within specific communities. Local councils also provide information on health and housing. In addition, practice-based information, such as immunisation rates or quality outcomes framework data, which are practice-specific and can be compared with other areas in the UK, might be useful. For health visitors involved in doing a needs assessment, there is now a Joint Strategic Needs Assessment (JSNA) Navigator (covering five domains), which provides information and data on children and young people for a specific locality in the following areas:

- population (e.g. demographics, ethnicity);
- social and place well being (e.g. homeless families);
- lifestyles and health well being status (e.g. smoking; obese & overweight children);
- health and well being status (e.g. developmental issues; accidents);
- service utilisation (e.g. outcomes for looked after children).

The Navigator can also be used to compare other areas (Public Health England, National Child & Maternal Health Intelligence Network, JSNA Navigator: www.chimat

.org.uk/jsnanavigator). This resource will be helpful to health visitors in meeting the public health focus on the six early years high impact areas (DH, 2014b):

- transition to parenthood;
- maternal (perinatal) mental health;
- breastfeeding;
- healthy weight, healthy nutrition (including physical activity);
- managing minor illness and reducing accidents;
- health, well being, and development of the child age 2.

All sources of routinely collected data have limitations and biases associated with them. Table 7.3 shows some of the sources of routinely collected information that are available. To gain experience in locating routine sources of information, complete Activity 7.5.

Structure, process, and outcome evaluation

In the context of health care evaluation, the classic reference of Donabedian (1969), a pioneer in this field, has not been superseded. He described three approaches to evaluation: structure evaluation, process evaluation, and outcome evaluation. Donabedian's approach to evaluation is as valid today as it was in the 1970s. The framework is also used as a basis for assessing quality of care (Donabedian, 1988). Others have built on his work (see QNI, 2008; Gardner et al., 2014; Walker et al., 2014), using slightly different language, although the approach to evaluation and assessing quality is the same.

Structure evaluation

Structure evaluation involves the study of factors in the organisation system, the availability of facilities and equipment, staffing levels, styles of management, and the characteristics of care givers. The assumption underlying this approach to evaluation is that if the facilities, staff, and equipment reach specified standards, then the care that follows will be 'good' and clients will benefit. In keeping with this approach, it is assumed that Trusts that have achieved their health visitor/client ratio target of 250–400 children per health visitor should be providing a better service than those which are not (Unite/CPHVA, 2009). Research by the Family and Parenting Institute (FPI, 2009) found from 165.00 to 894.25 children per health visitor in the Community Trusts it surveyed. The Community Practitioners and Health Visitors Association (CPHVA) and the union Unite recommend that the average caseload size for health visitors should be no more than 250, or much less for those working in areas of high vulnerability and that 400 should be the absolute maximum (Unite/CPHVA, 2009). The Institute of Health Visiting also recommends 1 health visitor to 250 families (iHV, 2014). With the increase in the number of health visitors and the strengthening of the health visiting service, further reduction in caseload size should occur, and evaluations of this structural change can then be undertaken.

Table 7.3 Routine sources of data and information.

Data and information	Source
Neighbourhood statistics:	Office for National Statistics (ONS)
Statistics about local areas of interest	http://www.neighbourhood.statistics.gov.uk
National statistics:	
Census data, population, health and care: health inequality, health expectancy, life expectancy, etc.	http://www.ons.gov.uk/ons/guide-method/census/index.html
Health profile of England: local indicators on breastfeeding, smoking, obesity, etc.; mortality target monitoring, health inequality data, etc.	Department of Health public health statistics: http://www.gov.uk/government/organisations/department-of-health/about/statistics
Hospital episode statistics: data on all admissions and outpatient appointments in the NHS	http://www.hscic.gov.uk/hes
Patient-related outcome measures (PROMS): data on health gains after e.g. surgical treatment with pre- and postoperative measures	Health & Social Care Information Centre (HSCIC): http://www.hscic.gov.uk/proms
GP data: quality & outcomes framework (QOF) of the GP contract – provides disease prevalence across the UK or by local GP practice	QOF database: http://www.gpcontract.co.uk
HSCIC: useful data on health and lifestyles, primary care, prescriptions, etc.	http://www.hscic.gov.uk
National guidelines, relating to public health and management of specific diseases	National Institute for Health and Care Excellence (NICE): http://www.nice.org.uk Scottish Intercollegiate Guidelines Network (SIGN): http://www.sign.ac.uk Social Care Institute for Excellence (SCIE): http://www.scie.org.uk/
Public Health England	http://www.gov.uk/government/organisations/public-health-england
NHS England and Child and Maternal Health Intelligence Network: knowledge hub around topics of safeguarding children, child health profiles, infant mortality profiles, healthy schools profiles, needs assessment tools – breastfeeding data, obese children data, etc. (can compare with localities)	http://atlas.chimat.org.uk/IAS/dataviews/earlyyearsprofile

(Continued)

Table 7.3 *(Continued)*

Data and information	Source
Scottish Public Health Observatory	http://www.scotpho.org.uk
Public Health Wales Observatory	http://www.wales.nhs.uk/sitesplus/922/home
Ireland & Northern Ireland Population Health Observatory	http://www.inispho.org
Joint Strategic Needs Assessment (JSNA) – for Children and Young People	http://www.chimat.org.uk/jsnanavigator
Association of Public Health Observatories	http://www.apho.org.uk/

Process evaluation

In a recent publication, the Medical Research Council (MRC) provided guidance on process evaluation, suggesting that in the context of complex interventions, the aim of process evaluation is to provide a more detailed understanding of the context, implementation process, and mechanisms of impact or change of behaviour (Moore *et al.*, 2014). However, this guidance is aimed at researchers who are seeking to design and evaluate complex interventions rather than practitioners. Process evaluation in the context of health visiting practice focuses on the staff providing care to clients in terms of whether or not the care they provide is appropriate and carried out in the correct manner. The emphasis is firmly on what the health visitor does; it may also include decision making. This may be considered as the traditional or taken-for-granted approach to evaluation.

In health promotion interventions, process evaluation enables questions such as: Was the intervention applied in the manner intended? Did other factors come into play that might have affected the result? What did the participants think about the process? (Speller *et al.*, 1997; Saunders *et al.*, 2005). An example of a large process evaluation can be found in a European multicentred health promotion intervention for the prevention of obesity in early childhood (Androutsos *et al.*, 2014). This intervention was school- and home-based, targeted at pre-school children, and focused on key behaviours related to early childhood obesity (drinking, eating and snacking, physical activity, and sedentary behaviour) and their determinants (see www.toybox-study.eu).

If we ask health visitors about the effects of their work, they usually begin by telling us what they do. Hence, the success of a visit is measured in terms of whether the health visitor has achieved what she or he set out to do: for example, did she successfully complete the health needs assessment, carry out a developmental assessment on a 2-year–old, or identify and support a mother with postnatal depression? This emphasis on what the health visitor does can be partially accounted for by reflecting on the type of information that health visitors are required to keep, although this now varies by Trust. The DH used to publish national statistics on health visiting activity, but it is now up to local services to collect this information. Often there are problems with recording activity, due to the complexities of health visiting. Each Trust tends to have its own system for recording information. A health visitor will usually complete several records as part of the child health recording system. Universally, the Personal Child Health Record, known as the 'Red Book', is the primary record for information pertaining to a child's health and development. Other forms of record keeping involve health care needs analysis, family assessment, care planning and evaluation, and identification of the needs of individual families (in order to achieve the best outcomes of care). These may be recorded on a family record or active intervention card. Computerised systems also vary by Trust, but client contacts (either face-to-face or by telephone) are recorded, and information on health checks and immunisations are often entered into a child health information system (CHIS) or something similar. Yet, despite these systems, few outcome data are available.

In the future, there will be more of a focus on enabling individuals to have control of their own health records. Initially this will be through access to their general practitioner (GP) record, but eventually it will extend to records held by other health care providers. Clients/patients will be able to give permission to other agencies to view their GP records in order to assist with their care (DH, 2010a). Future plans include the digitisation of the Personnel Child Health Record (NIB, 2014).

A further example of process evaluation is an audit of records. This is sometimes confused with evaluation research, but here the focus is not just on what the health visitor does, but may also include some notion of how well she or he performs in her or his role, as evidenced in record keeping or by observation at work. In the context of health visiting, an audit to evaluate the performance of students or health visitors can be developed from the skills outlined in a validated curriculum (NMC, 2004). For example, if we look at the skills involved in interviewing, we see that the 'attitudinal set' for this skill can be itemised as follows:

- be nonjudgmental both orally and nonverbally;
- be willing to listen and empathise;
- value objectivity, as appropriate;
- value subjectivity, as appropriate (show human warmth);
- value clients' rights to privacy and confidentiality;
- value the goal of clients having independence;
- value one's own listening role;
- affirm the principles of the practice of health visiting.

As a manager, community practice teacher, or mentor involved in the appraisal of health visitors or students, we could use this as a checklist against which to evaluate interviewing skills. The assumption underlying process evaluation is that what the health visitor *does* is of primary importance, and evaluations are made concerning health visitor (rather than client-orientated) objectives. Furthermore, the examples in this list exemplify the subjective nature of evaluation and the value judgments that are made.

Outcome evaluation

Outcome evaluation, on the other hand, refers to the end result of intervention or care in terms of its effect upon the client. In brief, a judgment is made about the achievement of client-orientated goals/objectives, with no regard as to the reason why the observed outcome occurred. The assumption underlying outcome evaluation is that the care a person receives is of secondary importance to its effects – hence, the emphasis is placed upon the client and not the health visitor or another health practitioner.

Outcome evaluation is implicit in care planning where client-orientated goals or objectives are set and act as the criteria against which the success or failure of an intervention is evaluated. Having clear goals is an essential requirement for achieving high quality of care (Dixon-Woods *et al.*, 2013). In the context of health visiting, it is usually assumed that the goals of care are commonly understood, but this is seldom the case. Where possible, the expected outcome of an intervention should be written down in the client or family record. Such an expected outcome can take many forms. It might relate to the acquisition of new knowledge as a result of a one-to-one teaching, or to a behavioural change (e.g. potty training, visiting the family planning clinic). Whatever the expected outcome, it should be clearly stated so that what constitutes success or failure can be readily understood by any practitioner. For example, all newborn babies are at risk of developing gastroenteritis. This risk is increased if the infant is bottle-fed, if the bottle is made up for two feeds and then reheated, and if the parents have little understanding of the need for sterilisation. In such circumstances, the health visitor may list gastroenteritis as a potential problem.

> *Goal statement A*: The mother/father will demonstrate that they understand the preparation of bottle feeds and the way to sterilise bottles.

This statement has limitations because it does not indicate how the parents will demonstrate their understanding and it does not set a time limit. Must this goal be achieved at the next visit, next feed, or for the next baby? Goal statement B gives us this additional information.

> *Goal statement B*: The mother/father will discuss the way in which they make up the bottle feeds and their method of sterilisation and will give a practical demonstration at the next visit, which has been arranged for (say) 10.00 hours on 23 October 2015.

The process of goal setting can be further explored in Activity 7.6.

In the context of outcome evaluation, it can be argued that in some respects health visiting is rather more complex to evaluate than hospital nursing. In the community, we are dealing with families, not individuals (this is not intended to imply that hospital nurses do not consider the family as important). The initial reason for a visit might be a referral from a GP reporting a family's difficulties in managing a pre-school disabled step-child. Despite the fact that the child is in one sense the client, it may well be that the health visitor directs most of her or his intervention towards the step-mother, who feels that she cannot go on indefinitely caring. In the context of hospital nursing, a care plan is usually only made for the patient – that is, the person who occupies the bed in the ward. Hence, the outcome of care is only evaluated in this context. In health visiting, it is not always so clear cut as to who the client is, and it may well be necessary to make more than one care plan. Similarly, goals may be in conflict with one another, and many compromises will need to be made. If, for example, a woman feels she can no longer care for her 4-year-old step-child with severe learning disabilities because she is getting little or no support from her husband, there are three individuals to consider. Any attempt to evaluate the outcome of an intervention will have to take into account the conflicting needs of all three. In order to begin to deal with this problem, the health visitor might initially try to uncover the reason for the apparently sudden feelings of not being able to cope on the part of the step-mother. The health visitor will have certain beliefs and values about the function of the family and about male and female roles within it, acquired for her or his role as a nurse, her or his education as a nurse and a health visitor, and perhaps from her or his own role as a carer.

Let us say that on taking a family history from the mother, we learn that she used to work as a cleaner and gave up work 6 months ago to be at home with her step-child. She has in many respects been happily married for 18 months, but considers that her husband has put pressure on her to give up work to take care of his child. She feels that her husband is rather old-fashioned about women working and prefers her to be at home. The husband has never helped in the house, but he does do all the gardening and decorating. The situation in this household was tolerable until the child began getting up in the night and wandering around the house. Because the husband has to be at work by 8 am each morning, the wife felt it was her duty to get up to keep an eye on the child. This practice has resulted in her feeling very tired and unable to cope with the housework, shopping, cooking, and caring. The problem has been further compounded by the recent onset of head banging and screaming; it was when this happened that the wife went to her GP. Towards the end of the interview, the husband returns from work and makes it quite plain that he has no intention of letting his child go to residential care. He also considers that his wife exaggerates the problem.

Clearly, there is no right or obvious answer to this family's problems. Indeed, it would be interesting to identify the actual and potential problems of each family member and try to write goal statements for each. Let us say that we believe that it is the step-mother who has the most dominant or pressing needs: what can we do to ameliorate the situation? Decisions concerning intervention are not made in a social vacuum; they are made in the context of service cutbacks and an awareness of the constraints of time. Let us say that it is decided that a possible solution would be a full-time day nursery (something the husband agrees to for a trial period). The problem then becomes one of getting the placement and the transport. In the first instance, there may be no vacancy at all. As an interim measure, we must somehow offer support to the step-mother to enable her to carry on a little longer. This support might be giving her an opportunity to talk about how she feels, both about her marriage and about caring for her step-child. In addition, we might spend time with the husband to try to give him some insight into his wife's situation, in the hope that he will be willing to help more in the house. We might also provide some practical advice and assistance with the management of the child's behavioural difficulties. The family may be entitled to benefits and support from other agencies, as well.

Obviously, there are a number of other interventions that we might try, but our intention here is not to provide an exhaustive list but instead to provide some insight into the complexities of dealing with families. An example of this nature introduces another problem in the context of evaluation, insofar as it is not possible to evaluate what cannot be provided: in this case, a full-time nursery place and transport. Nevertheless, all health practitioners are in a position to collect data on existing services that fall short in meeting the needs of the community. We contend that all practitioners have a moral responsibility to collate this information if they are serious about meeting community needs, and for health visitors, this information provides the evidence required to fulfil one of the principles of health visiting: influencing policies affecting health.

Summary

It is incumbent upon the evaluator to decide whether to use structure, process, or outcome criteria, or a combination of the three. In choosing a particular approach to evaluation, certain assumptions have to be made. If it is possible in terms of time and financial resources, it may be advantageous to attempt an evaluation incorporating structure, process, and outcome goals, and it might be expected that there would be a positive correlation between the three approaches.

Against the background of resource constraints in the NHS and the embedding of the evidence-based practice movement, it is expected that a greater emphasis will be placed on outcome evaluation as evidenced by health gain. The DH (2009b) emphasises the need for measurement and evaluation in achieving continuous improvement. As previously stated, NHS Trusts and local authorities are charged with the responsibility of assessing the health needs of their resident populations. Priorities will be set and services targeted accordingly. Performance will be measured by comparing health outcomes within and between health providers. By focusing on client or patient outcomes, the contributions of individual practitioners in the primary health care team are made less important, since it is the collective effort that is the measurable input in most cases. However, if health visiting and community services are to develop and expand, it is essential that individual practitioners are in a position to identify, quantify, and evaluate their own input in terms of client outcomes.

The care planning process

It would appear that the goal-attainment approach towards evaluation is applicable to health visiting at an individual and family level, since goal setting and evaluation are operationalised through the care planning process. Fundamentally, care planning is a problem-solving or needs-led approach to care. This approach enables a record of action plans (see Figure 7.2). There is also a focus on taking a strengths-based

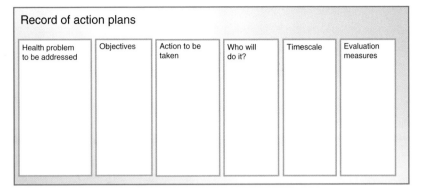

Record of action plans					
Health problem to be addressed	Objectives	Action to be taken	Who will do it?	Timescale	Evaluation measures

Figure 7.2 Record of action plans.
Source: DH (2001), used under OGL 2.0.

approach; that is, identifying the strengths and resources a family or individual has and how these can be used/built upon or supplemented, for example by attending a group at a children's centre. Pattoni (2012) discusses strengths-based approaches as building on the strengths and capabilities of those who are supported by services in order to assist them in resolving issues and finding their own solutions.

Activity 7.7 provides you with an opportunity to start using a record of action plans.

Other approaches to care planning involve: identifying the needs of both child and family; agreeing actions; setting expected outcomes; setting the timescale; and identifying actual outcomes (see Figure 7.3). Care planning is a continual process. The SMART approach, described previously, can be used to ensure activities are directed towards achieving the required outcome.

Using these or similar measures enables a systematic approach to the care planning process and to what needs to done in order to tackle the issues/problems

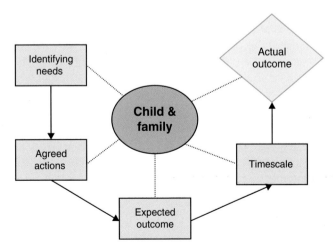

Figure 7.3 Care planning.

identified. It's important to ensure there are regular reviews of the progress. The evaluation process will determine whether objectives are being met and if amendments are required, but will also provide evidence in terms of the success of the plan of action. Gaining experience in using the SMART approach is explored in Activity 7.8.

Actual and potential problems

In the past, health visitors were reluctant to consider themselves as involved in dealing with clients' health problems. Instead, they asserted their uniqueness in that they visited families many of which had no apparent health problems. The role of the health visitor has become more defined with the provision of the four levels of health visiting service (community, universal, universal plus, and universal partnership plus) and the five key contacts in the HCP. The focus on 'proportionate universalism' ensures that health visitors provide a service according to need at a neighbourhood and individual level, achieving improved equity of outcomes for all children (DH, 2007, 2010b; Marmot et al., 2010).

Those families with greater risks and needs will receive more health visiting input. The word 'problem' is often associated by many health visitors with that nebulous term 'problem family'. However, in this context, a health problem or health need, following a health care needs analysis, is defined as a matter which concerns the health visitor or client with respect to the client's health at the time of the visit or assessment. Actual problems are those which are present at the time of the assessment or at follow-up visits. Potential problems are not present; instead, there are indicators or cues which suggest that an actual problem may develop if no action is taken.

Examples of actual problems at an assessment visit include a baby with a sore eye, a baby who refuses to suck at the breast, and a child who has regressed to soiling her/himself. Health visitors address actual problems, but they are also concerned with potential problems (i.e. preventing actual problems occurring). An example of a potential problem for a couple expecting a baby who already have a 2-year-old child might be jealousy on the part of the toddler after the baby is born. The health visitor would be keen to assist the parents in preventing this problem occurring. She or he would, therefore, discuss ways in which the family might begin to prepare the 2-year-old for the birth of the new baby. Discussion might follow concerning the management of the toddler during her or his first separation from the mother, which is, of course, inevitable if the birth is to take place in hospital. By intervening before there is an actual problem, the health visitor tries to promote the well being of the whole family. This is getting back to the core health visiting functions of early intervention and prevention.

Health visitors used to visit families from conception to the grave, but this is no longer the case. The main focus of the health visitor's work today is on the pre-school child and the family, although in many parts of the UK it may be that it is largely around child protection issues. There is a refocus now for health visitors on addressing public health issues, concerning six areas of high importance which impact on the health of communities (DH, 2014b). If we view life as a developmental timespan then, theoretically, it can be argued that the younger one is, the more potential health problems one has, and the fewer actual problems; conversely, the older one is, the more actual problems one experiences and the lower the relative risk of potential problems developing. A potential problem is usually only considered by a health visitor if it has a higher than average probability of becoming an actual problem. For example, all babies are at risk of developing obesity, but the infant whose siblings or parents are obese has a greater risk of becoming obese her or himself. Only babies with such confounding factors will be considered by health visitors to have a potential problem in this area. Similarly, all mothers may be considered at risk of postnatal depression, but this will only be recorded as a potential problem if there are factors present which suggest that there is an above average risk of developing it, such as previous postnatal depression or high anxiety. There are many tools available to assess a mother's risk of postnatal depression, and a number are recommended by NICE (2014a), such as the Edinburgh Postnatal Depression Scale (EPDS) (Cox *et al.*, 1987). The Boots Family Trust has developed a well being plan to help mothers prepare their support requirements for their mental health (Boots Family Trust, 2013).

Problem solving

The care planning process is made up of a number of components:

- data collection;
- goal setting;
- care planning;
- intervention;
- evaluation.

It is noteworthy that problem solving is subjective and can be value-laden. However, there is now a stronger evidence base underpinning the decisions that health visitors make, and families now bring more evidence themselves (e.g. acquired from the Internet), such that health visitors can more readily identify problems which they or the recipients of their care consider to be important, and hence act accordingly. Alternatively, where commissioners have identified important areas of practice, such as uptake of immunisations and breastfeeding rates, health visitors can work with families to achieve targets. Hence, the care planning process, like the evaluative process, begins with recognition of values (see Figure 7.4). It also makes use of available evidence from the family, from policy, and from research.

Additional issues in evaluating the practice of health visiting

When seeking to evaluate health visiting practice, a basic problem is that the goals of health visiting are broadly stated and as such cannot easily act as criteria against

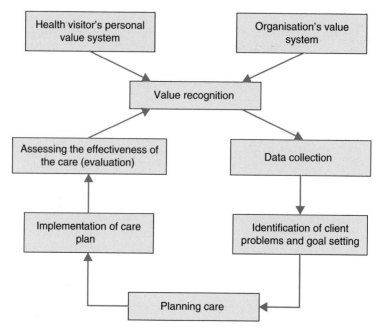

Figure 7.4 Evaluating practice.

which to measure it. A review of the role of health visitors (DH, 2007) described a renewed role that:

- delivers measurable health outcomes for individuals and communities and provides a rewarding and enjoyable job for nurses;
- has the support of families and communities;
- will be commissioned by commissioners;
- delivers government policies for children and families, improving health and reducing inequalities and social exclusion;
- fits the new system of providing choice and contestability through new providers, and promoting self-care, service integration, improved productivity, and local decision making;
- can adapt and respond to changing needs and aspirations;
- attracts a new generation to the profession.

The significance of this focus is the priority given to evaluation in terms of measurable outcomes. The core elements of health visiting were identified in the same report and provide an extended role, as discussed in earlier chapters. The overall goal of health visiting remains as 'the promotion of health and prevention of ill-health' in its broadest sense and embraces the principles of public health. However, this is too broad and unrealistic a goal to be considered as a single outcome criterion for health visiting practice.

Health visiting places an emphasis on prevention, and therefore it shares the problems inherent in the evaluation of all preventive techniques or programmes: namely, if something does not occur because it has been prevented, how can it be measured?

'Prevention' embraces a wide variety of programmes and activities. Some community health programmes, such as sewage disposal or screening for phenylketonuria, can be said to be highly effective, or at least cost-effective. Some programmes, on the other hand, such as screening for breast cancer, are controversial with respect to target population and efficacy. Programmes which depend for their success on the adherence or compliance of the client may in some circumstances not be effective. The importance of lifestyle is pre-eminent in the promotion of health (Bandura, 2004). Health visitors are involved in health promotion at both a group and an individual level. They engage in one-to-one health education when they visit people in their own homes or see individual clients at the clinic, but when they participate in antenatal classes, for example, they teach groups rather than individuals – this requires a different set of skills. Very little evidence exists concerning the effectiveness of teaching undertaken by health visitors. Hobbs, as long ago as 1973, commented on the lack of evidence regarding the effectiveness of one-to-one teaching undertaken by the health visitor (Hobbs, 1973); over 40 years later, we are no further forward. It can be argued that the successful outcome of the health visitor's work depends to a large extent upon cooperation and partnership with the client. The extent to which patients follow doctors' orders has been investigated, but little or no work has been carried out concerning clients' concordance with health visiting advice.

In the context of medicine, the adherence studies carried out have usually focused on the extent to which patients have followed their drug prescription. Since nonadherence has been a problem to GPs insofar as it has hindered the efficacy of their drug treatments, the quest has been to search out the potential nonadherer so that she or he can be encouraged to comply. The emphasis in these studies is on seeing the problem (i.e. nonadherence) from the doctor's point of view, rather than the patient or client's. Over the years, however, there has been a shift in emphasis from the practitioner's viewpoint to that of the patient or service user. It is now accepted that patients/service users make decisions about whether or not to follow advice in the light of the discussions they have with people who share their own social and cultural background, and we still need to know more about how to influence the lifestyle choices of at-risk groups. Whilst, to the best of our knowledge, no work of this nature has been carried with respect to advice given by health visitors, intuitively we feel that there is a high incidence of noncompliance with health visitors' advice. It would be interesting to investigate clients' perceptions of health visitor advice, since this might assist in improving the service given to them.

In the days of the sanitary missionary who engaged in primary prevention, it was possible to lower infectious disease mortality and morbidity rates. Today, we are in the position of choosing amongst interventions that have much lower levels of effectiveness. The reason for this is that we now have more problems whose resolution can only be achieved by a fundamental change in client lifestyle or behaviour. The example of obesity makes this point. In order to lose weight, it is necessary to alter one's eating patterns and consequently one's shopping and exercise habits. Food and the sharing of food have social meaning, and, therefore, reducing weight may require an adjustment in many aspects of everyday life. Few people are willing to alter their behaviour to this extent. The apparent lack of dramatic opportunities to measure the effects of prevention is one estimate of how far we have come in community health, although there are underserved groups within society who still exhibit disproportionate levels of ill health: a review of deaths between 1921 and 2007 shows inequality increasing, with the poorest people more likely to die prematurely than the more affluent (Thomas *et al.*, 2010). There is now a major policy drive to tackle inequalities in health (DH, 2009c, 2012c; Marmot *et al.*, 2010). In discussing a possible model for assessing the work of the health visitor over 35 years ago, Luker stated:

> Some health visitors believe that the effects of health visiting are too subtle, intangible or elusive to be realistically assessed. If this were so there would be little reason for health visitors to offer a service, since no one, including the client, would be aware of its effects. Intangible and elusive changes can hardly be worthwhile goals or a reason for continuing professional practice. Moreover in the context of the present economic climate it would seem urgent to assess the care given by health visitors in order to demonstrate its effectiveness and to justify the provision of the service.
>
> (Luker, 1978: p. 1257)

Health visitors have been content to avoid studying the process of health visitor intervention in terms of its benefit to the client by dismissing it as methodologically impractical. Researchers have focused instead on describing health visiting in terms of what health visitors say they do. The result has been that the number of health visitors has fallen over the last 30 years and the shortfall had hardly been commented upon, possibly because the impact had not been monitored closely enough. However, with the advent of the coalition government early years initiative, it was realised that there were insufficient health visitors available to deliver the programme, and the numbers of health visitor training places and actual health visitors were increased (DH, 2015). Clearly, given the increase in the workforce numbers, there is now an urgent need to demonstrate impact (or its lack) through an evaluation of effectiveness if we are to maintain and grow the health visiting workforce. This, and the earlier lack of focus on outcome evaluation, has given the government – via the DH – the opportunity to reconstruct health visiting and reconfigure its boundaries: see *Facing the Future* (DH, 2007), *Getting It Right for Children and Families* (DH, 2009b), *Healthy Child Programme* (DH, 2009d), *Health Visitor Implementation Plan 2011–15* (DH, 2011), and the *2015–16 National Health Visiting Core Service Specification* (NHS England, 2014a). These reports clearly set out the direction of travel, much of which has been discussed in earlier chapters. The health visitor's contribution falls into three main areas: (i) needs assessment; (ii) programme delivery (delivery of the HCP); and (iii) a wider public health function, including supplying information on vulnerable groups, in order to enable commissioners to create services (DH, 2009c). This is similar to that of health visitors working in Northern Ireland, whose contribution falls into: (i) delivery of the child health promotion programme; (ii) increased intensive home visiting across the 0–19 age range, with the implementation of appropriate evidence-based parenting programmes; and (iii) a mental health focus, including identifying and addressing mental health issues in families with children through case management interventions (DHSSPS, 2010). All this is underpinned by the best evidence and the demonstration and measurement of achievement.

The preventive aspects of health visiting are still important, but are difficult to measure because of the long-term nature of the work and the lack of data other than for specific programmes, such as immunisation and developmental screening. However, health visitors do deal with clients and families who have tangible problems, which are amenable to short-term intervention. In attempting to solve short-term problems, health visitors may affect the future health of the client or family in an unknown way, since problems which are prevented from developing because of health visitor intervention cannot readily be assessed. Nevertheless, it is thought that evaluation of health visitor intervention in terms of its effect upon the client might begin in the area of tangible problems. There have been some attempts to evaluate the effectiveness of health visitor intervention, but the studies that have been done are likely to be viewed as no longer relevant given the changing focus of health visiting (Luker, 1978; Elkan et al., 2000; Watson et al., 2004). Getting health visitors involved in 'new' activities, such as identifying postnatal depression using validated tools and then delivering a psychologically informed intervention to postnatal mothers, has been found to be effective (Morrell et al., 2009), but not all health visitors employ this approach. A review around health visiting interventions, processes, and outcomes for children and families found some evidence of outcomes with the work that health visitors do, for example, in structured home visiting programmes. However, there was a lack of evidence for some of the work, with only small-scale studies conducted in the areas of, for example, nutrition and obesity prevention (Cowley et al., 2013).

In fact, little research effort in nursing generally has been directed at evaluation, possibly because of the difficulties involved in demonstrating a cause-and-effect relationship. Ethical issues are often raised when considering the design of a study into cause and effect. The usual scientific approach is to use an experimental method such as an RCT, but this can necessitate denying a control group access to the service being evaluated, and health visitors have been reluctant to deny their service in the interest of scientific enquiry. This reluctance to evaluate practice, in addition to the methodological and ethical problems, raises the question, 'Can health visitor intervention be evaluated?'

Attempts have been made in North America to evaluate the effects of 'public health nurse' interventions (Brooten et al., 1986; Casiro et al., 1993; Olds et al., 1986, 1997; Macmillan et al., 2005) and home visiting programmes (LeCroy & Krysik, 2011; Lowell et al., 2011) using RCTs of new interventions, such as parenting programmes, intensive home visiting to reduce child physical abuse and neglect, and rehospitalisation of low-birth-weight babies. Work by McLennan & Lavis (2006) evaluating 12 parenting interventions in Canada found that only three had been evaluated by at least one RCT. There was a distinct lack of evidence supporting these interventions, but no doubt parenting interventions continue to be a regular feature of health visiting work. A recent systematic review investigating the effectiveness of home visiting programmes on child outcomes, which included 21 studies, largely RCTs and most from the USA, found some positive benefits of home visiting programmes in the prevention of child abuse – particularly when the intervention commenced in the antenatal period – and some development benefits in socially high-risk families (Peacock *et al.*, 2013). So, better evidence is emerging for home visiting programmes – including, in the UK, for the FNP programme (see Chapter 4) (Robling *et al.*, 2015).

The problems of evaluating social casework are similar to the problems involved in evaluating health visiting. Social workers initially were somewhat more adventurous than health visitors in using the experimental methods. Goldberg *et al.* (1970) attempted the first controlled field experiment in Britain in the complex and diffuse area known as 'social casework'. The target population was elderly people, and the study involved a comparison of the outcome of one group of clients who received the services of a trained social worker with that of another group who received the services of an untrained social worker. Goldberg *et al.* addressed some of the key problems in evaluation, which are shared by health visitors and other community nurses, namely:

- What constitutes success?
- How might success be measured?
- What is an improvement or deterioration, and who is it found in: the client or their family?
- Over what timescale should the effects of intervention be assessed?
- Whose judgment should be final: the client's or the professional's?

The questions posed by Goldberg are central to any attempt at evaluation. They have no straightforward answers, but could usefully form the basis of seminar or group work for both students and experienced health visitors. To date, there is little evidence to suggest where health visitors might most usefully be deployed. It is suggested here that the opinions of experienced health visitors, concerned with where they consider they have been the most and the least successful in realising their objectives, might shed some light on the goals of health visiting practice at an individual level. Evaluation is an important part of the health visitor's role, and given the growth in the number of health visitors, it may become more of a focus in the future.

Summary

This chapter has provided insight into some of the ways that health visitors might approach evaluation. It has highlighted some key sources of evidence available to health visitors in evaluating their practice, including suggested ways to approach evaluation, such as the care planning process and target setting using the SMART approach.

In the context of the commissioner–provider relationship, value for money as evidenced by health gain is the currency in the marketplace. Health visitors have thus been required to reflect on their contribution to health care. It is evident that in the past, health visitors were reluctant to evaluate their work. Instead, they were content to claim that a meaningful evaluation was impossible due to the individual nature of client problems and the centrality of the relationship with the client. Now, however, owing to competing demands on services and restricted financial resources at a national and local level, there is a danger of health visitors being replaced by other workers due to the lack of evidence to support the contention that health visiting makes a difference to the health of the population that could not be achieved using less well-qualified workers.

With the health needs of the population rising and the health differential between social classes increasing, the DH's implementation plan to increase the health visitor workforce in England by 37.5% by the end of March 2015 (DH, 2011) was timely. This has nearly been achieved, with 3985 additional full-time health visitors in practice at the time of writing (the target having been 4200), making 12 707 in total working in the UK (DH, 2015; HSCIC, 2015). Historically, health visitors have been spread thinly across a range of client groups, minimising their visibility and potential impact. Latterly, however, health visitors have been redeployed to work with high-risk families, which in some respects minimises their preventive health function and makes their work difficult to differentiate from that of other groups, such as social workers. Whilst health visitors might believe that they do 'good work', this is no longer sufficient evidence for others, who may be sceptical about the benefit of the service. In order to secure continued or additional resources, all health visitors should be prepared to generate information about what they do and the outcome of their work.

References

Androutsos, O., Apostolidou, E., Iotova, P., Socha, P., Birnbaum, J., Moreno, L., De Bourdeaudhuij, I., Koletzko, B. & Manios, Y.; ToyBox-study group (2014) Process evaluation design and tools used in a kindergarten-based, family-involved intervention to prevent obesity in early childhood. The ToyBox-study. *Obesity Reviews*, **15**(S3), 74–80.

Appleton, J.V., Harris, M., Oates, J. & Kelly, C. (2013) Evaluating health visitor assessment of mother –infant interactions: a mixed methods study. *International Journal of Nursing Studies*, **50**, 5–15.

Bandura, A. (2004) Health promotion by social cognitive means. *Health Education & Behaviour*, **31**(2), 143–64.

Barts Health NHS Trust (2014) Burdett Trust for Nursing Empowerment Health Visiting Toolkit Project Report. Barts Health NHS Trust, London.

Bleich, S.N., Segal, J., Wu, Y., Wilson, R. & Wang, Y. (2013) Systematic review of community-based childhood obesity prevention studies. *Paediatrics*, **132**(1), e201–10.

Boots Family Trust (2013) My Pregnancy & Post-Birth Wellbeing Plan. Boots Family Trust, London. Available from: http://everyonesbusiness.org.uk/wp-content/uploads/2014/06/Boots-Family-Trust-Wellbeing-Plan.pdf (last accessed 30 March 2016).

Bovend'Eerdt, T.J.H., Botell, R.C. & Wade, D.T. (2009) Writing SMART rehabilitation goals and achieving goal attainment scaling: a practical guide. *Clinical Rehabilitation*, **23**, 352–61.

Brain J., Schofield, J., Gerrish, K., Mawson, G., Mabbott, J., Patel, D. & Gerrish, P. (2011) A Guide for Clinical Audit, Research and Service Review – An Educational Toolkit Designed to Help Staff Differentiate between Clinical Audit, Research and Service Review Activities. Sheffield Teaching Hospitals NHS Trust, Sheffield. Available from: http://www.worcester.ac.uk/documents/HQIP_A-Guide-for-Clinical-Audit-Research-and-Service-Review.pdf (last accessed 30 March 2016).

Brooten, D., Kumar, S., Brown, L.P., et al. (1986) A randomized clinical trial of early discharge and home follow-up of very-low-birth-weight infants. *New England Journal of Medicine*, **315**, 934–9.

Bryar, R., Anto-Awuakye, S., Christie, J., Davis, C. & Plumb, K. (2013) Using the Delphi approach to identify priority areas for health visiting practice in an area of deprivation. *Nursing Research and Practice*, **2013**:780315.

Bull, J., McCormick, G., Swann, C. & Mulvihill, C. (2004) Ante- and Post-Natal Homevisiting Programmes: A Review of Reviews: Evidence Briefing. NHS Health Development Agency, London.

Casiro, O.G., McKenzie, M.E., McFadyen, L., Shapiro, C., Seshia, M.M., MacDonald, N., Moffatt, M. & Cheang, M.S. (1993) Earlier discharge with community-based intervention for low birth weight infants: a randomized trial. *Paediatrics*, **92**, 128–34.

CETHV (1977) An Investigation into the Principles of Health Visiting. Council for the Education and Training of Health Visitors, London.

Ciliska, D., Mastrilli, P., Ploeg, J., Hayward, S., Brunton, G. & Underwood, J. (2001) The effectiveness of home visiting as a delivery strategy for public health nursing interventions to clients in the prenatal and postnatal period: a systematic review. *Primary Health Care Research & Development*, **2**(1), 41–54.

Cowley, S., Whittaker, K., Grigulis, A., Malone, M., Donetto, S., Wood, H., Morrow, E. & Maben, J. (2013) Why Health Visiting? A Review of the Literature about Key Health Visitor Interventions, Processes and Outcomes for Children and Families. National Nursing Research Unit King's College London, London.

Cox, J.L., Holden, J.M. & Sagovsky, R. (1987) Detection of postnatal depression. Development of the 10-item Edinburgh Postnatal Depression Scale. *British Journal of Psychiatry*, **150**(6), 782–6.

DH (2001) Health Visitor Practice Development Resource Pack. Department of Health, London.

DH (2005a) Self-Care: A Real Choice. Department of Health, London.

DH (2005b) Choosing Health: Making Healthy Choices Easier. Department of Health, London.

DH (2007) Facing the Future: A Review of the Role of Health Visitors. Department of Health, London.

DH (2008a) High Quality Care for All: NHS Next Stage Review Final Report. Department of Health, London.

DH (2008b) Guidance on the Routine Collection of Patient Reported Outcome Measures (PROMs). Department of Health, London.

DH (2009a) Your Health Your Way – A Guide to Long Term Conditions and Self-Care. Department of Health, London.

DH (2009b) Getting it Right for Children and Families: Maximising the Contribution of the Health Visiting Team: 'Ambition, Action, Achievement'. Department of Health, London.

DH (2009c) Tackling Health Inequalities: 10 Years On. Department of Health, London.

DH (2009d) Healthy Child Programme: Pregnancy and the First Five Years of Life. Department of Health, London.

DH (2010a) Equity and Excellence: Liberating the NHS. Department of Health, London.

DH (2010b) White Paper – Health Lives, Healthy People: Our Strategy for Public Health in England. Department of Health, London.

DH (2011) Health Visitor Implementation Plan 2011–15: A Call to Action February 2011. Department of Health, London.

DH (2012a) Public Health Outcomes Framework 2013–2016. Department of Health, London.

DH (2012b) NHS Patient Experience Framework. Department of Health, London.

DH (2012c) Equality Objectives Action Plan: September 2012–December 2013. Department of Health, London.

DH (2014a) Co-morbidities: A Framework of Principles for System-Work Action. Department of Health, London.

DH (2014b) Overview of the Six Early Years High Impact Areas. Department of Health, London.

DH (2015) Health Visitor Programme: Position Statement & Key Achievements 2011–March 2015. Department of Health, London.

DHSSPS (2010) Healthy Futures 2010–2015. The Contribution of Health Visitors and School Nurses in Northern Ireland. Department of Health, Social Services and Public Safety, Belfast.

DHSSPS (2015) Patient Education/Self Management Programmes for People with Long Term Conditions (2013/14). Department of Health, Social Services and Public Safety, Belfast.

Derryberry, M. (1939) Nursing accomplishments as revealed by case records. *Public Health Report*, **54**(46), 2035–43.

Dixon-Woods, M., Baker, R., Charles, K., Dawson, J., Jerzembek, G., Martin, G., McCarthy, I., McKee, L., Minion, J., Ozieranski, P., Willars, J., Wilkie, P. & West, M. (2013) Culture and behavior in the English National Health Service: overview of lessons from a large multimethod study. *BMJ Quality and Safety*, **23**(2), 106–15.

Donabedian, A. (1969) Some issues in evaluating the quality of nursing care. *American Journal of Public Health*, **59**(10), 1833–6.

Donabedian, A. (1988) The quality of care: how can it be assessed? *Journal of the American Medical Association*, **260**, 1743–8.

Donetto, S., Malone, M., Hughes, J., Morrow, E., Cowley, S. & Maben, J. (2013) Health Visiting: The Voice of Service Users – Learning from Service Users' Experiences to Inform the Development of UK Health Visiting Practice and Services. National Nursing Research Unit, King's College London, London.

Doran, G.T. (1981). There's a S.M.A.R.T. way to write management's goals and objectives. *Management Review*, **70**(11), 35–6.

Elkan, R., Kendrick, D., Hewitt, M., Robinson, J.J., Tolley, K., Blair, M., Dewey, M., Williams, D. & Brummell, K. (2000) The effectiveness of domiciliary health visiting: a systematic review of international studies and a selective review of the British literature. *Health Technology Assessment*, **4**(13), 1–339.

Evans, W.D., Wallace J.L. & Snider J. (2012) Pilot evaluation of the text4baby mobile health program. *BMC Public Health*, **12**, 1–10.

FPI (2009) Health Visitors: A Progress Report. Family and Parenting Institute, London.

Gardner, G., Gardner, A. & O'Connell, J. (2014) Using the Donabedian framework to examine the quality and safety of nursing service innovation. *Journal of Clinical Nursing*, **23**(1–2), 145–55.

Goldberg, E.M., Mortimer, A. & Williams, B. (1970) Helping the Age: A Field Experiment in Social Work. Allen & Unwin, London.

Health Foundation (2015) Evaluation: What to Consider. The Health Foundation, London.

Hobbs, P. (1973) Aptitude or Environment. Royal College of Nursing, London.

HSCIC (2015) Health Visitor Minimum Dataset (March 2015). Health & Social Care Information Centre, London.

Hunt, C. & Rudolf, M. (2008) Tackling Child Obesity with HENRY: A Handbook for Community and Health Practitioners. Unite/Community Practitioners and Health Visitors Association, London.

iHV (2014) Press Release Institute calls for Government Commitment to Maximum Ratio of 1 : 250 Health Visitors to Families. Institute of Health Visiting, London.

Kane, G.A., Wood, V.A. & Barlow, J. (2007) Parenting programmes: a systematic review and synthesis of qualitative research. *Child: Care, Health & Development*, **33**(6), 784–93.

LeCroy, C.W. & Krysik, J. (2011) Randomized trial of the healthy families Arizona home visiting programme. *Children and Youth*, **33**(10), 1761–6.

Lowell, D.I., Carter, A.S., Godoy, L., Paulicin, B. & Briggs-Gowan, M.J. (2011) A randomized controlled trial of Child FIRST: a comprehensive home-bases intervention translating research into early childhood practice. *Child Development*, **82**(1), 193–208.

Luker, K.A. (1978) Goal attainment: a possible model for assessing the work of the health visitor. *Nursing Times*, **75**(35), 1257–1259.

MacMillan, H.L., Thomas, B.H., Jamieson, E., Walsh, C.A., Boyle, M.H., Shannon, H.S. & Gafni, A. (2005) Effectiveness of home visitation by public-health nurses in prevention of the recurrence of child physical abuse and neglect: a randomized controlled trial. *The Lancet*, **365**, 1786–93.

Marmot, M., Atkinson, T., Bell, J., Black, C., Broadfoot, P., Cumberlege, J., Diamond, I., Gilmore, I., Ham, C., Meacher, M. & Mulgan, G. (2010) Fair Society, Healthy Lives: The Marmot Review. Marmot Review Team, University College, London. Available from: http://www.instituteofhealthequity.org/projects/fair-society-healthy-lives-the-marmot-review (last accessed 30 March 2016).

McDonald, K.M., Sundaram, V., Bravata, D.M., Lewis, R., Lin, N., Kraft, S.A., McKinnon, M., Paguntalan, H. & Owens, D.K. (2007) Care Coordination. Vol. 7 of: Closing the Quality Gap: A Critical Analysis of Quality Improvement Strategies, Technical Review 9 (eds K.G. Shojania, K.M. McDonald, R.M. Wachter & D.K. Owens). Prepared by the Stanford University-UCSF Evidence-Based Practice Center under Contract 290-02-0017, AHRQ Publication No. 04(07)-0051-7, Agency for Healthcare Research & Quality, Rockville, MD.

McHugh, G. & Luker, K. (2002) Users' perceptions of the health visiting service. *Community Practitioner*, **75**(2), 57–61.

McLennan, J.D. & Lavis, J.N. (2006) What is the evidence for parenting interventions offered in a Canadian community? *Canadian Journal of Public Health*, **97**(6), 454–8.

Moore, G.F., Audrey, S., Barker, M., Bond, L., Bonell, C., Hardeman, W., Moore, L., O'Cathain, A., Tinati, T., Wight, D. & Baird, J. (2014) Process Evaluation of Complex Interventions: Medical Research Council Guidance. MRC Population Health Science Research Network, London.

Morrell, C.J., Slade, P., Warner, R., Paley, G., Dixon, S., Walters, S.J., Brugha, T., Barkham, M., Parry, G.J. & Nichol, J. (2009) Clinical effectiveness of health visitor training in psychologically informed approaches for depression in postnatal women: pragmatic cluster randomised trial in primary care. *British Medical Journal*, **338**, a3045.

Muir Gray, J.A. (2004) Evidence based policy making: Editorial. *British Medical Journal*, **329**, 988–9.

NCCPC (2006) Routine Postnatal Care of Women and their Babies. NICE Clinical Guideline 37. NICE, London.

NHS England (2013) The NHS Belongs to the People: A Call to Action. NHS England, London.

NHS England (2014a) 2015–16 National Health Visiting Core Service Specification. NHS England, London.

NHS England (2014b) Commissioning for Quality and Innovation (CQUIN) 2014/15 Guidance. NHS England, London.

NHS England (2015) Health Visitor Service Metrics Commentary Q2 2013–14 to Q2 2014–15. NHS England, London.

NIB (2015) Personalised Health and Care 2020: A Framework for Action. National Information Board, London.

NICE (2008a) Community Engagement. National Institute for Health and Care Excellence, London.

NICE (2008b) Maternal and Child Nutrition. National Institute for Health and Care Excellence, London.

NICE (2009a) Reducing the Differences in the Uptake of Immunisations. National Institute for Health and Care Excellence, London.

NICE (2009b) Reducing the Differences in the Uptake of Immunisations: Audit Support. National Institute for Health and Care Excellence, London.

NICE (2014a) Addendum to Clinical Guideline 37, Postnatal Care. National Institute for Health and Care Excellence, London.

NICE (2014b) Behaviour Change at Population, Community and Individual Levels: Public Health Guidance 6. National Institute for Health and Care Excellence, London.

NICE (2014c) Health Visiting. National Institute for Health and Care Excellence, London. Available from: http://publications.nice.org.uk/lgb22 (last accessed 30 March 2016).

NICE (2015) Maintaining a Healthy Weight and Preventing Excess Weight Gain among Adults and Children. National Institute for Health and Care Excellence, London.

NICE & SCIE (2010a) Looked-After Children and Young People. National Institute for Health and Care Excellence, London.

NICE & SCIE (2010b) Strategies to Prevent Unintentional Injuries among Children and Young People Aged Under 15. National Institute for Health and Care Excellence, London.

NMC (2004) Standards of Proficiency for Specialist Community Public Health Nurses. Nursing and Midwifery Council, London.

Olds, D.L., Henderson, C.R., Chamberlin, R. & Tatelbaum, R. (1986) Preventing child abuse and neglect: a randomized trial of nurse home visitation. *Pediatrics*, **78**, 65–78.

Olds, D.L., Eckenrode, J., Henderson, C.R. Jr,, Kitzman, H., Powers, J., Cole, R., Sidora, K., Morris, P., Pettitt, L.M. & Luckey, D. (1997) Long-term effects of home visitation on maternal life course and child abuse and neglect. Fifteen year follow-up of a randomized trial. *Journal of the American Association*, **278**(8), 637–43.

O'Mahen, H.A., Woodford, J., McGinley, J., Warren, F.C., Richards, D.A., Lynch, T.R. & Taylor, R.S. (2013) Internet-based behavioural activation – treatment for postnatal depression (Netmums): a randomized controlled trial. *Journal of Affective Disorders*, **150**, 814–22.

O'Mahen, H.A., Richards, D.A., Woodford, J., Wilkinson, E., McGinley, J., Taylor, R.S. & Warren, F.C. (2014) Netmums: a phase II randomized controlled trial of a guided Internet behavioural activation treatment for postpartum depression. *Psychological Medicine*, **44**, 1675–89.

Pattoni, L. (2012) Insights 16: Strengths-Based Approaches for Working with Individuals. Institute for Research & Innovation in Social Sciences, Scotland.

Peacock, S., Konrad, S., Watson, E., Nickel, D. & Muhajarine, N. (2013) Effectiveness of home visiting programmes on child outcomes: a systematic review. *BMC Public Health*, **13**, 17.

Public Health Wales NHS Trust (2014) Raising the Profile: The Public Health Wales Nursing and Midwifery Strategy Working towards a Healthier, Happier and Fairer Wales. Public Health Wales, Wales.

QNI (2008) Briefing: Evaluating Outcomes. Queen's Nursing Institute, London.

Rees, R., Oliver, K., Woodman, J. & Thomas, J. (2009) Children's Views about Obesity, Body Size, Shape and Weight: A Systematic Review. EPPI-Centre, London.

Robling, M., Bekkers, M-J., Bell, K., Bulter, C.C., Cannings-John, R., Channon, S., Martin, B.C., Gregory, J.W., Hood, K., Kemp, A., Kenkre, J., Montgomery, A.A., Moody, G., Owen-Jones, E., Pickett, K., Richardson, G., Roberts, Z.E., Ronaldson, S., Sanders, J., Stamuli, E. & Torgerson, D. (2016) Effectiveness of a nurse-led intensive home-visitation programme for first-time teenage mothers (Building Blocks): a pragmatic randomised controlled trial. *The Lancet*, **387**(10014), 146–55.

RCN (2012) Paying for Quality-Commissioning for Quality and Innovation (CQUIN). Royal College of Nursing, London.

Rudolf, M. (2010) Tackling Obesity through the Healthy Child Programme: A Framework for Action. University of Leeds & Leeds Community Healthcare NHS Trust, Leeds. Available from: http://www.noo.org.uk/uploads/doc/vid_4841_rudolf_TacklingObesity1_200110.pdf (last accessed 30 March 2016).

Russell, S. & Drennan, V. (2007) Mothers' views of the health visiting service in the UK: a web-based survey. *Community Practitioner*, **80**(8), 22–6.

Saunders, R.P., Evans, M.H. & Joshi, P. (2005) Developing a process-evaluation plan for assessing health promotion program implementation: a how-to guide. *Health Promotion Practice*, **6**(2), 134–47.

Schaffer, M.A., Goodhue, A., Stennes K. & Lanigan, C. (2012) Evaluation of a public health nurse visiting program for pregnant and parenting teens. *Public Health Nursing*, **29**(3), 218–31.

Sidhu, M.S., Daley, A., Jordan, R., Coventry, P.A., Heneghan, C., Jowett, S., Singh, S., Marsh, J., Adab, P., Varghese, J., Nunan, D., Blakemore, A., Stevens, J., Dowson, L., Fitzmaurice, D. & Jolly, K. (2015) Patient self-management in primary care patients with mild COPD – protocol of a randomized controlled trial of telephone health coaching. *BMC Pulmonary Medicine*, **15**, 16.

Shaw, E., Levitt, C., Wong, S. & Kaczorowski, J.; The McMaster University Postpartum Research Group (2006) Systematic review of the literature on postpartum care: Effectiveness of postpartum support to improve maternal parenting, mental health, quality of life, and physical health. *Birth*, **33**(3), 210–20.

Skills for Health (2008) Public Health Skills and Career Framework. Skills for Health, Bristol.

Speller, V., Learmonth, A. & Harrison, D. (1997) The search for evidence of effective health promotion. *British Medical Journal*, **315**, 361–3.

St Leger, A.S., Schnieden, H. & Walsworth-Bell, J.P. (1992) Evaluating Health Services' Effectiveness. Open University Press, Buckingham.

Suchman, E.A. (1967) Evaluation Research. Russell Sage Foundation, New York.

Thomas, B., Dorling, D. & Davy Smith, G. (2010) Inequalities in premature mortality in Britain: observational study from 1921 to 2007. *British Medical Journal*, **341**, C3639.

Twinn, S. & Cowley, S. (1992) Principles of Health Visiting: A Re-examination. Community Practitioners and Health Visitors Association, London.

Unite/CPHVA (2009) What Size Caseload Should a Health Visitor Have? Unite/Community Practitioners and Health Visitors Association, London.

Walker, D.M., Robbins, J.M., Brown, D. & Berhane, Z. (2014) Improving processes of care for overweight and obese children: evidence from the 215-GO! program in Philadelphia health centers. *Public Health Reports*, **129**(3), 303–10.

Waters, E., de Silva-Sanigorski, A., Hall, B.J., Brown, T., Campbell, K.J., Gao, Y., Armstrong, R., Prosser, L. & Summerbell, C.D. (2011). Interventions for preventing obesity in children. *Cochrane Database of Systematic Reviews*, **7**(12):CD001871.

Watson, M., Kendrick, D., Coupland, C., Woods, A., Futers, D. & Robinson, J. (2004) Providing child safety equipment to prevent injuries: randomised controlled trial. *British Medical Journal*, **330**(7484), 178.

While, A., Forbes, A., Ullman, R. & Murgatroyd, B. (2005) The Contribution of Nurses, Midwives and Health Visitors to Child Health and Child Health Services: A Scoping Review. NCCSDO, London.

Whitlock, E.P., O'Connor, E, A. , Williams, S.B., Beil, T.L. & Lutz, K.W. (2008) Effectiveness of Weight Management Programs in Children and Adolescents. Agency for Healthcare Research & Quality, Rockville, MD.

Whitlock, E.P., O'Connor, E.A., Williams, S.B., Beil, T.L. & Lutz, K.W. (2010) Effectiveness of weight management interventions: a targeted systematic review for the USPSTF. *Paediatrics*, **125**(2), e396–418.

Activities

Activity 7.1

Using guidelines

- Visit the following websites: www.nice.org.uk and www.scie.org.uk.
- Select a guideline which is of relevance to your practice.
- Compare this national guidance to the local guidelines in your workplace (if they exist) or to your own current practice and identify any similarities and differences.
- What recommendations would you make for changing your current practice after reading the national guideline?

Activity 7.2

Locating sources of evidence

Take the opportunity to explore the following websites:
- NHS Evidence: www.evidence.nhs.uk
- NHS Improving Quality: www.nhsiq.nhs.uk
- Effectiveness Matters: http://www.york.ac.uk/crd/publications/effectiveness-matters/
- *Effective Health Care Bulletin*: http://www.york.ac.uk/crd/publications/archive/
- CRD publications: http://www.york.ac.uk/crd/publications/
  - CRD database: http://www.crd.york.ac.uk/CRDWeb/
  - HTA: www.hta.ac.uk

Activity 7.3

Thinking about your practice

- Think about a specific area of your practice. What are its aims?
- How do you know the aims are being met?

(Continued)

Activity 7.3: *(Continued)*

- After integrating new guidance or research evidence (if available), is there anything you would change about this area of practice?
- How would you go about assessing whether the change has had any impact on improving your practice or service delivery?

Activity 7.4

Developing new programmes

- Design a programme which could be delivered in your practice (e.g. weight management, weaning programme, behaviour management).
- Start to identify the evaluation criteria. (What are the aims of the programme? What do you want to achieve? How do you know it is of benefit?)

Activity 7.5

Locating sources of information

The Association of Public Health Observatories (APHO; now part of NHS Public Health England), the Scottish Public Health Observatory, Pubic Health Wales Observatory, and Ireland and Northern Ireland Population Health Observatories provide useful data for assessing health needs and planning resources for a range of public health issues. Visit the National Child and Maternal Health Intelligence Network (www.chimat.org.uk) and see if you can locate the child health profiles for your specific area (click on *Tools and Data*, then *Interactive Child Health Profiles*, then on your *geographical region* then on *area*). This can also be done to find out the *breastfeeding profiles* in your area (see http://atlas.chimat.org.uk/IAS/dataviews/breastfeedingprofile).

Activity 7.6

Developing goals

Imagine a visit to a new mother who has sore breasts. Set two goals for this visit: goal A is the more general goal and goal B will help you specify the activities by which success will be measured (e.g. watch how baby latches on to nipple). This activity will help you to understand how specific goals must be in order to be achievable and evaluable.

Activity 7.7

Action planning

- Think of a health problem(s) to be addressed with one of your families.
- Complete a record of action plans (Table 7.4).

Table 7.4 Record of action plans.

Health problem to be addressed	Objectives	Action to be taken	Who will do it?	Timescale	Evaluation measures
1					
2					
3					
4					

Activity 7.8

Using the SMART approach

Think of a common issue you encounter in practice and complete the SMART approach to goal setting. An example is provided in Table 7.5 for a mother who wishes to lose weight. Use Table 7.6 to complete your own example.

Table 7.5 SMART Example of weight loss

SMART	Client problem
Specific goal	Mother will lose half a stone
Measurable goal	Mother will lose 3 lb in a month and a further 4 lb 2 months later
Achievable goal	Mother will weigh herself fortnightly Mother will follow diet plan provided
Realistic goal	By the end of the year, mother will be able to fit into pre-pregnancy clothes
Time-bound	Mother will have lost half a stone within 3 months

(Continued)

Activity 7.8: *(Continued)*

Table 7.6 SMART Template

SMART	Client problem
Specific goal	
Measurable goal	
Achievable goal	
Realistic goal	
Time-bound	

Index

Health Visiting: Preparation for Practice, Fourth Edition.
Edited by Karen A. Luker, Gretl A. McHugh and Rosamund M. Bryar.
© 2017 John Wiley & Sons, Ltd. Published 2017 by John Wiley & Sons, Ltd.